Occupational Toxicology

Edited by
Neill H. Stacey

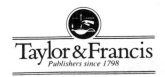

Taylor & Francis
Publishers since 1798

UK	Taylor & Francis Ltd, 4 John Street, London WC1N 2ET
USA	Taylor & Francis Inc., 1900 Frost Road, Suite 101, Bristol, PA 19007

British Library Cataloguing in Publication Data

A catalogue record for this book is available from the British Library
ISBN 0-85066-830-1 (cloth)
ISBN 0-85066-831-X (paper)

Library of Congress Cataloging-in-Publication Data are available

Cover design by Hybert Design & Type

Typeset in 10/12 Times by
Pure Tech Corporation, Pondicherry, India

Printed in Great Britain by Burgess Science Press, Basingstoke on paper which has a specified pH value on final paper manufacture of not less than 7.5 and is therefore 'acid free'.

Occupational Toxicology

£25·00
12|93

Contents

List of Contributors   vii
Preface   ix

Understanding Occupational Toxicology

1. Introduction to Occupational Toxicology   3
   N. H. Stacey
2. Basics of Toxicology   15
   N. H. Stacey

Targets of Chemicals

3. Systemic Toxicology   37
   N. H. Stacey, W. M. Haschek and C. Winder
4. Respiratory Toxicology   77
   G. Baker
5. Occupational Skin Disease   89
   E. A. Emmett
6. Reproduction, Development and Occupational Health   107
   C. Winder
7. Genetic Toxicology   123
   A. D. Mitchell
8. Carcinogenesis and its Prevention   149
   H. Vainio

Toxicity by Group of Chemical

9. Toxicity of Metals   165
   C. Winder
10. Toxicity of Pesticides   177
    A. Moretto and M. Lotti
11. Toxicity of Solvents   205
    N. H. Stacey

12. Toxicity of Plastics   213
    R. Drew
13. Toxicity of Gases   233
    C. M. Murdoch
14. Toxicity of Particulate Matter   251
    A. J. Rogers

Fields Interfacing with Toxicology

15. Occupational Hygiene—Interface with Toxicology   269
    C. Gray
16. Occupational Medicine—Interface with Toxicology   295
    W.O. Phoon
17. Occupational Epidemiology—Interface with Toxicology   305
    M. S. Frommer and S. J. Corbett

Uses of Toxicological Data

18. Managing Workplace Chemical Safety   329
    C. Winder and C. Vickers
19. Working Examples in Occupational Toxicology   349
    N. H. Stacey and C. Winder
20. Chemicals, Workplaces and the Law   367
    C. Winder and J. Barter

Index   391

List of Contributors

G. BAKER
General, Respiratory and
    Occupational Physician
Senior Lecturer in Occupational
    Medicine
Department of Occupational Health
The University of Sydney
Australia

J. BARTER
Manager, Environmental Affairs
Chemicals Group, PPG Industries Inc
Pittsburgh, PA
USA

S. J. CORBETT
Epidemiology & Health Services
    Evaluation Branch
New South Wales Health Department
Sydney
Australia

R. DREW
Research Associate in Toxicology
Toxicology Information Section
    Manager
ICI Australia Pty Ltd
Melbourne
Australia

E. A. EMMETT
Chief Executive
National Occupational Health and
    Safety Commission (Worksafe
    Australia)
Sydney
Australia

M. S. FROMMER
Epidemiology & Health Services
    Evaluation Branch

New South Wales Health Department
Sydney
Australia

C. GRAY
Associate Professor of Occupational
    Hygiene
Deakin University
Geelong
Australia

W. M. HASCHEK
Professor of Toxicology, College of
    Veterinary Medicine
University of Illinois
Urbana, IL
USA

A. D. MITCHELL
Genesys Research, Incorporated
North Carolina
USA

M. LOTTI
Professor of Industrial Toxicology
University of Padua Medical School
Padua
Italy

A. MORETTO
University of Padua Medical School
Padua
Italy

C. M. MURDOCH
Scientific Officer
Occupational Hygiene and Safety
    Engineering Unit
National Occupational Health and
    Safety Commission (Worksafe
    Australia)

Sydney
Australia

W. O. PHOON
Professor and Head, Department of
  Occupational Health, University of
  Sydney
Director, Professional Education
  Program and Head, Occupational
  Medicine Unit
National Occupational Health and
  Safety Commission (Worksafe
  Australia), and
Consultant in Occupational Medicine
  to Sydney, Royal Prince Alfred
  and Westmead Hospitals
Sydney
Australia

A. J. ROGERS
Head, Occupational Hygiene and
  Safety Engineering Unit
National Occupational Health and
  Safety Commission (Worksafe
  Australia), Sydney and Senior
  Lecturer
The University of Sydney
Sydney
Australia

N. H. STACEY
Executive Director

Research and Scientific Division
National Occupational Health and
  Safety Commission (Worksafe
  Australia), and
Associate Professor (in Toxicology)
The University of Sydney
Sydney
Australia

H. VAINIO
Chief, Unit of Carcinogen
  Identification and Evaluation
International Agency for Research
  on Cancer
Lyon
France

C. VICKERS
Manager, Agricultural and
  Veterinary Chemicals Section
National Occupational Health and
  Safety Commission (Worksafe
  Australia)
Sydney
Australia

C. WINDER
Senior Lecturer in Chemical Safety
Department of Safety Science
University of New South Wales
Kensington
Australia

Preface

Occupational health and safety is a field that involves many disciplines. Interaction amongst these fields is essential in dealing with workplace problems making it a truly multidisciplinary endeavour. Chemicals are found in many if not all workplaces and require careful attention to avoid overt acute poisoning as well as the longer term more insidious adverse health effects that may occur. Toxicology is a specialty in its own right with its attendant jargon and complexities. As many people involved in occupational health and safety must deal with chemical issues from time to time, but do not necessarily have a stong background in toxicology, it is an aim of this book to provide such people with the opportunity to understand the basis of this science and how toxicological information is used. Thus the book is directed towards occupational health and safety personnel at different levels to allow them to attend to chemical-related issues with greater understanding and confidence.

The book is structured to provide, in addition to an understanding of what toxicology is about, an overview of the effects of chemicals on target tissues, with emphasis on those more often affected by workplace exposures. Following this, the agents most often associated with occupational diseases are dealt with so that the reader can be alerted to the types of substance of most concern. It is not intended that the reader be able to use this as a reference source to look up the toxic effects of various chemicals. There are many texts and databases devoted to this sort of information. Rather, it is intended to give an overview of the class of agents with one or two examples in more detail. The important fields interacting with toxicology are then covered to help the reader understand just what these fields involve and how they all interrelate. Finally, systems for managing workplace chemicals are detailed and some working examples requiring the use of toxicological information are provided. This is meant to allow the reader to appreciate how information is used and some of the difficulties and uncertainties involved in the interpretation and decision-making with toxicological data. The legal aspects of chemical use complete the book.

Overall this book covers the field of occupational toxicology and is intended to serve as a valuable guide for those involved with dealing with workplace chemicals.

Understanding Occupational
Toxicology

Chapter 1

Introduction to Occupational Toxicology

N. H. Stacey

The science of toxicology has many applications. One of these, which is the topic of this book, relates to exposure of people to noxious agents during the course of their work. In order that one may understand and use toxicity information on workplace chemicals, it is necessary to obtain a grounding in the basic principles and concepts of toxicology. Chapter 2 of this book covers these aspects in some detail, while a more comprehensive coverage may be found in the fundamental textbook of toxicology, *Casarett and Doull's Toxicology. The Basic Science of Poisons* (Amdur *et al.*, 1991). Although the basic principles and concepts of toxicology relating to particular organs and/or groups of chemicals are similar across different fields of toxicology, many of the details are deserving of different emphasis with regard to the occupational setting, and this is a focus of this book. Furthermore, there are specific uses of toxicological data particularly related to managing workplace chemicals and these are dealt with in detail in our final section.

What is occupational toxicology?

Occupational toxicology is the study of the adverse effects of agents that may be encountered by workers during the course of their employment. The adverse effects may be in the workers themselves or in experimental animals or other test systems used to define and/or understand the toxicity of the agent of interest. The term 'occupational' is used in preference to 'industrial' because the latter term may have the connotation of chemical exposures in factories. This would not necessarily include work such as farming with potential exposure to pesticides or office work with issues such as photocopiers in enclosed spaces.

Why is occupational toxicology required?

In recent years public awareness of health effects of chemicals has risen considerably due to events such as the thalidomide tragedy and environmental

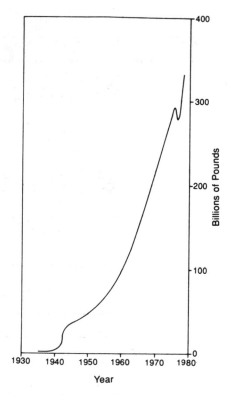

Figure 1.1. The production of synthetic organic chemicals. (From the National Toxicology Program, US Department of Health and Human Services.)

contamination with chemicals. Recognition of workplace exposures resulting in health effects has been part of this. A cursory glance at the Group 1 carcinogen list of the International Agency for Research on Cancer (IARC) should be evidence enough from this perspective. The current epidemic of asbestos related cancer in Australia and other countries might suggest that there is no room for complacency in our efforts to curb chemical-related ill health.

Since the 1940s the production of synthetic organic chemicals has risen dramatically (Figure 1.1) which indicates that there are now many more chemicals to which people are likely to be exposed. Of the 10 million or so chemical entities that are in existence, it is estimated that there are about 60 000 that have reasonable potential for human exposure. An investigation into the data available on these that would allow health-hazard assessments of varying degrees to be undertaken was approved by the National Research Council in the USA (1984). This provided the documented information that most believed to be the situation as illustrated in Figure 1.2. That is, there is a great lack of toxicity data available to do comprehensive risk assessments by contemporary standards.

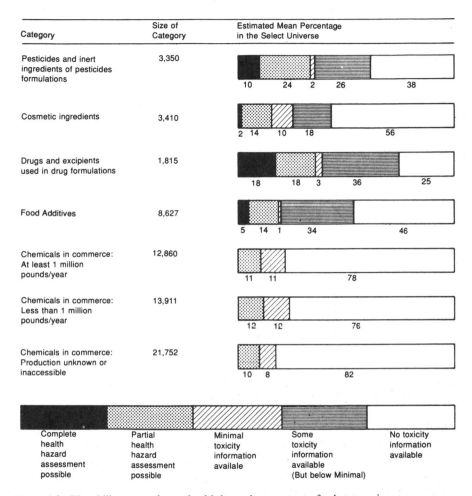

Figure 1.2. The ability to conduct a health-hazard assessment of substances in seven categories of a select universe. (From *Toxicity Testing. Strategies to Determine Needs and Priorities*, 1984. Washington, DC: National Academy Press.)

The true extent of work-related chemical-associated ill health in both human and economic terms is unknown. Estimates for occupational diseases have given figures like 5000 to 7000 deaths per year from occupational cancer, pneumoconioses, cardiovascular diseases, chronic respiratory diseases, renal diseases and neurological disorders in New York State, which had a workforce of between 7 and 8 million at about that time (Markowitz and Landrigan, 1989). The same report estimated that 35 000 new cases of occupational disease would develop each year in New York State. Their estimate for the cost of just occupational cancer in New York State amounted to approximately US$500 million.

Thus there remains much work to be done in the area of workplace chemicals and other agents of toxicological concern. Not only is there a lack of data on existing chemicals, but new ones are also continually becoming available. Furthermore, the methods used for carrying out risk assessment are by no means perfect and there is great scope for advances in this field.

How is occupational toxicology used?

The primary goal of occupational toxicology is to protect the health of workers. Application of toxicological information in this way is one component of the overall strategy in achieving this end. Other components are shown in Table 1.1.

Table 1.1. Strategy for controlling exposures to hazardous substances in the workplace

Elimination
Substitution
Containment
Engineering controls, e.g. local ventilation
Safe work practices
Personal protective equipment

Role in decision-making within hierarchical control

Toxicology plays an important role in deciding on the appropriateness of some of these steps. For example, there may be a wish to find a substitute for a particularly toxic chemical currently used in a workplace. There may be one available, but the toxicity of the replacement also requires evaluation. It is not satisfactory to replace one chemical with a second of unknown toxicity just because the first is of toxicological concern. All those involved in occupational health need to be aware of this. It is not unheard of for the sole reason for request to register one product for use is on the basis that it will replace one known to be responsible for a particular toxicity.

Role in setting exposure standards for workplace chemicals

Apart from contributing to the above strategy for controlling exposure to workplace chemicals, toxicology is intimately involved in decision-making on what levels of human exposure are acceptable for chemicals that are in use; that is, the setting of exposure standards. Investigations into the toxicity of a chemical seek to define a level at which there are no toxic effects. Terms used to describe this are shown in Table 1.2.

Table 1.2. Terms describing a no toxic effect level in experimental animals

NEL	No effect level
NOEL	No observed effect level
NOAEL	No observed adverse effect level

These terms warrant some explanation. NEL describes the dose level used in the animal experiment where no effect was noted. NOEL goes a step further including the word 'observed' to indicate that only a finite array of possible toxic end-points was investigated and therefore acknowledges that some form of toxicity may have been present but that the appropriate test was not employed to detect it. It also allows for other uncertainties such as differences among species and so on. NOAEL is designed to accommodate the possibilty that an effect may have been observed but it may be one that is not deemed to have toxicological significance for the organism. An example of one such effect that is considered by some not to be of import-ance in setting acceptable exposure limits is an increase in liver weight of the exposed animals. Many chemicals are known to do this by increasing the amounts of the enzyme system responsible for biotransformation and this is often considered to be an 'adaptive response'.

Once the level of no effect of toxicological significance has been derived it can be used to decide upon what constitutes an acceptable level to which humans may be exposed. Often this is done by incorporating a *safety factor* or *uncertainty factor* the latter being a more contemporary term and one which better reflects why this factor is used. It is used because of our uncertainty in this process due to aspects such as extrapolation across species, differing sensitivities among individuals and so on. It cannot, however, guarantee that the level of exposure so chosen will protect every individual to each and every possible toxicological manifestation of that chemical. Nevertheless, it may be expected that below the chosen level it is most unlikely that any adverse effects of the chemical will be observed. Different factors have been employed under differing circumstances. While there is no set rule for deciding on the factor to be used there are guidelines that may be followed as outlined in Table 1.3.

Table 1.3. Guidelines for choice of uncertainty factors in setting exposure standards

Factor	Rationale
10	Suitable human data
100	Chronic data in animals
1000	Limited animal data

Apart from the safety factor approach, mathematical models have been used as a means by which to arrive at an exposure standard. They can be used to predict what level of exposure would result in an incidence of, say, one in a million. However, use of such models is contentious as they all depend on particular assumptions and can give final values that vary by orders of magnitude. Thus their use remains limited at this time.

It is important to recognise that toxicological data from experimental animals are not the only source of information used in setting exposure standards. Clearly any human data that are available must be included and are of great importance. Often, however, we find that these data are of limited use for a variety of reasons such as co-exposures in the workplace, the reports not being of satisfactory scientific rigour and so on. Nevertheless, well conducted positive epidemiological studies in humans will always outweigh analogous studies from experimental animals. Furthermore, other data, such as those from cells relating to the genotoxic effects of the chemical in question may be used. It is also important that data relating to the mechanism of toxicity be considered in reaching conclusions. The appropriateness of the study and quality of the data are other important factors that also must not be overlooked. Overall then, all available information must be considered in arriving at an acceptable value for the exposure standard.

The process for setting exposure standards for workplace chemicals has been somewhat different to that for chemicals found in other settings over the last 40 or so years. Since many workplace chemicals were already in use when standards were first set, information was already available on effects in exposed humans. Thus the setting of exposure limits often relied heavily on this information. Furthermore, there was likely to be little toxicological data from experimental animals available for consideration since detailed animal testing has only been required in more recent years. In comparison, for pesticide residues considerable animal data have been a requirement before registration and marketing for many years. Thus standards setting for pesticide residues has relied more heavily on animal data gathered before any human exposure. It should be the end result of toxicological testing, of course, that positive human toxicity data for that chemical are never obtained. This view sometimes seems to arouse some condescension in colleagues during committee meetings to decide on acceptable practices for using chemicals in the workplace. For example, should a genotoxic aromatic amine with clear and strong evidence of causing urinary bladder cancer in dogs not be treated as a human carcinogen? In asserting that it should, one often hears that there are no human data to support this. The author's response to that is 'Aren't we fortunate that this is so?' It is of interest to consider the IARC list of Group 1 carcinogens (proven human carcinogens) in this context where many are related to occupational (as compared with environmental) exposures (IARC, 1987).

Over recent years the process of setting standards for exposure to workplace chemicals has received considerable criticism (Castleman and Ziem, 1988; Halton, 1988; Roach and Rappaport, 1990). One reason for this has been the use of uncertainty factors to a much lesser extent than as applied to other chemical groups. Nevertheless, it should be appreciated that the process began because there was a clear void that required attention and this gap was filled due to the efforts particularly of the American Conference of Governmental and Industrial Hygienists (ACGIH). This does not mean that the process should remain unchanged, however, as more and newer chemicals are brought into the workplace or existing ones are re-evaluated. There are now increasing requirements for toxicological information on new chemicals before they may be brought into the workplace. However, it should also be recognised that the extent of information is not as great as that for pesticides, for example.

Role in biological monitoring for chemical exposure

Biological monitoring is the measurement of a substance, its metabolites or its effects in body tissues, fluids or exhaled air of exposed persons. Consideration of biological monitoring is an interesting exercise because it is a topic that clearly exemplifies the interdisciplinary nature of protecting workers from the deleterious effects of exposure to chemicals.

There is usually a relationship between workplace air levels of substances and their levels actually in the workers. Determination of the air levels is largely the domain of the occupational hygienist while information about levels in the body requires the biological component. Information from experimental animals is very useful if not essential in regard to the latter, especially in the initial considerations of what may be the most suitable entity to determine. Thus the involvement of the occupational toxicologist is required.

Then we have the issue of biological exposure and biological effect. A metabolite of a chemical in the urine can be considered an index of

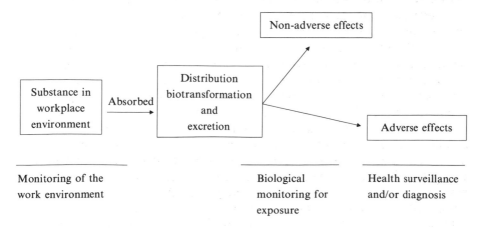

Figure 1.3. Scheme to show the relationships between monitoring of the environment, biological monitoring and health surveillance and/or diagnosis.

exposure but is cholinesterase depression in serum or red blood cells an indicator of exposure or effect? It is a biological effect but is used as a marker of exposure at the early stages of its depression. With DNA adducts they are certainly related to exposure and provide a measure of internal dose at a critical site, but do we have sufficient information at this time to consider them as an effect as such? Here the three disciplines of occupational toxicology, medicine and hygiene meet.

Lastly, when there is evidence of organ dysfunction related to chemical exposure we move into the domain of the occupational physician. These interrelationships are represented schematically in Figure 1.3.

When resolving problems such as evidence of an adverse health effect it is appropriate for the occupational physician to consult a hygienist for advice on ventilation controls and/or a toxicologist for advice on the toxicity of alternatives, for example. Thus a team approach is very much called for to obtain the best end result. The same view is promulgated by Lauwerys (1991).

Comparison with chemicals in the general environment

Having referred to pesticides above, it is interesting to compare exposure to chemicals in the environment with that in the workplace. Exposure at a workplace is often to higher concentrations of the chemicals than in the environment, although the duration of the exposure will be limited to the time at work while exposure in the environment could be 24 hours per day, 7 days per week. Another difference is the size of the exposed population which will be limited to the particular workforce in the occupational setting, while environmental exposures would include larger numbers depending on the spread of the chemical in question. It is perhaps easier to investigate occupational toxicological problems because of the generally higher concentrations and a more defined exposed population. Then it must be considered that there may be exposure to the chemical in both the workplace and the environment as well as to multiple chemicals. Perhaps passive smoking or exposure to diesel emissions may be suitable examples. It is of interest to consider a recent study of DNA adducts in this regard. Hemminki *et al.* (1990) found that workers at the site and people in the surrounding community had similar levels of adducts, while those in a rural population had much lower levels.

Relationship of occupational toxicology to other disciplines relating to workplace chemicals

As apparent from preceding sections, the overall management of workplace chemicals requires input from various disciplines. These include occupational toxicology, hygiene, medicine and epidemiology. Each are specialties in their own right, but each is required for satisfactory attention to this important endeavour. For this reason individual chapters have been included on each of these. The practising occupational toxicologist must have an appreciation of these other areas if the most meaningful input into the overall deliberations on issues involving occupational exposure to chemicals is to be made. As alluded to above, necessity for consideration of information emanating from each of these fields becomes particularly apparent during the standards setting process for chemical exposures and during resolution of workplace problems involving chemicals.

Future directions and challenges for occupational toxicology

Continued vigilance and improvement in the safety of chemical products should be a goal for those of us working in the area of occupational toxicology. There are some particular issues that are deserving of and will receive increasing attention over the coming years. Some are issues relating to toxicology in general, while others are more specific to occupational toxicology.

The continued development of *in vitro* tests should be a priority because this will have both humane and economic benefits once successfully established. It will also allow a more rapid procedure for assessing the toxicity of chemicals. While there have already been some considerable achievements in the area of *in vitro* toxicology (Tyson and Stacey, 1992) it must also be appreciated that there is much work to be done and that human health must not be compromised.

The toxicity of *mixtures* has received some attention over recent years as it has become more widely appreciated that people are exposed to many chemicals simultaneously and that the vast majority of toxicological data are on the individual chemicals. This presents a massive problem as it would not be possible to test all permutations and combinations of chemicals to which humans may be exposed. Here there may be a more interim role for *in vitro* systems as a screen for likely problem mixtures (that is, those with more than additive effects) so that more comprehensive investigations can target these.

The greater application of *molecular biological* tools to aid in toxicological assessment is gradually emerging. One example is the use of transgenic mice so that genotoxic chemicals can be identified in multiple organs with all body systems interacting so that a more reliable indication of likely applicability to the human can be obtained. A second application which is already having an impact on toxicological matters relating to the workplace is to be found with the identification of adducts to cellular macromolecules as indicators of carcinogen exposure. These adducts, especially those to DNA, the genetic material, are thought to reflect exposure at the critical site of action of the chemical. Thus there is the promise of being able to monitor workers for exposures at a site where differences in disposition *and* interaction at the molecular target *and* repair mechanisms in that individual are no longer an unaccounted for entity.

There will also be increasing attention to the *detection of toxicity that may have been unappreciated in the past* due to inadequate measurement techniques. Examples of these can be found with investigations into neuro-behavioural effects of solvents and greater emphasis on immunological alterations induced by chemicals *and* the relevance of such changes to the organism as a whole. Another improvement in monitoring for what may be subtle hepatic effects of solvents can be found in recent studies on serum bile acids in both exposed workers and experimental animals (Franco, 1991; Bai *et al.*, 1992a, b; Driscoll *et al.*, 1992).

It might also be anticipated that with the passage of time there will be an *improvement in data* used for hazard assessment for occupational chemicals. Toxicology in general would also benefit substantially from *improvements in models* used for hazard assessment. This is exemplified by the increasing use of the pharmacokinetic modelling approach in recent times (Clewell and Andersen, 1989; Conolly and Andersen, 1991). However, it must be remembered that substantial amounts of data are required in the first instance to allow the successful application of such models.

Three final issues are deserving of special mention because of their importance and because they are not really the province of the occupational toxicologist but impinge greatly on our efforts. Firstly, it is apparent that even the existing toxicological knowledge is not always transmitted and disseminated as well as it should be. Efforts to improve this should be continued. Secondly, it would seem that chemical-related injury in the workplace may be reduced by invoking programmes to change attitudes with regard to exposure to occupational chemicals. It seems as if even when the knowledge is there it is sometimes ignored for questionable reasons. Finally, it will be difficult to evaluate the benefits of such programmes because our baseline knowledge of the extent of workplace chemical-related injury is unknown. While it should be appreciated that this is a difficult problem, it will be essential to have such knowledge in the future to determine the areas where resources should be concentrated.

References

Amdur, M. O., Doull, J. and Klaassen, C. D. (Eds), 1991, *Casarett and Doull's Toxicology. The Basic Science of Poisons*, 4th Edn. New York: Pergamon Press.
Bai, C., Canfield, P. J. and Stacey, N. H., 1992a, Effects of hexachloro-1, 3-butadiene and 1,1,2,2-tetrachloroethylene on individual serum bile acids, *Toxicol. Indust. Health*, **8**, 191–203.

Bai, C., Canfield, P. J. and Stacey, N. H., 1992b, Individual serum bile acids as early indicators of carbon tetrachloride- and chloroform-induced liver injury, *Toxicology*, **75**, 221–34.

Castleman, B. I. and Ziem, G. E., 1988, Corporate influence on threshold limit values, *Am. J. Indust. Med.*, **13**, 531–59.

Clewell, H. J., III and Andersen, M. E., 1989, Improving toxicology testing protocols using computer simulations, *Toxicol. Lett.*, **49**, 139–58.

Conolly, R. B. and Andersen, M. E., 1991, Biologically based pharmacodynamic models: tools for toxicological research and risk assessment, *Ann. Rev. Pharmacol. Toxicol.*, **31**, 503–23.

Driscoll, T., Hamdan, H., Wang, G. F., Wright, P. F. A. and Stacey, N. H., 1992, Concentrations of individual serum or plasma bile acids in workers exposed to chlorinated aliphatic hydrocarbons, *Br. J. Indust. Med.*, **49**, 700–5.

Franco, G., 1991, New perspectives in biomonitoring liver function by means of serum bile acids: experimental and hypothetical biochemical basis, *Br. J. Indust. Med.*, **48**, 557–61.

Halton, D. M., 1988, A comparison of the concepts used to develop and apply occupational exposure limits for ionizing radiation and hazardous chemical substances, *Reg. Toxicol. Pharmacol.*, **8**, 343–55.

Hemminki, K., Grzybowska, E., Chorazy, M., Twardowska-Saucha, K., Sroczynski, J. W., Putman, K. L., Randerath, K., Phillips, D. H., Hewer, A., Santella, A. M. and Perera, F. P., 1990, DNA adducts in humans related to occupational and environmental exposure to aromatic compounds, in Vainio, H., Sorsa, M. and McMichael, A. J. (Eds) *Complex Mixtures and Cancer Risk*. Lyon: IARC.

International Agency for Research on Cancer, 1987, *IARC Monographs on the Evaluation of Carcinogenic Risks to Humans*, Supplement 7. Lyon: IARC.

Lauwerys, R. R., 1991, Occupational toxicology, in Amdur, M. O., Doull, J. and Klaassen, C. D. (Eds) *Casarett and Doull's Toxicology. The Basic Science of Poisons*, 4th Edn. New York: Pergamon Press.

Markowitz, S. and Landrigan, P., 1989, The magnitude of the occupational disease problem: an investigation in New York State, *Toxicol. Indust. Health*, **5**, 9–30.

National Research Council, 1984, *Toxicity Testing. Strategies to Determine Needs and Priorities*. Washington, DC: National Academy Press.

Roach, S. A. and Rappaport, S. M., 1990, But they are not thresholds: a critical analysis of the documentation of threshold limit values, *Am. J. Indust. Med.*, **17**, 727–53.

Tyson, C. A. and Stacey, N. H., 1992, *In vitro* technology, trends and issues, in Frazier, J. M. (Ed.) *In Vitro Toxicity Testing. Applications to Safety Evaluation*, pp. 13–43. New York: Marcel Dekker.

Chapter 2

Basics of Toxicology

N. H. Stacey

Introduction

The intention of this chapter is to provide an outline of the basic aspects of toxicology to enable the reader to appreciate and understand the principles of the science when using toxicological information in a workplace situation. Furthermore, areas that are pertinent to toxicology in general will be covered in a broad sense so that the reader is aware of their existence and how they are integrated into toxicology overall. Thus a framework for the field of toxicology will be provided for future application by the reader.

It is perhaps of interest to mention some of the difficulties experienced by those working in the field of toxicology at this introductory stage. They relate primarily to the perceptions of others about toxicology and the general concern about chemicals amongst the public at large. In an address to the Society of Toxicology meeting in the USA in 1987, press referred to the difficulties of science due to the uncertainties in particular areas such as the interpretation of some experimental animal carcinogenicity data. It is often inappropriate if not incorrect to make unequivocal pronouncements on such matters but this is often interpreted by others as evasiveness. Dayan (1981) has raised similar issues in pointing out that the toxicologist is often lauded for preventing harm but attacked for failing to prevent all undesired effects of chemicals and disparaged as a source of delay and cost to the industry concerned. He goes on to indicate that many industrial toxicologists are troubled by the impossibility of their work ever meeting public and managerial expectations. The media also play an important role in the perception and appreciation of toxicology by the general public. One example that illustrates the point very clearly to the author, concerns the issue of beef meat contaminated with pesticide residues. Recently this became an issue and many media communications over several days addressed the matter expressing great concern over the impact on the export market. For weeks nothing was published on possible health effects on local consumers. If there had not been a significant export market at stake and the story was followed up by the media the slant would have been different and could well have focused on the long-term health implications of the local consumer. The point is that the media play an important role in the public perception of toxicological matters by the manner in which they present material.

Terms and definitions

'Toxicology' and other associated terms have been defined in various ways by different experts. The definitions used here are believed to be the most appropriate, but the reader should be aware that others will present slightly different views. Where it is felt necessary and/or beneficial, explanations relating to differences or confusion in terminology will be provided.

Toxicology is the study of the adverse effects of agents on living organisms. This definition will benefit from some expansion. *Study* refers to various aspects such as experimentation, collection, collation, evaluation and review of toxicological material. *Adverse* refers to unwanted effects— these are usually overt but may also include more subtle effects. The adverse nature of an effect may be contentious (as referred to in Chapter 1) in that an effect may be considered adverse by some but not others. Then there will be other effects about which it may be uncertain as to whether they are truly adverse to the homeostasis of the organism as a whole. *Agent* is used because, even though it is chemicals that are most often dealt with, other entities such as radiation and dusts fall within the bounds of toxicology. *Living organisms* indicates that the target of concern spans plants through lower animals through to humans. In different branches of toxicology any one of these may be the target of concern.

It is now worth defining a **toxicologist**, who may be considered as an individual with expertise in the nature of the adverse effects of agents on living organisms and the assessment of the probability of their occurrence. While this may appear somewhat repetitive, it highlights one very important aspect. That is, once the process of assessment involving humans is being undertaken there is the opportunity for subjectivity to become a factor in any final decisions. This relates very much to what some have described as the art and the science of toxicology (Doull, 1984). That is, the science is the hard data upon which assessments are made, while the art is the less certain process of decision-making which will often involve subjective and/or arbitrary components. One example of this is the choice of a safety or uncertainty factor when deciding on an acceptable exposure standard.

Now that a definition of toxicology has been given and the extra dimension that the toxicologist brings to the science has been explained, it is pertinent to split toxicology into different divisions in order to understand better what toxicology involves. A convenient breakdown is provided in Figure 2.1.

It can be seen that the first two areas in Figure 2.1 can be collectively viewed as generator areas of toxicology, while the latter two can be

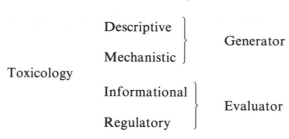

Figure 2.1. Breakdown of toxicology into divisions.

regarded as evaluator divisions. That is, descriptive and mechanistic toxicology are involved in actually generating the required information while the latter two are primarily involved in using and evaluating the information for particular purposes. A toxicologist may work in any of these divisions or across these divisions, as is often the case. Needless to say, a mix of expertise brings advantages to activities in any particular area. It should also be appreciated that others have used different terms such as 'testing', 'research' and 'safety evaluation' (Malmfors, 1981), but the meaning is essentially similar.

Descriptive toxicology involves the undertaking of experiments or test procedures to provide standard toxicological data for the assessment of the safety of a chemical. This includes various protocols from acute to chronic toxicity testing, which will be detailed later. Thus the outcome is data that describe the toxicity of the chemical under test.

Mechanistic toxicology involves the study of mechanisms by which chemicals exert their toxic effects. While it seems that this has been regarded by some in the past as an academic pursuit, it is becoming increasingly realised just how important understanding the mechanism of action is if a meaningful risk assessment for humans is to be undertaken.

Informational toxicology involves the collection, collation and dissemination of toxicological information. It increasingly includes some interpretation and summarising of data as, for example, is seen in the provision of material safety data sheets for chemicals. This area of information provision has been overlooked by others but it is one of developing importance and visibility, particularly in the application of toxicological knowledge. It is crucial that those involved in the area have an adequate background in toxicology so that their efforts are not thwarted by misinterpretation of often complex material.

Regulatory toxicology involves the evaluation of the available data for an agent and decision-making about its application. A clear example of this is the setting of workplace exposure standards. As outlined earlier, tasks like this bring another dimension to toxicology in that there is much more scope for subjectivity and opinion to have an influence on outcome. The final decision may often be based on factors in addition to the toxicological information. This is not to say that the toxicological information is disregarded but a recognition that socio-economic factors as well as differing opinions among experts have been involved in the final decision on how a chemical may or may not be used.

Other terms that are intimately involved in toxicology and the application of data also require attention as follows.

● *Toxicity* is the intrinsic capacity of an agent to adversely affect an organism.

● *Hazard* is the potential for the toxicity of an agent to be realised in a particular situation.

● *Risk* is the probability that a hazard will be realised.

● *Safety* is the probability that a hazard will not be realised.

Again, one may find that others define these terms a little differently, so it is worth explaining them further by way of example. Consider a chemical that has a known acute toxicity in that y mg kg^{-1} will result in death. It is to be used in a factory for the production of a certain material in a fully enclosed process. Before it is delivered to the factory it presents no hazard to the workers at that plant. Once it has been delivered there is potential for exposure during procedures such as handling, accident during operation, during maintenance procedures, and so on. Thus there is a certain hazard now present. However, the toxicity of the chemical (its inherent properties) belong to the chemical itself and remain unchanged irrespective as to whether it is in the supply house, on the delivery truck or at the plant. Risk is when one quantitates the likelihood of a hazard being realised— that is, an estimate of the likelihood of an event occurring is given in numerical terms.

Consideration of these terms highlights a very important aspect of toxicology, in that for a toxic response to be manifest exposure must occur. That is, not only is the toxicity of the chemical of importance but so are the conditions under which it is used, which relate to the exposure that occurs. If there is no exposure there can be no toxicological effects.

Empirical truisms in toxicology

There are two fundamental aspects of toxicology that are critical to its functionality and application. They are usually described as basic assumptions or tenets, but empirical truisms may better represent their origins. These are the relationship between dose and response or effect and the validity of extrapolation of data from experimental animals to humans.

Dose response and dose effect

As the dose of a chemical is increased the response or effect also increases. The first formal recognition of this relationship is attributed to Paracelsus (also known as Philippus Theophrastus Aureolus von Hohenheim) of the sixteenth century. Interestingly, his reason for espousing the relationship was to justify his use of a remedy of recognised toxicity for treatment of the Great Pox. As a justification for his use of this poisonous remedy he was informing those concerned about its use that it was the dose that was important in determining whether or not a toxic reaction occurs. Thus he was indicating that if the appropriate dose was given the therapeutic benefit could be obtained without the toxicity being expressed. The obvious relationship to concerns over exposures to workplace chemicals is that it should be possible to determine an exposure level below which a response or effect will not be seen. Thus an acceptable exposure level should be attainable. It is worth noting at this stage that this is an area of uncertainty and debate for carcinogenic effects of chemicals.

The terms 'response' and 'effect' require some clarification because they are used differently in different areas of occupational health. *Response* is used to mean the proportion of a population showing a specified change. *Effect* is the actual magnitude of the change in the parameter. An example

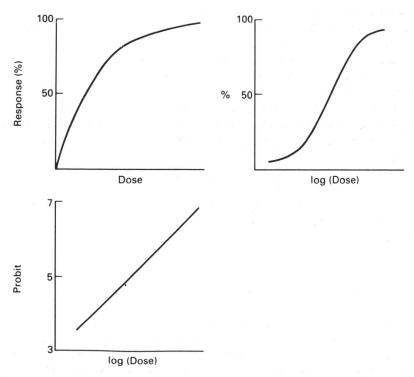

Figure 2.2. Examples of the relationship between dose and response using different scales.

will help to explain the difference. If there is evidence of liver damage in response to exposure to different levels of a particular agent the data could be presented as the number of individuals as compared with the total with a serum alanine aminotransferase level over, say, 100 IUl^{-1} at the different exposure levels. This would be the response. Alternatively, the data could be presented as the actual enzyme measurements at the different exposure levels, say 95 or 870 IUl^{-1}. This would be the effect. These terms will be used differently and often interchangeably by others. This is most probably related to the use in pharmacology of the terms 'quantal response' and 'graded response' as equivalent to 'response' and 'effect', respectively, as defined above.

The relationship between dose and response or effect is often depicted graphically using log(dose) against response or effect arithmetically or using a probit scale. Return to arithmetic versus arithmetic is also useful in dealing with extrapolation from high to low dose levels. Examples of plots using these scales are shown in Figure 2.2. The use of log scales has facilitated calculation of values such as the dose calculated to cause lethality in half the exposed population (LD_{50} value), that calculated to cause a certain toxic outcome in 1% of those exposed (TD_1 value), and so on. However, such scales have not proved useful when it is necessary to extrapolate from the high doses used experimentally in small numbers of animals to the low doses experienced by humans where it is desirable to be able to predict response rates of down to 0.0001%. This remains a contentious issue in contemporary toxicology and is of primary concern when dealing with end-points such as carcinogenicity as there is debate about the existence of a threshold for this event. The existence of a *threshold* means that there is a dose below which there will be no effect. However, when there may be no threshold there is a need to extrapolate to very low exposure levels and the shape of the curve is unknown at this point. Figure 2.3 illustrates some possible alternatives. In order that experimental data are accurate from a statistical point of view, huge numbers of experimental animals would be required—tens or hundreds of thousands for each

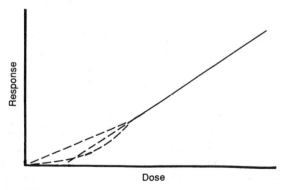

Figure 2.3. Possible alternative ways of extrapolating to very low levels of response.

chemical. The only alternative that seems to be available currently is to continue to use the high dose protocol and extrapolate cautiously due to the added uncertainty. If known, factors relating to non-linear kinetics due to saturation of metabolic pathways must be incorporated into the evaluation process as these may be important in allowing a more accurate determination of appropriate exposure levels.

Extrapolation across species

Extrapolation of data from experimental animals such as rats to humans is central to the use of toxicological data. However, there are undoubtedly many exceptions to this association and one must be circumspect in extrapolating without giving due thought to the undertaking. In fact there have been so many differences documented that there is serious reservation by some about accepting any animal data for extrapolation to humans. While, as noted above, caution is required in undertaking the process, one should not lose the overall perspective. In this regard the author challenges the sceptic to think of general groups of chemicals, pick one or two chemicals at random and compare toxicity in rats and humans along the lines shown in Table 2.1.

Table 2.1. Extrapolation across species

	Consider:
Metals	Cadmium
Solvents	Trichloroethane
	n-Hexane
Pesticides	Organophosphate
Plastics	Vinyl chloride

It is interesting to do this, and to illustrate the point the examples in Table 2.1 will be used. More details on these are given in subsequent relevant chapters. Therefore, only general aspects are raised here to draw out the general similarities.

Cadmium is recognised as causing nephrotoxicity as one of its main toxic end-points on long-term exposure of humans. In rats, the toxic response is also found to involve the kidneys. In both rats and humans evidence of kidney damage is first seen from protein in the urine once kidney cortex cadmium concentrations reach around $180\,\mu g\,g^{-1}$ wet weight.

With 1,1,1-trichloroethane, as with most organic solvents, the toxic response of primary concern in humans relates to their effects on the central nervous system, especially for high levels of acute exposure where deaths have occurred. Similar observations are made in experimental animals where at high doses the narcotic effects of 1,1,1-trichloroethane are evident. With *n*-hexane the toxicity of concern is one of peripheral neuropathy, which was found in exposed workers. Similar effects occur in exposed rats with clear biochemical and morphological correlates.

The mechanism by which organophosphates kill their target species, insects, is by inhibition of cholinesterases. In humans, decreases in workers' blood levels of cholinesterase are used to determine when workers should be removed from exposure to these chemicals. Thus the same biochemical effect is being observed across species.

Vinyl chloride is the monomer used to make the very common plastic PVC (polyvinyl chloride). In the early 1970s PVC was found to cause cancers in rats. About 3 years later haemangiosarcomas were found in livers of workers exposed to vinyl chloride during PVC manufacture. In 1975 the same very rare tumour was detected in rats as well (see Chapter 12).

It should be reiterated that there are many examples where there are important differences across species and the possibility of such differences must be considered when applying animal data. Nevertheless, these differences should not detract from the continued recognition of the predictive ability of data from experimental animals to humans. It should also be appreciated that, while there are often qualitative similarities across species for chemical toxicity data, there are often quantitative differences. This is one sound reason for the inclusion of safety or uncertainty factors when using animal data to determine acceptable exposure levels for humans.

How the body affects chemicals and influences toxicity

As previously mentioned, in order that a toxic response be manifest there must first be exposure to the chemical. Then, unless the toxic response is local in nature (that is, at the point of first contact) the chemical will need to move to the site within the body where the toxic response occurs. Once in the body further events may be required for the toxic response such as biotransformation, depletion of critical protective body molecules, interaction with key components in the cells and so on. Elimination of the chemical will be necessary, otherwise it will build up to toxic levels eventually. Then there will be other variables that may influence the toxic response. This section deals briefly with how the body affects chemicals, especially with respect to the toxicity that they may incur. Figure 2.4 schematically represents the major relevant influences of the body on chemicals.

Exposure

Both the route and duration of exposure are important with regard to toxicity. Major routes of exposure are shown in Figure 2.4. Those of primary concern in the workplace are inhalation and dermal. Ingestion can be of importance if hands are contaminated, as can swallowing respiratory

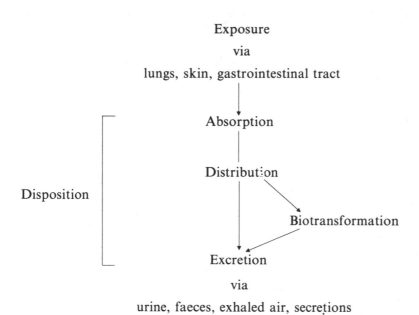

Exposure

via

lungs, skin, gastrointestinal tract

Absorption

Distribution

Disposition

Biotransformation

Excretion

via

urine, faeces, exhaled air, secretions

Figure 2.4 Schematic representation of the passage of chemicals through the body.

secretions after inhalational exposure. Inhalation of dusts, gases, vapours and aerosols from the workplace air is an obvious way of exposure by breathing, while the dermal route is less obvious. There are examples of situations where repeated air monitoring shows undetectable levels of a chemical, while urinary monitoring continually presents positive results (see MOCA exercise Chapter 19). Not all chemicals cross the skin, however. Indeed, the skin is generally a very efficient barrier to chemicals but there are some that cross readily and those people responsible for workplace health and safety need to be aware of this possibility.

When testing chemicals for their toxic properties the route of exposure chosen should reflect the most likely route by which humans would be exposed. This is not always the case as can be appreciated from the earlier section on comparison of routes. In experimental toxicology it is often convenient to use routes that are quite unusual such as intravenous, subcutaneous or intraperitoneal. The reader should especially be familiar with the last of these (the intraperitoneal route is by injection into the peritoneal cavity) as it is quite often used as a convenient way of administering a chemical that will result in high absorption.

Duration of exposure needs to be considered from two aspects. Firstly, whether the exposure is one that occurs on a single occasion or whether there is an ongoing day-by-day exposure to (presumably) low levels of the chemical. Table 2.2 presents these types of exposure with examples.

It should be noted that the terms used are similar to those for the test methods outlined for Toxicity resting-descriptive toxicology, in the section on Terms and Definitions.

Table 2.2. Duration of exposure

Nature	Example
Acute	Accident; maintenance in enclosed space
Subchronic	Worker on process for 1 year
Chronic	Worker on process for 20 years; pesticide in food

Secondly, duration of exposure in an acute situation is particularly important in some workplace situations. For example, it may be possible to be exposed to a certain concentration of a chemical in the inspired air for, say, 15 min without serious health effects, but exposure for, say, 2 h to the same concentration may have serious consequences. Thus, in such situations the duration of exposure becomes critical. This is, of course, related to the actual dose that the individual is exposed to. It should be noted that one way of expressing toxic or lethal concentrations in air is by using toxic time (TT) or lethal time (LT) values. For example, a LT_{50} of 60 min means that at the designated concentration of that chemical in air exposure for 1 h would be expected to result in death of 50% of those exposed.

When gathering toxicity information it becomes clear that much more acute toxicity data exist for oral exposures than for other routes such as inhalational or dermal. This can be limiting when preparing information about chemicals for which the likely exposure route is via the lungs or the skin. Some extrapolation across routes can be undertaken, however, as determined by Agrawal (1993), who comprehensively compared acute toxicity by different routes of administration. Table 2.3 shows comparative classifications for acute toxicity for the three major routes of exposure.

Table 2.3. Classification system for acute toxicity

Classification	Oral LD_{50} ($mg\,kg^{-1}$)	Dermal LD_{50} ($mg\,kg^{-1}$)	Inhal LC_{50} ($mg\,m^{-3}$)
Supertoxic	< 5	< 250	< 250
Extremely toxic	5–50	250–1000	250–1000
Very toxic	50–500	1000–3000	1000–10 000
Moderately toxic	500–5000	3000–10 000	10 000–30 000
Slightly toxic	> 5000	> 10 000	> 30 000

Disposition

Once there has been exposure to a chemical other factors become involved in the processes that relate to the eventual expression of a toxic response. Collectively these are often referred to as 'disposition', which includes absorption, distribution, biotransformation and excretion of chemicals. These are included in Figure 2.4 as a general outline of the interaction between the body and chemicals. For each of the processes of absorption, distribution and excretion there are certain common aspects that govern the movement of the chemical molecules. These relate directly to the passage of the molecules across cellular membranes which relate to the composition of the membranes which are made up of a lipid bilayer containing protein molecules. Both play a role in the passage of molecules across the membrane to the inside of cells which is the site of most crucial interactions for the actual toxic event. Those chemicals that are readily soluble in oils (which is reflected in their oil/water partition coefficient) are able to easily dissolve in the lipid of the membrane which is in a fluid state. The chemical molecules can then move in the lipid and cross to the inside of the cell. This process is generally referred to as simple diffusion. Factors affecting this simple diffusion apart from the oil/water partition coefficient of the chemical in question include the concentration gradient and the area and thickness of the membrane. This process will only occur down a concentration gradient—that is from high to low concentration. This raises another important concept for this process, however, in that the overall movement is dynamic and will occur in both directions across the membrane. Thus it is net movement down a concentration gradient that is being referred to. It should be appreciated that many chemicals exist in both ionised and non-ionised forms and it is the latter that are more lipid soluble. Thus the degree of ionisation under body conditions will be important with regard to the amount to cross membranes. There is also some passage by aqueous channels and by endocytosis, but these are relatively minor pathways. Some protein components of the cell membrane are also involved in the movement of molecules to the interior (or exterior) of the cell. They act as carriers for the passage of particular chemical molecules across the membrane. The process is subject to saturation and to competition by like molecules (competitive inhibition). Both facilitated diffusion and active transport have these characteristics, being differentiated by the requirement of metabolic energy for active transport and the ability of this process to result in net movement against a concentration gradient.

Absorption

Absorption is essentially the passage of chemical molecules across the membranes of the cells that separate internal and external aspects of the body. Once across these cell membranes the molecules enter the blood which will then distribute the chemical to other parts of the body. While there are similarities for absorption at the major sites—gastrointestinal tract, lungs and skin—there are also some important differences. Absorption from the gastrointestinal tract occurs along its entire length although mostly in the upper parts. As there is varying pH from, for example, 1–2 in the stomach to about 8 in the small intestine, chemicals that exist in an ionised/non-ionised equilibrium will be differentially absorbed. Other factors include the amount of surface area available and the effects of digestive enzymes and intestinal flora on chemicals. As has been mentioned already, the lungs are the most important site for absorption of chemicals from workplace exposures. Factors that predispose to rapid absorption in the lungs include their large surface area, the high blood flow to them and the close proximity of the alveolar air to the blood. Other factors such as size and dimensions of dusts and aerosols are important with regard to how far into the respiratory system they penetrate which affects their absorption substantially. These aspects in particular will be covered in greater detail in the chapters on the respiratory system (Chapter 4) and particulate matter (Chapter 14). Similarly, further information on dermal absorption is to be found in Chapter 5. Suffice to reiterate here that the skin presents a considerably greater barrier to absorption than do either of the other two routes outlined above. The molecules need to pass a large number of cells to reach the blood which inhibits the process.

Distribution

Distribution is the movement of the chemical molecules around the body from the site of absorption to the various tissues. Factors influencing this process include the blood supply to the tissue, movement across capillary beds and, of course, movement across the cell membranes. Concentration in different tissues will depend on factors such as binding to cellular constituents (for example, metallothionine), exchange into the tissue (for example, accumulation of lead and fluoride in bone), active transport in that tissue, and high fat solubility. It should be appreciated that the brain is protected by extra barriers which inhibit access by many chemicals. Once an initial distribution has occurred there will be ongoing redistribution back to the blood to other tissues and so on, as the situation is dynamic with some movement/exchange always occurring. Redistribution is readily apparent in the kinetics of some chemicals such as lead which has an initial distribution to red blood cells but later is concentrated in bone.

Excretion

Excretion serves to remove chemicals from the body. This is important because if this did not occur chemicals would accumulate in the body until toxic and/or lethal levels were reached. The main routes of excretion are via the kidney in the urine, via the gastrointestinal tract in the faeces (from non-absorbed material or the bile), via the expired air or to a minor extent via other bodily secretions such as sweat, saliva, semen and milk. These are included in Figure 2.4. The urine is the most important route of excretion as many chemicals and/or their metabolites are eliminated in this way. The blood is filtered at the glomerulus of the nephron with the plasma minus high molecular weight proteins forming the filtrate. This fluid passes to the tubules where components are subject to reabsorption across the membranes of the cells lining the tubules. If this happens as it will with liposoluble compounds the chemical re-enters the blood and will not be excreted. If the molecules are not reabsorbed they will remain in the urinary fluid, pass to the bladder and eventually be voided with the urine and hence excreted. Thus the more water soluble the molecule is at this stage the more likely it is that it will be excreted. This is an important factor when considering biotransformation (next section) as one overall outcome of biotransformation is to make metabolites more water soluble and thereby promote excretion from the body. Some molecules are actively secreted by the cells of the kidney tubules, but this is not an important aspect of excretion in general. It should be noted that the pH of urine is variable and that the excretion of chemicals that are subject to an equilibrium of ionised to non-ionised molecules will thus be affected. The other routes of excretion are of lesser importance, although for some metals the biliary route is important and for some volatile chemicals excretion across the lungs is a major elimination pathway.

Biotransformation

This process, which is also sometimes called 'metabolism', is being dealt with a little separately from the other components of disposition because it is rather distinct from them. While molecules must attain certain intracellular sites to undergo biotransformation the process is biochemically quite different. However, it should be noted that biotransformation is an important component in the handling of chemicals by the body because it can eliminate the parent molecule by changing its structure. This performs a similar function to excretion because that parent molecule no longer exists in the body. Nevertheless, the metabolite is still present and still needs to be dealt with.

Further to the elimination of a molecule by changing its structure to a metabolite, the advantage to the body of the process of biotransformation is to change the parent molecules to forms that are more readily excreted. Overall, biotransformation can be viewed as turning liposoluble compounds into more water soluble forms. As noted above, this promotes the excretion of the chemicals from the body which is necessary so that they do not build up to toxic levels. Thus in general terms biotransformation may be regarded as a detoxifying process.

The enzyme systems responsible for biotransformation are found primarily in the liver, although lesser amounts exist in several other organs including lung, small intestine, adrenal cortex and kidney. They not only biotransform exogenous chemicals but various endogenous moieties such as steroidal hormones, bile acids and fat-soluble vitamins, to name a few. The

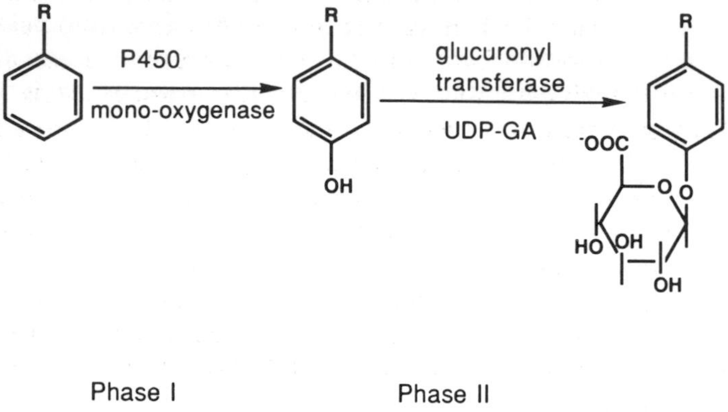

Phase I   Phase II

Figure 2.5 Representative example of phase I and phase II biotransformation

main site and disparate function of these enzyme systems may relate (in an evolutionary sense) to the wide range of chemical structures found in the foods we eat, remembering that blood containing absorbed foods goes through the liver before reaching the general circulation.

Biotransformation is usually separated into two parts—phase I and phase II. The two phases are generally regarded as being linked in that the products of phase I often provide substrates for phase II. A representative example of this process is shown in Figure 2.5.

Phase I biotransformation is mainly carried out by a family of enzymes known as the 'cytochrome P450 system' which is also referred to as the 'P450 mono-oxygenases' or the 'mixed function oxidases'. They are found mainly in the endoplasmic reticulum of the liver but are in lesser amounts in other organs. They consist of many similar proteins with varying substrate specificities and, as the name implies, catalyse largely oxidative reactions. This is not always the case, however, as some reactions are reductive. The enzymes are subject to induction by a variety of chemicals and to inhibition also. While the process of biotransformation is generally one of advantage to the organism from the toxicity point of view, there are also many examples of toxicity where it is the metabolite that is the offending moiety rather than the parent molecule. One example of this is with the formation of epoxides (an oxygen bridge across two carbon atoms) which are very reactive and have been implicated as important in the process of carcinogenicity. The genotoxicity of 1,3-butadiene, for example, involves the formation of epoxide metabolites. Other phase I biotransformations are carried out by enzymes other than those of the P450 system such as the flavin-containing mono-oxygenase, epoxide hydrolase, esterases, amidases and alcohol and aldehyde dehydrogenases. Some substrates are also metabolised by a peroxidase-dependent co-oxidation. To extend the above example with epoxides the epoxide hydrolase enzyme may biotransform the epoxide to a dihyrodiol which may be further biotransformed to the diol epoxide which may play a critical role in carcinogenesis. As can be appreciated from this one example, biotransformation can be a complex process with many steps to either detoxification or, in some cases, to toxic moieties.

Phase II biotransformation generally results in the addition of a relatively large moiety to the substrate, which is often the product of a phase I reaction. Examples of the different sorts of phase II biotransformation reactions are shown in Table 2.4. An example of the most common of these reactions, glucuronidation, is shown in Figure 2.5. The products of phase II reactions are often much more water soluble than the substrates, thereby promoting the overall excretion of the chemical. The glucuronidation process uses uridine-5'-diphospho-α-D-glucuronic acid (UDP-GA) as a cofactor and is carried out mainly in the endoplasmic reticulum of the liver.

Table 2.4. Examples of phase II biotransformation processes

Glucuronyl transferase
Glutathione *S*-transferase
Sulphotransferase
Amino acid conjugase
Methyl transferase
N-Acetyl transferase

Another common phase II reaction is via the enzyme glutathione *S*-transferase which is actually a family of enzymes responsible for the eventual formation of mercapturic acid or thioether metabolites. These have been determined in urine in biological monitoring for exposure to some chemicals. As the name implies, the cofactor for the enzyme is the tripeptide, reduced glutathione. This is a widely studied reactant in the detoxification of a variety of chemicals. If its supply is limited, increased toxicity may be observed.

While it has been stated that the biotransformation of chemicals is overall a detoxification process, it must be remembered that many chemicals are toxic because they are biotransformed. It is the metabolites of some chemicals that actually cause the toxicity. This has been extensively studied and the reader is referred to other texts for further information. As it is important to understand how biotransformation can result in a toxic product and as it is also important that the reader appreciates the value of such knowledge, a salient example using *n*-hexane is given in Chapter 11 on solvents.

Toxicokinetics

The quantitative study and mathematical description of the disposition of chemicals related to their toxic effects is termed 'toxicokinetics'. Thus the amount absorbed, the relative distribution to different tissues, the rate of

removal by biotransformation and/or excretion are all included in a toxico-
kinetic appraisal of the movement of a chemical through the body. While
there will be no attempt to detail the field of toxicokinetics in this text, it
should be appreciated by the reader that important information is attainable from understanding the kinetics of chemicals in the body. For example,
the amount absorbed will be a factor in the toxicity of a chemical—if none
is absorbed then there will be no systemic toxicity at a site removed from
the portal of entry. The reader should be warned not to oversimplify this,
however, as lack of absorption of particles like nickel subsulphide from the
lung may in fact be a major factor in the toxicity expressed at that site. That
is, no absorption does not simply equate to no toxicity.

Knowledge of the toxicokinetics of a chemical also allows prediction of
body burdens of a chemical, both temporally and quantitatively even after
exposure has stopped. It is also crucial to know about the kinetics (and
biotransformation) of a chemical when planning or implementing urinary
monitoring programmes. This can be clearly appreciated by considering this
aspect in the chlordimeform exercise given in Chapter 19.

The application of toxicokinetics is also important in the risk assessment
process both in extrapolating from high dose to low dose and across species.
Knowledge of saturation of kinetic processes at high doses as compared with
low doses must be integrated into the risk assessment process if it is known
to occur. Similarly, differences in the quantitative handling of chemicals
across species can be crucial to a meaningful risk assessment for a chemical.
It should be appreciated, however, that often critical pieces of data, such as
the kinetics in humans, may not be readily available or obtainable for
ethical reasons.

How chemicals affect the body

There are different types of toxic effects that chemicals have on the body;
these are listed in Table 2.5.

Table 2.5. Types of effects of chemicals

Local vs. systemic
Acute vs. chronic
Immediate vs. delayed
Reversible vs. irreversible
Cellular vs. molecular
Allergic
Idiosyncratic
Carcinogenic/genotoxic
Developmental

Local as opposed to *systemic* effects are discussed in Chapter 3. The
differences between *acute* and *chronic* exposure have been addressed earlier

in this chapter. This generally relates to effects where there may be a reaction due to a single one-off exposure, perhaps to a high amount of a chemical. On the other hand, a toxic response to another chemical may be seen after repeated long-term low-level exposures, as is the case with carcinogenic effects. Most chemicals will result in *immediate* effects, but for some there will be a delay before the toxicity is manifest. An example of both can be found with paraquat where at a high enough dose death will be immediate, but at a moderate dose death is delayed until about 2 weeks after intoxication. The delayed death is due to pulmonary insufficiency related to fibrosis in the lungs. Many toxic effects, like death, are *irreversible*, while others may be *reversed*—for example by regeneration of liver tissue after toxic insult to that organ. While ultimately all toxicity is related to interactions at the *molecular* level the result may be visible only at the *cellular* level. For example, liver toxicity may be seen as death of the parenchymal cells, but may be related to destruction of cellular lipids or covalent binding of chemical molecules to cellular macromolecules.

There are also specific types of effect that require some attention. *Allergic* reactions are not uncommon and are of concern with workplace chemicals such as toluene diisocyanate (TDI). Here one individual may become extremely sensitive to TDI, reacting to very low levels, while the workmate remains unaffected. *Idiosyncratic* responses are those seen in particular individuals and are related to some underlying metabolic abnormality. They occur at exposure levels below those at which the 'normal' population would respond. The term is often used to account for otherwise inexplicable observations in particular people. *Carcinogenic, genotoxic* and *developmental* effects are specific types of effects that are dealt with in other chapters.

There are a number of other variables that can influence the toxic response to a chemical and that should be kept in mind. These include impurities in the chemical in question, especially if it is a commercial formulation, the vehicle that may be used in the formulation, characteristics of the individual such as sex, age, disease and immunological status, and other environmental factors.

Toxicity testing—descriptive toxicology

In order that information on the toxicity of chemicals is available for the risk assessment process, tests need to be carried out. These are discussed only superficially here and the reader is referred to other sources for further information—in particular, the Organisation for Economic Co-operation and Development guidelines for testing of chemicals. These are detailed procedures covering the tests required for general marketing of chemicals. In addition to these there will be requirements in individual countries which may vary among jurisdictions. This is covered in more detail in Chapter 20. The reader will also need to become familiar with any special requirements that their country may have. The information that is usually required includes that shown in Table 2.6.

Table 2.6. Information required for chemical assessment

Physical and chemical properties
Production, use and disposal
Ecotoxicological data
Toxicological (mammalian) data

It is toxicological data which are our concern here—that is, a description of the toxicity of the chemical in mammals with the most common test species being the rat. The major general testing protocols are related to the duration of exposure (see Table 2.7), with duration given in terms as related to rats.

Table 2.7. Testing protocols for mammalian toxicity

Name	Duration (for rats)
Acute	single
Short-term repeated dose (STRD)	14–28 days
Subchronic	90 days
Chronic	6 to 30 months

It should be noted that there is some confusion in the use of the terms given in Table 2.7, which are consistent with their use by the OECD. 'Subacute' has also been used—in some instances as the equivalent to 'subchronic' and by others to mean the same as 'STRD'. Thus care is required when considering data of this nature. The safest approach is to refer to the actual duration of exposure to the chemical.

The general information sought under the acute toxicity testing protocols includes that listed in Table 2.8. Thus the information will include estimates of the amount of chemical that might result in death of exposed individuals by various routes, an indication as to how damaging skin or eye contact of the chemical would be, and determination of the possibility that a chemical may result in sensitisation of individuals. It should be noted that these last tests are not well developed, and it is not common to test specifically for the potential for respiratory sensitisation; however, it is included here because of its importance to the workplace.

Table 2.8. Acute toxicity testing

Lethality	Oral
	Inhalational
	Dermal
Irritation	Skin
	Eye
Sensitisation	Skin
	Respiratory

While details of the tests are not provided it should be appreciated that there is a single administration of chemical for the acute lethality studies (for a stated duration for inhalation) with subsequent observation of the animals for 7–14 days.

The STRD, subchronic and chronic protocols all involve administration of the test chemical repeatedly for the time specified. The route of exposure should be that likely in humans and there should be a control group plus groups exposed to increasing doses. There should be several animals per group with larger numbers in the chronic protocols. Animals are assessed for parameters such as those shown in Table 2.9.

Table 2.9. Assessment of treated animals

Mortality
Physical examination
Body weight
Diet consumption
Haematology
Clinical chemistry
Gross and microscopic pathology (including organ weight)

It should also be noted that it is a prudent use of resources to combine chronic toxicity studies with studies to determine the oncogenicity of chemicals. The tests cost some millions of dollars so it is economically rational to do this. However, it must also be appreciated that the aims of the two are somewhat different. The protocol for chronic toxicity seeks primarily to determine a level of exposure at which no toxic effects are observed—that is, a no observed effect level (NOEL)—while that for oncogenicity seeks to push the dose as high as practicable without other toxic effects to provide the best chance of detecting an oncogenic effect.

As well as the standard test protocols that have been outlined above there are some speciality tests that require individual test procedures. These are listed in Table 2.10. There will be still more information on certain chemicals used for particular purposes that may be appropriate. Thus it should be remembered that the assessment of the toxicity of chemicals is more than a routine check-list approach. Flexibility should be retained to allow for the provision of additional information as appropriate. Similarly, there may be occasions when information for one or other aspect is unnecessary.

Table 2.10. Specialty tests

Reproduction and fertility
Developmental toxicity (including teratogenicity)
Genotoxicity
Behavioural toxicity
Immunotoxicity
Toxicokinetics

Toxicological information

One aspect of toxicology that everyone involved in the science needs is information. The researcher must be aware of what is already known, the regulator of the extent of information available for assessment, and so on.

There are several levels of toxicity information available. These include the primary literature, reviews, books and computerised databases. Less available, for reasons of confidentiality, are data in government or company files. The primary literature consists of reports of original research published in scientific journals. Reviews are generally found in journals both as covering articles and in publications dedicated to reviewing information in particular fields. There are now several textbooks in the field of toxicology —some covering the science in general, others focusing on one or other aspect of toxicology. The most comprehensive for toxicology in general remains *Casarett and Doull's Toxicology. The Basic Science of Poisons* (Amdur *et al.*, 1991). *Patty's Industrial Hygiene and Toxicology* (1981) consists of several volumes and contains a large amount of toxicological information on chemicals. Several computerised databases are also available for seeking toxicological data on chemicals. While they were once mostly available through substantial libraries, they are now being marketed for more personal use. Some of the useful databases include RTECS, TOXNET, TOXLINE, HSELINE, NIOSHTIC, CISDOC and CCINFO.

For a comprehensive listing of sources of toxicological information the reader is referred to a publication by Wexler (1988) which is dedicated to this topic.

References

Agrawal, M., 1993, Acute toxicity rating charts: the inter-relationship between acute oral, dermal and inhalational toxicities, Master of Occupational Health and Safety Treatise, The University of Sydney.

Amdur, M. O., Doull, J. and Klaassen, C. D. (Eds), 1991, *Casarett and Doull's Toxicology. The Basic Science of Poisons*, 4th Edn. New York: Pergamon Press.

Dayan, A. D., 1981, The troubled toxicologist, *Trends Pharmacol. Sci.*, **2**, 1–4.

Doull, J., 1984, The past, present, and future of toxicology, *Pharmacol. Rev.*, **36**, 15S–18S

Malmfors, T., 1981, Toxicology as science, *Trends Pharmacol. Sci.*, **2**, I.

Patty's Industrial Hygiene and Toxicology, 1981, Clayton, G. D. and Clayton, F. E. (Eds) 3rd Edn. New York: Wiley.

Wexler, P., 1988, *Information Resources in Toxicology*, 2nd Edn. New York: Elsevier.

Targets of Chemicals

Chapter 3

Systemic Toxicology

N. H. Stacey, W. M. Haschek and C. Winder

Introduction

This chapter deals with the important effects of chemicals on various organs or tissues within the body. The toxic responses in the different organs are referred to as *target organ toxicity* or *systemic toxicity*. This type of effect needs to be distinguished from what is known as *local toxicity*. This latter type of toxicity occurs at the site of exposure or first contact, as happens with chemicals that have an irritant or corrosive action on the skin, eye or respiratory tract. Local toxicity commonly occurs with workplace chemicals due to the pattern of usage and hence likely routes of exposure. For systemic toxicity to occur, absorption and distribution of the agent are required so that the effect may be expressed at a site distant from the exposure or contact.

The term 'primary target organ' refers to the organ directly or most severely affected by the toxicant, while 'secondary target organs' are those less severely or indirectly affected. Chemicals are sometimes grouped with respect to their primary target organ for classification purposes. This is one convenient way of splitting the toxic properties of chemicals into manageable and meaningful subunits. Furthermore, this has a useful purpose clinically in that specific organ dysfunction is the most likely clinical presentation. In conjunction with a good occupational history it should be possible to determine if the injury is related to workplace exposure to a chemical. However, chemical-induced organ dysfunction must be differentiated from that due to other causes. The most diagnostic test in most cases is the detection of the chemical or metabolite in body fluids or tissues.

The ultimate expression of toxicity at any particular target depends on a variety of factors, as discussed in some detail in Chapter 2. These include the nature of the chemical itself, the route of exposure, the disposition of the chemical, including any biotransformation, and the sensitivity of the exposed organ or tissue.

Any organ of the body is a potential target for injurious effects from chemicals. Some organs are more susceptible to adverse effects than others. In the workplace setting, the skin and respiratory tract are the two systems most commonly affected, and therefore individual chapters have been devoted to them. Reproductive and developmental toxicity is also dealt with in a separate chapter as this has particular requirements in comparison with other organs or tissues. This chapter provides an overview of the liver and kidney and the nervous, haematopoietic, immune, cardiovascular and gastrointestinal systems. Clearly, each of these is a topic in its own right. For a more detailed coverage of these target organs the reader is referred to texts such as the Target Organ Toxicology Series (Dixon, 1981–), *Casarett and Doull's Toxicology. The Basic Science of Poisons* (Amdur *et al.*, 1991), *Handbook of Toxicologic Pathology* (Haschek and Rousseaux, 1991), or specific references used in the following sections.

Another potential target for chemicals is the genetic material. Interaction with DNA may result in cancer, which is of major concern with workplace chemicals as several have been associated with cancer in workers. Thus Chapters 7 and 8 are devoted to this very important aspect of occupational toxicology.

Liver (N. H. Stacey)

Introduction

The liver is a very important organ for chemical-induced toxicity as it is rather vulnerable to attack by chemicals. Reasons for this include its anatomical location and its ability to concentrate, biotransform and excrete some chemicals via the bile. The first of these, anatomical location, relates especially to ingested chemicals and is therefore less relevant to workplace exposures which occur mainly by inhalation or skin. Nevertheless, it should be appreciated that chemicals absorbed across the gastrointestinal mucosa will then be delivered directly to the liver via the portal blood supply. Thus the liver will be exposed to the highest concentrations of these chemicals and on this basis alone could be expected to exhibit toxicity more often than other organs. Chemicals encountered by other routes of exposure may also reach the liver, through its blood supply from the hepatic artery as well as the portal vein. The second reason listed for susceptibility of the liver to chemical-induced injury is its ability to concentrate, biotransform and excrete chemicals, irrespective of the route of exposure. Chemicals may be toxic as the parent compound or may be biotransformed to reactive metabolites for expression of toxicity. When the metabolite is formed in the liver this organ will again be exposed to the highest concentrations of the toxic moiety with the associated likelihood of being injured. Furthermore, the liver has the greatest amounts of the biotransformation enzymes which also predisposes this organ to injury by reactive metabolites.

Structure and function of the liver

Within the liver, the hepatic artery and portal vein branches, together with the bile collecting system, the bile duct, form the portal triad. The blood entering the liver travels from the portal triad through the sinusoids to the terminal hepatic venule (or central vein) and is thence returned to the systemic circulation via the hepatic vein. Figure 3.1 depicts the structure of the liver. The functional unit of the liver is the acinus, which is divided into zones 1, 2 and 3 (Rappaport, 1980). The area around the portal triads is called 'zone 1' (or 'periportal' according to an old classification), while that around the central vein is 'zone 3' (or 'centrilobular'). Zone 2 (or 'midzonal') lies between zones 1 and 3. When a section of liver is viewed under the microscope the classical hexagonal lobule can be seen as shown in Figure 3.1. The structure can be easily recognised by locating the central vein and portal triads. Knowledge of the structure of the liver is important because a widely used classification of hepatotoxic reactions is based on histological location and appearance. Injury such as necrosis around the central vein is termed 'centrilobular' (sometimes 'pericentral'), while that in the area of the portal space is called 'periportal' (or 'periacinar'). Liver cell damage in between is described as 'midzonal'.

In general terms, the liver is a vital metabolic organ which is essential to the organism's survival. It is singly responsible for the synthesis of many

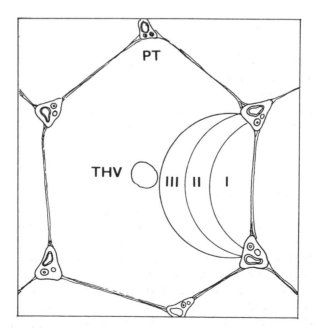

Figure 3.1. Schematic representation of the main structural elements of the liver. PT, portal triad; THV, terminal hepatic venule (or central vein).

proteins, for energy storage in the form of glycogen, for the majority of biotransformation of exogenous chemicals by the body, and the excretion of some chemicals through the bile to name a few. For details on the functions of the liver the reader is referred to other texts such as *The Liver—Biology and Pathobiology* (Arias *et al.*, 1988).

Classification of chemical-induced injury

Liver injury can be classified in various ways. Zimmerman (1978, 1982) may be consulted for greater detail in this field. Firstly, on the basis of its *histological change* or morphological or microscopic appearance with respect to the site within the lobule and with respect to the nature of the alteration; secondly, on the *predictability* of the lesion; and thirdly, with regard to the *organelle* primarily affected.

Histological change

Chemicals can be classified based on the region within the lobule that is damaged. It may be centrilobular as with the classical hepatotoxicant carbon tetrachloride, midzonal as with beryllium, or periportal as exemplified by phosphorus.

The appearance of changes induced in the liver on microscopic examination is varied, as shown in Table 3.1.

Table 3.1. Histological classification of liver injury

Lesion type	Examples
Necrosis	Carbon tetrachloride Beryllium
Steatosis	Carbon tetrachloride Ethanol
Cholestasis	Organic arsenicals
Apoptosis	Uncertain
Immune cell infiltrate	See text
Fibrosis/cirrhosis	Carbon tetrachloride Trinitrotoluene
Neoplasia	Carbon tetrachloride Vinyl chloride
Mixed	Carbon tetrachloride

Necrosis, which is one type of cell death, is a common effect of acute exposure to a hepatotoxic agent. It may be zonal or diffuse. If the insult is not lethal the liver is usually able to undergo complete repair after an episode of acute necrosis. *Steatosis*, or intracellular fat accumulation, is also a common change that is generally reversible on removal of the offending chemical. *Cholestasis*, which means cessation or slowing of bile flow, is another type of injury often encountered. Bile stasis can be observed histologically. More recently, the term 'cholestasis' has been used to describe any interference with biliary function, as this may occur with some chemicals without there necessarily being a clear histological equivalent. *Apoptosis* is a more recently described type of cellular event being important in physiological cell deletion as well as some forms of tissue injury such as chronic active hepatitis. It is usually associated with immune cell-induced cytotoxicity and remains to be convincingly ascribed as a sole cause of chemical-induced damage. *Immune cell infiltrate* is observed in conjunction with chemical-induced cell injury, but it can be unclear if some immune cells are present as a causative factor or as a response to tissue injury to remove cellular debris. Nevertheless, there is a number of chemicals (mainly therapeutic agents) that have a definite association with the presence of immune cells other than in a debris removal function (see Predictability).

Fibrosis and *cirrhosis* are the end result of ongoing liver injury, generally following long-term exposure. Collagen is deposited in the liver leading to a disruption in normal architecture and function. Occupational exposure to carbon tetrachloride and trinitrotoluene has been implicated in this liver condition (Table 3.1). *Neoplasia* may also ensue from such ongoing occupational exposures, with hepatic carcinoma being the most common type of cancer. Other types of cancer have also been recorded with the outstanding example being angiosarcoma following exposure to vinyl chloride. As is apparent from Table 3.1, some chemicals produce more than one type of histological alteration so that the pattern is a *mixed* response.

Predictability

Many chemicals cause liver injury in a manner that is normally expected— that is, in a predictable way with clear evidence of a dose–effect relationship. However, other chemicals do not and, in recognition of this, Zimmerman (1978, 1982) has proposed a classification scheme on this basis. The features of the two types of reaction are shown in Table 3.2.

Table 3.2. Features of predictable and non-predictable hepatotoxicity

	Predictable	Non-predictable
Histology	Distinct	Diffuse/immune cells
Extrahepatic allergy	No	Yes
Dose effect	Yes	No
Latent period	Regular	Varied
Incidence	High	Low
Reproducible in test animals	Yes	No

Non-predictable hepatotoxicity has also been referred to as an 'idiosyncratic response' which may have either an immunological basis resulting in a hypersensitivity type reaction or may be due to a metabolic abnormality.

Organelle

A less commonly used method of classifying hepatotoxicants is according to the organelle primarily affected. Nevertheless, chemicals have been termed as 'primarily injurious' to mitochondria, endoplasmic reticulum, plasma membrane, lysosomes or cytoskeleton. If serious injury does occur to one or other of these organelles then death of the cell may result. Again there may be a mixture of effects, with carbon tetrachloride being a good example, having been associated with damage to all of the above except the cytoskeleton.

Detection and evaluation of liver injury

Acute hepatotoxicity can be detected with commonly used non-invasive tests; detection of subacute and chronic hepatic damage is more difficult. The methods for testing for liver damage in response to chemical exposure are listed in Table 3.3

Table 3.3. Methods for detecting liver injury

Physical examination

Clinical chemistry:
  Enzymes
  Bilirubin
  Bile salts
  Proteins

Histopathology:
  Light microscopy
  Electron microscopy

Organ function test:
  Dye excretion
  Drug biotransformation

Blood sampling followed by analysis of various serum constituents is employed in the first instance as the sampling of liver tissue (biopsy) for microscopic examination is an invasive procedure which can have complications. However, the histological appearance of the liver remains the most definitive indicator of liver injury. The nature of such changes has been outlined above. Biopsy in humans for confirmation of diagnosis is usually employed when there is any uncertainty.

Hepatocytes contain many enzymes that may be released into the blood if the cell membranes are damaged. An elevation of serum enzymes such as alanine aminotransferase and aspartate aminotransferase reflect damage to the hepatic parenchymal cells, while elevated levels of alkaline phosphatase indicate injury to the biliary apparatus of the liver. The enzyme γ-glutamyl transpeptidase is often found to be increased with excessive alcohol consumption. Bilirubin, bile salts and proteins such as albumin and clotting factors are also serum indicators of liver dysfunction. Thus they can be regarded as tests of liver function using endogenous markers. The organ function tests listed in Table 3.3 require administration of exogenous chemicals such as the dye indocyanine green or the drug antipyrine. Neither of these are used routinely in animal experimentation, but they do have (or have had) some application in the evaluation of liver injury in humans and in experimental animal investigations. The use of individual serum bile acids, which seem to provide a very sensitive index of liver injury, may serve as a useful indicator of chemical-induced damage as well as organ dysfunction (Bai *et al.*, 1992). Such dysfunction may be detected prior to release of cytoplasmic enzymes into the blood.

Mechanisms of hepatic injury

The mechanisms by which chemicals cause liver injury are deserving of mention because this knowledge is important in the prevention and treatment of injury. The liver has received more attention than other organs in this regard, probably due to the number of chemicals which have the liver as their primary target. This in turn may be related to the high levels of biotransformation enzymes located in the endoplasmic reticulum. Another factor may be the greater availability of hepatic *in vitro* preparations that retain *in vivo* characteristics for studies relating to mechanism of action of the toxic agent. The various mechanisms that have been implicated in chemical-induced liver injury are listed in Table 3.4.

Table 3.4. Mechanisms of hepatic injury

Lipid peroxidation
Covalent binding
Alteration of calcium homeostasis
Alteration of protein synthesis
Depletion of protein thiols
Mitochondrial dysfunction
Immune mediated
Endonuclease and apoptosis
Interference with triglyceride secretion
DNA damage

Although thousands of papers have been published on these proposed mechanisms over the last 30 years, there is still no comprehensive unified understanding of the steps involved in cell death after exposure to the toxic agent. Each of the mechanisms has considerable evidence supporting its role, but there is also conflicting evidence which is difficult to reconcile with that mechanism bang causally linked to the ensuing cell death. For example, the theory that lipid peroxidation is the cause of liver injury due to some chemicals has a lot of appeal due to the autocatalytic nature of the process once it is initiated. However, some experimental evidence exists that shows that the peroxidation of the lipids can be inhibited without stopping cell death. This clearly suggests that the peroxidation is not directly responsible for the death of the cells induced by that chemical. Similarly, covalent binding of reactive metabolites to cellular macromolecules and disturbance in the homeostasis of the calcium ion have a lot of experimental support. Some critical evidence also disallows unequivocal acceptance of these as the key events in cell death. Inhibition of protein synthesis is an older hypothesis that lost support when the timing of the inhibition did not coincide well with other observations in the process leading to cell destruction. The involvement of mitochondria as a key and causative event also lost favour on consideration of the timing of events. However, more recently there has been a renewed interest in the role of the mitochondrial damage as being directly responsible for cell death. The immunological component relates to the hypersensitivity reactions referred to earlier. It is possible that some chemicals act as haptens by binding to tissue components, thereby presenting an antigenic stimuli which elicits an immune response. This may lead to cell destruction. It is possible that apoptosis could be involved in this process as there are now several reports associating apoptosis with lymphocytotoxicity. It is also possible that some chemicals may activate endonuclease(s) that seem to be involved in the process of apoptosis, which could result in the cell being destroyed. The inhibition of triglyceride secretion is listed last because, although it is one of the mechanisms responsible for steatosis, the cellular accumulation of fat does not necessarily predispose to hepatocyte death.

Overall then, a common component in the pathway leading to liver cell death has yet to be identified. Each of the above proposed mechanisms is clearly involved in some way. With further investigation the current anomalies may be explained or perhaps the critical event that is the irreversible step leading to cell death has not yet been identified. It may also be possible that there is no single step common to all chemicals and that there may be different key effects with different chemicals.

Examples of hepatotoxicity from workplace exposures

There are many chemicals that have the potential to cause liver injury in workers. In the past, chemicals such as carbon tetrachloride have been associated with both acute and chronic liver injury in exposed workers. With increased knowledge and improved workplace conditions such examples are now less frequent. Nevertheless, they do continue to occur, as evidenced by case reports of workers experiencing liver damage after using various chemicals such as dimethyl formamide and methylene dianiline.

Although some examples of hepatotoxicants have already been listed in Table 3.1, it is worth considering such chemicals in greater detail and from the viewpoint of duration of exposure as shown in Table 3.5. In some cases, groups of chemicals, such as organic solvents, are listed because more than one chemical in the group has been associated with that response.

Table 3.5. Examples of workplace exposures that have resulted in hepatic toxicity*

Exposure	Agent	Type of lesion
Acute	Organic solvents	Mixed
STRD †	Tetrachloroethane Trinitrotoluene	Acute or ongoing necrosis. May progress to cirrhosis
Chronic	Arsenicals Vinyl chloride Organic solvents	Fibrosis, cirrhosis, cancer

* Adapted from Dossing and Skinhoj (1985).
† STRD, Short-term repeated dose.

Kidney (W. M. Haschek)

Introduction

It is estimated that nearly 4 million workers in the USA are exposed to chemicals that can be nephrotoxic at high concentrations (Landrigan *et al.*, 1984). Although the best documented toxic causes of renal failure are drugs, occupational exposure to chemicals, such as lead and cadmium, may also play a role in the development of chronic renal failure (Bernard and Lauwerys, 1992). Chemicals can induce renal injury due to a direct effect on the kidney, or indirectly through various systemic effects such as cardiac failure or intravascular haemolysis. In this section only direct toxic injury to the kidney will be considered.

Structure and function of the kidney

On gross dissection, the kidneys are clearly divided into an outer cortex and an inner medulla with papilla extending into the renal pelvis. The kidneys receive 25% of the cardiac output, with approximately 85% of the total renal blood flow distributed to the cortical region and the remainder to the medulla. Thus, most blood-borne chemicals enter the cortex.

The functional and structural unit of the kidney is the nephron, which is divided into the vascular and glomerular portions located in the cortex, and the epithelial tubular segment that extends from the glomerulus into the medulla opening into the pelvis (Figure 3.2). These elements are separated by a sparse but highly vascularised connective tissue, the interstitium.

Blood passes through the afferent arteriole into the glomerulus, where it is filtered by selective passage of water, electrolytes, low molecular weight proteins and other compounds, including waste products. Glomerular filtration is based mainly on molecular size, with retention of plasma proteins with a molecular weight higher than 40 000; net charge and shape also are factors in retention. Chemicals rarely injure the glomerulus, although damage through immune-mediated mechanisms has been reported. The filtrate (urine) passes into the tubule while filtered blood leaves the

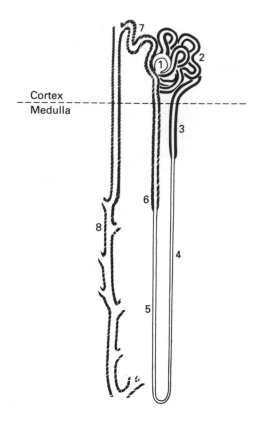

Figure 3.2. The nephron. Note the demarcation between cortex and medulla. (1) Glomerulus; (2) proximal convoluted tubule; (3) proximal straight tubule (pars recta); (4) descending limb of the loop of Henle; (5) thin ascending limb of the loop of Henle; (6) thick ascending limb of the loop of Henle; (7) distal convoluted tubule; (8) collecting duct. (From Hewitt *et al.* (1991: 355), with permission.)

glomerulus by the efferent arteriole, either entering the capillary network surrounding the adjacent nephron or the vasculature supplying the medulla. Therefore, chemicals that reach the glomerulus can be filtered into the urine which is in direct contact with the lumenal side of the tubular epithelium (Figure 3.3). Alternatively, the chemical can remain in the blood, and reach the basal side of the tubular epithelium via the capillary network or enter the medulla. The proximal tubule selectively reabsorbs most of the water, salts, sugars and amino acids from the filtrate. Active secretion by the tubular epithelium from the adjacent capillary network into the urine also occurs and is primarily responsible for excretion of certain organic compounds and for elimination of hydrogen and potassium compounds. The transport systems utilised for these physiological processes are also able to extract and/or concentrate toxic chemicals from the basolateral side of the tubule. The proximal tubule is the most common site of toxic injury due to

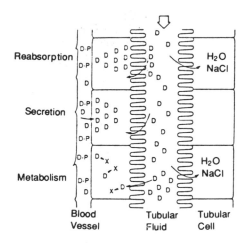

Figure 3.3. The proximal tubule. Chemicals or drugs (D) can reach the tubular epithelial cell either via the tubular fluid (urine) or blood. Once the chemical enters the cell it can remain unchanged, undergo metabolism to a metabolite (X), or be bound to protein (P). (From Hewitt *et al*. (1991: 357), with permission.)

concentration of transport systems in this region; sensitivity to ischaemia (lack of blood supply) because of high energy and substrate requirements, and presence of high concentrations of biotransforming enzymes.

The loop of Henle, which allows the kidney to concentrate urine by the countercurrent mechanism, can also result in concentration of chemicals, such as analgesics, in the deep medulla or papilla. Papillary necrosis is a well known sequela of analgesic abuse. The distal tubule and collecting duct additionally reabsorb sodium chloride and water, and acidify urine.

Classification of chemical-induced renal injury

Chemical-induced renal injury can be classified according to functional and structural characteristics of chemicals, mechanisms of injury (see below), or target sites within the kidney. The most useful classification for consideration of the functional consequences and therefore for clinical evaluation is classification according to target site. The primary target sites for chemicals found in the workplace are the proximal tubule and, less commonly, the glomerulus. The medulla and papilla are target sites of injury due to analgesic abuse and the use of non-steroidal anti-inflammatory drugs (NSAIDs). The proximal tubule is the most common site of chemical-induced injury, including injury from heavy metals, antibiotics, hydrocarbons, herbicides, and organic solvents. The type of injury is dependent on the conditions of exposure (dose and duration) and the properties of the toxicant. Acute injury generally results in tubular epithelial necrosis which may be reversible by epithelial regeneration, depending on the severity of the insult and persistence of the compound. Chronic injury presents as tubulointerstitial nephritis which is often irreversible and can progress to renal failure. Although most renal cancers arise from the proximal tubule, a role for workplace chemical exposure in renal cancer has not been demonstrated (Alden and Frith, 1991).

Injury to the glomerulus, characterised by inflammation (glomerulonephritis), can occur due to immune-mediated mechanisms that result in the deposition of circulating or *in situ* formed immune complexes in the glomerulus. This results in abnormal loss of protein in the urine, predominantly albumin. Gold, mercury, and D-penicillamine have been incriminated in this type of injury (Bernard and Lauwerys, 1992).

Detection and evaluation of renal injury

Clinical signs in patients with renal injury may include oliguria (decreased urine output), oedema from severe hypoalbuminaemia due to glomerular dysfunction (nephrotic syndrome), hypertension, anaemia, and abnormalities of the urine. Examination of the urine (urinalysis) may reveal the presence of blood (haematuria), protein (proteinuria), and/or casts of sloughed tubular cells, clotted blood or inflammatory exudate. Proteinuria is often an early and sensitive indicator of renal injury. High molecular weight proteins in the urine indicate glomerular dysfunction, while low molecular weight proteins indicate tubular dysfunction. If large-scale loss of function has occurred (>67–75% of renal mass) serum concentrations of small molecules such as urea, creatinine, or low molecular weight proteins such as β_2-microglobulin, may be elevated. Other methods that can be used in the detection and evaluation of renal injury are listed in Table 3.6 (Bernard and Lauwerys, 1992).

Table 3.6. Methods for detecting and evaluating chemical-induced renal injury

Urinalysis and microscopy

Estimation of glomerular filtration rate:
  Plasma creatinine
  Blood urea nitrogen
  Clearance of creatinine, inulin, or labelled compounds

Assessment of tubular function:
  Urine acidification and concentration ability
  Phosphate clearance

Radiographic and radioisotopic investigations

Examination of renal biopsy:
  Light microscopy
  Electron microscopy
  Immunofluorescence

Because of the marked improvement of workplace hygiene, most patients with chemical-induced renal injury due to workplace exposure present with mild abnormalities such as proteinuria. History of exposure to known nephrotoxicants and the confirmation of the exposure by detection of the chemical in blood, urine, or tissues, are the most diagnostic tests. It is important to rule out other causes of renal injury, including non-workplace exposures to chemicals, particularly drugs, and non-toxic causes such as infection and metabolic abnormalities.

Mechanisms of chemical-induced renal toxicity

Renal injury may occur as a result of biochemical, haemodynamic, or immunological mechanisms, as listed in Table 3.7. Biochemical mechanisms are important in chemical-induced tubular injury. The toxic chemical generally enters the tubular epithelial cell by physiological transport processes. Toxicity usually develops in a dose-dependent fashion once a critical concentration of the chemical has accumulated in the cell. There the chemical may be metabolically activated and then bind to cellular macromolecules. Direct perturbation of subcellular organelle function can then occur. For example, aminoglycoside antibiotics result in lysosomal overload and dysfunction, while heavy metals, such as lead, cadmium and mercury cause a more general perturbation of cell function. Bioactivation of most organic chemicals, such as chloroform, is required for toxicity. Chloroform is biotransformed by the cytochrome P450 enzyme system to phosgene, a reactive compound that depletes glutathione (GSH) and covalently binds to tissue macromolecules. Perturbation of renal haemodynamics can lead to ischaemia or hypoxia, which may rarely initiate or, more frequently, exacerbate chemical-induced renal injury. As stated above, immune-mediated injury is a primary mechanism for chemical-induced glomerular injury.

Table 3.7. Mechanisms of renal injury

Biochemical
Direct perturbation of cellular or subcellular organelle function, e.g. heavy metals, aminoglycoside antibiotics
Reactive intermediate formation and/or oxidative stress, e.g. organic solvents, halogenated alkenes
Perturbation of endogenous or nutritive substrate, e.g. iron, zinc, ethylene glycol

Haemodynamic
Perturbation of renal haemodynamics, e.g. hypertension

Immunological
Immune-mediated injury, e.g. mercury

Examples of renal toxicity from workplace exposure

Many chemicals have been reported to cause renal toxicity following workplace exposure. Examples are given in Table 3.8. Classification of these chemicals according to structural or functional characteristics of the chemical can be useful since members of such classes often act through similar mechanisms. The most important nephrotoxic chemicals in the workplace are metals, hydrocarbons and organic solvents.

Table 3.8. Examples of workplace exposures that have resulted in renal toxicity

Metals
Arsenic
Cadmium
Gold
Lead
Mercury

Organic solvents
Carbon tetrachloride
Chloroform
Toluene
Trichloroethylene

Glycols
Ethylene glycol
Diethylene glycol

Industrial chemicals involved in plastics and resin manufacture
Acrylonitrile
Hexachloro-1,3-butadiene
Styrene

Herbicides
Diquat
Paraquat

The nervous system (C. Winder)

Introduction

The nervous system comprises the central and peripheral nervous systems. While the structure of nervous system is quite complex, at the cellular level the components are:

● The neurons—the nerve cells, which themselves comprise the cell body, several short processes (dendrites), and one long process (the axon).

● Support cells—these are called 'glial cells' in the central nervous system and 'Schwann cells' in the peripheral nervous system.

● Other cells—such as endothelial cells and blood cells.

In occupational health the true importance of diseases of the nervous system is seldom recognised. Fortunately, improvement in hazard control has decreased the incidence of nervous lesions of toxic or traumatic origin, although borderline or 'subclinical' effects may occur and may often go undetected.

The central and peripheral nervous systems are dealt with separately in terms of their structure, function and classification.

The central nervous system

Structure and function

The central nervous system consists of the brain and the spinal cord. Further subdivisions of the brain include the cerebral cortex (which regulates many higher brain functions, including body movement and long-term memory), the hippocampus and limbic systems (which control 'strong emotions' and short-term memory) and the cerebellum (which coordinates movement).

Behaviour, which is governed by the brain, has been shown to be sensitive to the effects of a number of chemicals.

Classification and detection with examples

The predominant *brain* and *spinal cord* disorders are shown in Table 3.9.

Table 3.9. Occupational diseases—brain and spinal cord

Neurological effect	Agent(s)
Toxic encephalopathy	
Acute	Organochlorine pesticides; arsenic (and arsine)
Damage to basal ganglion	Carbon monoxide; manganese; carbon disulphide
Damage to cerebellum	Organic mercury
Damage to occipital cortex	Organic mercury
Intracranial pressure	Lead Organotins
Chronic	Carbon disulphide Organic solvents Lead Inorganic mercury Arsenic Manganese
Encephalic syndromes	
Parkinsonism movement disorders	Carbon monoxide; manganese; carbon disulphide;

Table 3.9. (*Contd.*)

Neurological effect	Agent(s)
	methylphenyltetrahydropyridine
Dyskinesia and tremors	Methyl bromide
Toxic tremors	Mercury; organophosphorus compounds; tetrachloroethane; hexacyclohexane
Isolated convulsive crises	Organochlorine pesticides; carbon tetrachloride; nitrophenols; nitrocresols; lead
Bulbar (brain stem) syndromes	Hydrocyanic acid
Spinal cord syndromes Polyneuritis	Thallium; triorthocresol phosphate
Cancer	See text

Cancer can arise as a result of occupational exposures. However, epidemiological associations of primary brain tumours to specific agents is undetermined, with the possible exception of ionising radiation. However, an increase in brain cancer in a number of occupations has been reported (see Table 3.10). The results of animal studies also suggest that a number of agents cause cancer of the brain (see Table 3.11).

Table 3.10. Occupations associated with an excess of brain cancer

Aluminium workers	Oil refinery workers
Chemists	Petrochemical workers
Lead smelter workers	Pharmaceutical workers
Machinists	Rubber workers
Medical personnel	Veterinarians
Dentists	Vinyl chloride workers

Table 3.11. Agents capable of producing brain cancer in experimental animals

2-Acetylaminofluorene	Elaiomycin
Acrylonitrile	Ethyl methanesulphonate
1-Aryl-3,3-dialkyltriazenes	Ethylnitrosobiuret
Azoxyethane	Ethylnitrosourea
Azoxymethane	1-Methyl-2-benzylhydrazine
Butylnitrosourea	Methylnitrosourea
Cycasin	Methylnitrosourethane
1,2-Diethylhyrazine	Procarbazine
Diethylnitrosamine	Propane sulphone
Diethyl sulphate	Propylene imine
Dimethylbenzanthracene	Pyrrolizidine alkaloids
Dimethyl sulphate	Vinyl chloride

Mental disorders without pathological correlates have been reported to occur in response to occupational exposure to chemicals. These are listed in Table 3.12.

Table 3.12. Occupational diseases—mental disorders

Neurological effect	Agent(s)
Toxic psychoencephalopathies	Organic solvents
	Alkyl lead compounds
	Chemicals that cause
	methaemoglobinuria
	Carbon monoxide
	Cyanides
Confusional states	Organic solvents
	Asphyxiant gases
	Insecticides
	Manganese
	Organotins
Pantophobia	Methyl bromide
Hallucinations	Carbon disulphide
Subjective and behavioural toxic syndromes	See text
Psychotic effects	Organophosphorus compounds

Toxic psychoencephalopathies may be caused by exposure to a wide range of materials, including most solvent vapours, alkyl lead compounds, chemicals that cause methaemoglobinuria, carbon monoxide and cyanides. This intoxication can be resolved by removal from exposure, although a state of confusion may be a temporary effect.

Confusional states result from a deeper and more prolonged acute action and include pantophobia (methyl bromide), hallucinations (carbon disulphide), schizoid reactions, Korsakoff's syndrome and *delerium tremens*. The role of alcohol in the production of these signs and symptoms varies, and there may even be interaction with other exposures.

Subjective and behavioural syndromes comprise a complex of non-specific disorders such as headache, mental fatigue and personality changes, which some have associated with exposure to chemicals. A condition described as 'chronic fatigue syndrome' has received attention recently, but it remains a contentious issue.

Psychotic effects may be induced by organophosphorus compounds, although the mechanism of action remains inhibition of nervous system cholinesterases.

The *autonomic nervous system* is divided into the *sympathetic* and *parasympathetic* systems. These can be affected by a number of occupational chemicals.

The specific inhibitory action of organophosphorus and carbamate compounds on cholinesterases, leading to postsynaptic excitation of cholinergic systems, explains their very homogeneous parasympathetic effects, including muscular fibrillation, severe muscular clonus, tonic contractions of limb and trunk muscles, and motor incoordination.

Acroparaesthesia, Raynaud's phenomenon, and intense sweating of the hands are caused by vibration (operation of vibrating tools).

Tachypnoea, tachycardia, hypertension, vasoconstriction of the extremities, and diminution of intestinal peristalsis are autonomic reactions caused by noise. Ultrasound may provoke hyper-reactions of the sympathetic nervous system and attacks of sweating.

Colic caused by a number of metals (notably lead) is thought to be a spasm of smooth muscles of the intestine, sometimes of the bladder, but also as a generalised arterial spasm, notably in the mesentary.

Some chlorinated solvents, such as trichloroethylene, dichloroethane, calcium cyanamide dust and dithiocarbamates produce effects on alcohol oxidation and result in a reddening of the face ('degreasers flush') and possibly arterial hypotension with a risk of collapse.

The peripheral nervous system

Structure and function

The peripheral nerves are composed mainly of the afferent (sensory) and efferent (motor) nerves. These perform the functions of carrying:

- Sensory information to the spinal cord, through the brainstem sensory tracts to the somoaesthesic area in the cerebral cortex, including:
  (a) mechanoreception (touch, pressure, kinaesthesia, proprioreception, posture),
  (b) thermoreception (heat and cold), and
  (c) pain reception.

- Motor impulses from the motor cortex of the brain through the spinal cord to their effects, that is the spinal muscles.

Classification and detection with examples

The types of effects on the peripheral nervous system are outlined in Table 3.13.

Table 3.13. Occupational diseases—peripheral nervous system

Neurological effect	Agent(s)
Toxic neuropathy (and polyneuropathy)	See text, Table 3.14
Traumatic injury	
Interstitial (vascular)	Vibration
Parenchymal	Compressive or entrapment neuropathy
Neuromuscular junction blockade	Organophosphorus compounds

Long- or medium-term exposure to neurotoxic substances may produce nerve fibre impairment with the clinical development of a *polyneuropathy* (damage to several nerves). Agents such as *n*-hexane, methyl-*n*-butyl ketone, acrylamide and carbon disulphide have been reported to cause polyneuropathy. However, this condition is quite uncommon in modern industry.

The features of polyneuropathy are segmental demyelination and axonal degeneration. Initially, the myelin sheath around the nerve (the axon) unravels and becomes 'leaky'. Degeneration of axons is a more severe neuropathy occurring at the distal segments of the nerve fibre, evolving to the more proximal segments (also called 'distal axonopathy').

Clinically, many nerves are involved simultaneously. Long-standing para-esthesias (tingling, pins and needles, coldness and cramping pain in the calves) may precede for years the appearance of clear-cut clinical findings. This leads to flaccid muscular weakness in the distal muscles and of stocking-glove sensory loss; the sense of position is occasionally altered with consequent ataxia (failure of muscular coordination; irregularity of muscular action). Motor impairment is generally prominent in the distal muscles of the limbs and in severe cases foot drop and wrist drop (lead poisoning) can occur. Proximal involvement is rare, but has been described in some glue neuropathies. Cranial nerves are occasionally affected, mainly the optic nerve (carbon disulphide, methanol and other solvents) and the cochlear vestibular nerve (trichloroethylene).

Sometimes purely motor neuropathies (lead, tri-*o*-cresol phosphate) or sometimes purely sensory neuropathies occur. However, in general, both sensory and motor nerves are affected.

Table 3.14 contains a list of substances for which peripheral nerve fibre damage in exposed workers has been recognised or suspected on clinical grounds. However, depending on dose and mode of exposure, a far greater number of chemicals can probably induce toxic lesions of both the central and peripheral nervous systems. In general, compounds that can damage the peripheral nervous system can also damage the central nervous system.

Table 3.14. Agents causing occupational neuropathy

Recognised neurotoxicants	Suspected neurotoxicants
Metals	
Arsenic	
Lead	
Mercury (organic)	
Organic solvents	
Carbon disulphide	Toluene
n-Hexane	
Methanol	
Methyl-*n*-butyl ketone	
Trichlorethylene	

Table 3.14. (*Contd.*)

Recognised neurotoxicants	Suspected neurotoxicants
Pesticides	
Lead arsenate	Cyclopentadienes (e.g. aldrin, dieldrin)
Organophosphorus compounds	
Organotin compounds	DDT
Thallium	Hexachlorobenzene
Chlorinated phenol derivatives (2,4-D)	
Chlodecane	
Gases	
Methyl bromide	
Carbon dioxide	
Other organic compounds	
Acrylamide	PBBs
o-Arylphosphates (such as TOCP)	PCBs
Dimethylaminopropionitrile	
Styrene	
TCDD	

DDT, dichloro-diphenyl-trichloroethane; PBBs, polybrominated biphenyls; PCBs, polychlorinated biphenyls; TCDD, 2,3,7,8-tetrachlorodibenzo-*p*-dioxin; TOCD, tri-ortho-cresyl phosphate; 2,4-D, 2,4-dichlorophenoxyacetic acid.

There has been growing concern over the occurrence of less severe cases, known as 'subclinical neuropathies'. These essentially consist of sensory symptoms and electromyographic anomalies which, if exposure continues, could eventually result in development of clinical signs of polyneuropathy. The main investigative tools of these effects are electromyography (EMG) and nerve conduction tests, also termed 'electroneurography' (ENG).

Electromyography measures the electrical potential in muscle in resting or contracted states, which are altered following denervation of muscle fibres resulting from axonal or Wallerian degeneration.

Electroneurography measures the conduction rate of the impulses of both motor and sensory nerves. The use of this technique has some problems. A drop in skin temperature of 1°C can cause a reduction in nerve conduction velocity of 2–2.4 ms^{-1}. Age, alcohol consumption, therapeutic drug use, and diabetes can all decrease nerve conduction rate. However, slowing of motor and sensory nerve conduction velocities is considered to be a sign of incipient neuropathy, or of incomplete recovery if it persists after clinical signs have regressed. The technique has been widely used in the screening of neuropathies in exposed groups, and it is believed that if interfering factors are taken into account, it can be useful in the prevention of industrial neuropathies. The technique has sufficient reliability that the results of electroneurographical studies can also contribute to the exposure standard setting process.

Basic mechanisms of neurological damage

Apart from damage by trauma, there are three basic pathophysiological processes that damage nerves.

● Damage to basic biochemical or neurochemical processes in nerve or support cells, such as damage to energy producing systems. Agents such as carbon disulphide and acrylamide act by interfering with enzymes of glycolysis, and methyl-*n*-butyl ketone reduces ATP levels in nerve tissue. The result of a lack of cellular energy is disruption to high energy demand systems like axonal transport and nerve fibre polarisation, which are essential for neurotransmission.

● Damage to the cell to cell connections, which is crucial for nervous system integrity. In particular:
  (a) the connection of the axons to the myelin sheath producing Schwann cell. Disruption to this connection will lead to breakdown of the myelin sheath (Wallerian degeneration). If the sheath degenerates, the nerve fibre degenerates as well, which may explain why damage occurs in the more distal parts of the limbs and the longest fibres ('dying back' neuropathies); and
  (b) the connection of the nerve fibre to the motor neurone (connection is essential for its survival).

● Specific neurotoxic mechanisms. The well-established polyneuropathy caused by organophosphorus compounds is due to phosphorylation and eventual modification of an enzyme in nerve cells, the 'neurotoxic esterase'. Also, paediatric lead encephalopathy is due to damage to the immature endothelial cells of the cerebellum (and eventually cerebrum).

Examples of neurotoxicity from workplace exposures

Although many examples have already been provided (Table 3.14), there are some chemical exposures including solvents, metals and pesticides that require specific attention as they have the nervous system as a primary target organ. These are considered in more detail in the chapters dealing with these groups of chemicals.

Haematopoietic system (W. M. Haschek)

Introduction

The incidence of chemical-induced injury to the haematopoietic system is low, even in populations chronically exposed to the well-documented haematotoxicant, benzene (Irons, 1992). However, when injury does occur, it can be life threatening because of the critical functions of the haematopoietic system. These include transport of oxygen, host resistance to infectious agents, and haemostasis. Chemicals reach the haematopoietic system through the circulation. Reasons for susceptibility to injury include heavy metabolic demands to meet the need for rapid production of cells, and the dependence of this system on small numbers of stem cells with limited proliferative activity.

There are two major classes of haemotoxic compounds, drugs and occupationally important chemicals. In the case of drugs, blood dyscrasias (abnormalities) other than cancer have been extensively studied, however, for occupationally important chemicals the major emphasis has been on their ability to cause cancer. In spite of extensive studies, benzene is the only major industrial chemical which is known to cause cancer of the hematopoietic tissue in humans (Irons, 1992).

Structure and Function

Hematopoiesis occurs in the bone marrow with differentiated cells entering the circulation to replace senescent cells. Within the bone marrow, haematopoietic cells are located extravascularly and are supported and regulated by stromal cells which produce a variety of growth factors. In addition, erythropoietin, produced by the kidney, is essential for erythropoiesis. The microenvironment of the haematopoietic cells is critical for their proliferation and differentiation. The pluripotent stem cell gives rise to the progenitor cells of all lineages; it has little proliferative capacity in

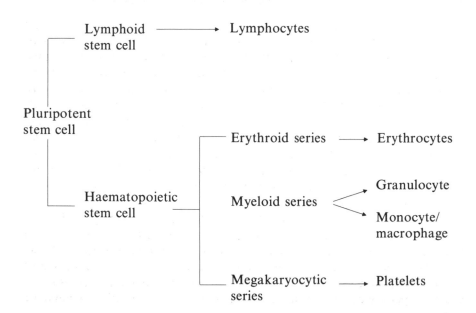

Figure 3.4. Haematopoiesis. Bone marrow differentiation into mature elements of peripheral blood.

spite of unlimited self-renewal. The progenitor cells have greater proliferative capacity but are committed to a limited number of lineages. The
proliferative precursors of each cell lineage give rise to the well differentiated end-stage cells that enter the circulation. These end-stage cells cannot
proliferate, except for monocytes and lymphocytes, and all have a finite
life span. The two basic cell lineages are the lymphoid (discussed under
the immune system) and haematopoietic, the latter differentiating into the
myeloid, erythroid and megakaryocytic series, as shown in Figure 3.4.
Differentiated cells released into the circulation consist of granulocytes
and monocytes (called macrophages in tissues) from the myeloid lineage,
erythrocytes (red blood cells) from the erythroid lineage, and platelets from
the megakaryocytic lineage.

Granulocytes play a major role in the non-specific host defence mechanisms due to their capacity for phagocytosis and release of inflammatory
mediators.

Monocytes/macrophages also play a role in non-specific host defences as
well as acting as regulatory cells in haematopoiesis and the immune
response. Erythrocytes provide haemoglobin for the transport and delivery
of oxygen to tissues and facilitate the removal of carbon dioxide. Platelets
have an important role in haemostasis.

Classification and mechanisms of chemical-induced haematotoxicity

Haematotoxicity can be targeted to cells of the bone marrow or those in the
circulation. Injury to the pluripotent stem cells or their microenvironment
can result in underproduction of all cell types. Once differentiation begins,
individual cell types can be affected, either in the bone marrow or in the
blood, leading to a decrease in cell numbers of a particular cell type or in
abnormal function of that cell type. Direct toxicity to circulating cells
results in an increased demand on the bone marrow with increased cell
proliferation (hyperplasia) and decreased differentiation time. Abnormal
cell function will not be discussed in detail, since the target organs lie
outside the haematopoietic system (see Smith (1991) for an in-depth
discussion). A decrease in erythrocyte numbers, mean corpuscular volume
(MCV), haemoglobin content (MCH), or any combination thereof, is
termed 'anaemia'. A decrease in white blood cells is termed 'granulocyto-
penia', 'lymphocytopenia', or 'pancytopenia', depending on the cell type(s)
affected; a decrease in platelets is termed 'thrombocytopenia'. Effects
will vary in severity and reversibility, depending on the chemical and
exposure conditions. Possible outcomes are recovery following cessation of
exposure, persistence of changes, or progression to aplastic anaemia or
leukaemia.

Classification of haematotoxicity is generally based on the type of injury
or the compartment affected, as shown in Table 3.15, rather than the
mechanism of injury.

Table 3.15. Classification of chemical-induced haematopoietic injury according to site and type of injury

---

Bone marrow
Suppression
    Red blood cells—anaemia, e.g. arsenic, lead
    Other cell types—cytopenia
    All cell types—pancytopenia, aplastic anaemia, e.g. benzene, trinitrotoluene, chemotherapeutic drugs, radiation
Carcinogenesis
    Any cell type—leukaemia, e.g. benzene, chemotherapeutic drugs, radiation
Blood
Direct toxicity leading to decreased numbers of circulating cells
    Red blood cells—haemolytic anaemia, e.g. arsine
    White blood cells—cytopenia
Functional impairment
    Red blood cells—methaemoglobinaemia, e.g. analine,
    nitrobenzene—carboxyhaemoglobinaemia, e.g. carbon monoxide
    Platelets—aggregation
    White blood cells—phagocytosis

Bone marrow suppression can be general or selective. General suppression at the stem cell level results in pancytopenia with decreased numbers of all cell types. If the marrow fails to respond, the condition is called 'non-regenerative' or 'aplastic' anaemia. Of the industrial chemicals, benzene is the best known cause; other causes include chronic mercury poisoning and radiation exposure. Selective suppression affects one of the more differentiated cellular elements, resulting in a specific cytopenia. Mechanisms by which chemicals can induce bone marrow suppression include selective toxicity to proliferating cells, as seen with chemotherapeutic drugs; and interference with RNA or DNA synthesis, or with cell division, as seen with folate antagonists.

Chemicals that cause severe bone marrow depression leading to aplastic anaemia have a well-established tendency to cause transformation of remaining stem cells resulting in cancer, especially acute leukaemia. This is well documented for chemotherapeutic drugs, radiation, and benzene. Although leukaemias can arise from any cell lineage, leukaemias associated with chemical and drug exposure are predominantly of the acute myeloid type (Irons, 1991).

Metabolism is a requirement for benzene-induced bone marrow toxicity. As in other organs, metabolic activation may play a role in some of the chemical-induced bone marrow toxicities. Primary metabolism of benzene to a phenol occurs in the liver. Phenol is further metabolised to a hydroquinone that reaches the bone marrow and is oxidised to 1,4-benzoquinone by the enzyme myeloperoxidase, found in high concentrations in granulocytes (Irons, 1992). Benzene cytotoxicity is cycle and phase specific, with dividing cells in G_2 and M phases of mitosis being targets. Progression to leukaemia is thought to be due to chromosomal abnormalities (Irons, 1992).

Another mechanism of toxicity is exemplified by lead which causes abnormal erythropoiesis by impairing a specific phase of the metabolic process so that the differentiated erythrocyte is abnormal. Lead induced anaemia is due to two major mechanisms: interference with erythropoiesis by the inhibition of heme synthetase and δ-aminolevulinic acid dehydrase, and direct binding of lead to the red blood cell membrane resulting in increased fragility (Irons, 1992). On cytologic examination, erythrocytes may exhibit basophilic stippling, which represents altered ribosomes. A mild normocytic hypochromic anaemia with elevation of reticulocytes (erythrocyte precursors) and basophilic stippling is an indicator of lead exposure.

Toxicity to circulating cells that results in decreased cell numbers increases the demand for formation of new cells in the bone marrow. For example, a decrease in red blood cells in the circulation due to haemolysis results in increased haematopoiesis in the bone marrow. Haemolysis may be caused by direct toxic damage to the erythrocyte membrane, oxidative injury to haemoglobin leading to its precipitation (Heinz body), or by immune mediated mechanisms. The best known example of an industrial chemical causing haemolytic anaemia is arsine gas. However, drugs are the most common cause, with people deficient in 6-phosphate dehydrogenase being especially susceptible to erythrocyte damage. Toxicity to circulating granulocytes can be caused by drug-induced immune mediated mechanisms.

Functional impairment of specific cell types without an actual decrease in cell numbers is also possible. This is especially common for red blood cells since many agents can affect oxygen transport or utilisation. For example, cyanide increases the affinity of haemoglobin for oxygen, while carbon monoxide causes carboxyhaemoglobinaemia (replacement of oxygen by carbon monoxide) with a decrease in total oxygen carrying capacity of blood. As discussed above, lead also causes erythrocyte abnormalities. Abnormalities in the function of white blood cells and platelets can also occur, such as inhibition of platelet aggregation by aspirin.

Detection and evaluation of chemical-induced haematopoietic injury

Most patients with acute blood dyscrasias tend to present with overt clinical signs and symptoms. In such cases, routine haematological examination and determination of haemoglobin concentration are adequate for diagnosis of a problem. To determine a role for occupational exposure, both the clinical course of the disease and the level of exposure should be considered. Most chemical-induced blood dyscrasias are transient and resolve following termination of exposure. In chronic poisoning, evaluation for Heinz bodies, basophilic stippling, and methaemoglobin are indicated. Another parameter that is now available for use as a diagnostic tool is the red cell distribution width (RDW), or coefficient of variation associated with the mean corpuscular volume (MCV) (Irons, 1992). Additional tools include bone marrow biopsy, with quantitation of cellularity, and flow cytometry which is beginning to be utilised in evaluation of leukaemias and lymphomas.

Examples of haematopoietic injury from workplace exposure

Although a wide variety of industrial chemicals have been implicated epidemiologically in haematopoietic toxicity, careful evaluation of the available data has narrowed the list of definite haematotoxicants to those listed in Table 3.16 (Irons, 1992). The difficulty in identifying haematotoxicants is mainly due to the difficulty in obtaining a reliable history of chemical exposure, simultaneous exposure to multiple potentially toxic chemicals, and the marked variability in individual responses.

Table 3.16. Examples of haematopoietic injury from workplace exposure

Definite haematotoxicants
Lead (anaemia)
Radium, radiation (leukaemia)
Trinitrotoluene (anaemia)
Benzene (anaemia, leukaemia)

Possible haematotoxicants
Arsenic
Ethylene oxide
Glycol ethers
1,3-Butadiene
Chlordane and heptachlor
Phenoxy herbicides, especially 2,4-D

Haemoglobin toxicants
Aromatic amino and nitro compounds (methaemoglobinaemia)
Carbon monoxide (carboxyhaemoglobinaemia)

2,4-D, 2,4-dichlorophenoxyacetic acid.

Chronic lead poisoning is an occupational hazard in painters, with anaemia as a late manifestation. Occupational exposures to radium and trinitrotoluene (TNT) are of historical interest only. Benzene is the only primary aromatic solvent with haemotoxic properties. It is an important industrial compound, with its production ranking among the top 10 commodity chemicals in the USA (Irons, 1992). Haematopoietic toxicity occurs with repeated exposure to high concentrations of benzene and can progress to acute myelogenous leukaemia.

Some recent well-documented studies show an association between the agricultural use of the herbicide, 2,4-dichlorophenoxyacetic acid (2,4-D) and the risk of non-Hodgkin's lymphoma (Irons, 1992). In addition, associations between certain occupations, such as the rubber and tyre industry, and increased risk of leukaemia or lymphoma are well known; however, the nature of the causative agent remains obscure.

Immune system (N. H. Stacey)

Introduction

Although the immune system has only recently been studied substantially from a toxicological perspective, immunotoxicity has now emerged as a formal field of toxicology. The evaluation of immunological function in routine toxicological screening is still not commonplace and the appropriate level of testing remains to be determined. The effects of chemicals on the immune system are potentially wide ranging and vary from the obvious to the subtle which requires careful investigation so that the effects are recognised. The end result of suppression of the immune system ranges from viral infections such as the common cold lasting a little longer than usual to increased incidence of tumour development. Chemicals can also initiate immune mediated disorders such as allergic reactions and the development of autoimmune conditions. As these immune mediated effects are most commonly manifested in the skin and the respiratory system, they will not be further discussed in any detail in this section.

It is worth noting that toxicity testing is done under specific pathogen-free conditions—that is, in animals that are protected from exposure to infectious agents. Thus effects on a system that normally protects against infectious organisms will not be observed unless specific functional assays are undertaken. In humans, the immune system differs from other organs in its accessibility; white blood cells from peripheral blood can be separated and studied, while tissues from other organs are much less accessible. This improves the investigator's ability to understand and interpret chemical-induced immune changes in humans.

The reader is referred to other sources (Dean and Murray, 1991) for detailed and comprehensive information on the effects of chemicals on the immune system. The purpose of this section is only to provide a broad outline of this area.

Structure and function

The immune system is a little different to other major organs from a structural point of view. It is rather diffuse in that it has a circulating component as well as a presence in other parts of the body. The circulating component originates from the *pluripotent stem cells*. Then there are the *primary lymphoid organs* which include the thymus where T cells mature and the bone marrow where B cells mature. The *secondary lymphoid organs* include the spleen, lymph nodes and mucosal associated lymphoid tissue.

From a functional aspect, the immune system plays a crucial role in the protection of the body against invading and potentially infectious organisms. It is also involved in a surveillance function for cancerous cells with the apparent ability to eliminate certain neoplastic cells as they arise. The immune system consists of many different cell types many of which are interactive with one another. Thus interference with one component of the immune system can affect other components.

The major cell types and their functions are shown in Table 3.17. Macrophages, granulocytes and lymphocytes can be distinguished from one another by their appearance under the microscope. Further morphological distinction, among the lymphocytes in particular, can be made by examination of surface markers using specific antibodies which are often attached to a fluorescent marker for identification by flow cytometry. This approach is applicable to other cell types as well and has become widely used.

Table 3.17. Cellular components of the immune system

Cell type	Function
Macrophage/monocyte	Phagocytose foreign material
Polymorphonuclear cells or granulocytes	Phagocytose foreign material
Lymphocytes	
T	Cell-mediated cytotoxicity (MHCr)*
T_H or T_S	Helper or suppressor
B	Antibody production
Natural killer (NK)	Cell-mediated cytotoxicity (non-MHCr)

* MHCr, major histocompatability complex, restricted.

Classification and detection of chemical-induced injury with examples

Classification and detection are considered together for the immune system as one is dependent upon the other. Table 3.18 lists the major types of chemical-induced interference with immune function. Chemicals can be further classified on the basis of the function with which they interfere. For example, a chemical (trichloroethylene) may be shown to inhibit natural killer cell function, but not T or B cell function.

Table 3.18. Types of immunotoxic reaction

Reaction	Example
Immunosuppression	Benzene, asbestos
Carcinogenicity	Cyclophosphamide*
Autoimmunity	Trichloroethylene, epoxy resins
Hypersensitivity	Nickel, di-isocyanates

*Cyclophosphamide is a cytotoxic drug used in chemotherapy. Workers preparing this and similar drugs require a high level of protection.

Many chemicals of occupational relevance have been shown to cause immunosuppression of one type or another in experimental animals. Often more than one function is affected. Considerable caution is required, however, in this emerging field because there are many conflicting reports for many chemicals. One particular example with cadmium highlights this point, as in 1984 this heavy metal was reported to increase, decrease and have no effect on one parameter of immune cell function. Interestingly, all three reports came from the one laboratory. This also brings out the issue of interpretation of interference with immune cell function in studies of this nature. At this stage it is apparent that not all aspects of inhibition can be ascribed the role of necessarily resulting in a clear compromise of the organism's homeostasis. Factors such as reserve capacity for parts of immune system function need to be borne in mind.

Functional assays performed after treatment with chemicals are a major way to detect an adverse effect on the immune system. The treatment may be *in vivo* or *in vitro*. The numbers of the various cell types can also be determined as an indication of the effects of a chemical. Other functions may also be evaluated, as indicated in Table 3.19 which displays the suggested tiered approach to screening for immunotoxic effects (Dean and Murray, 1991).

Table 3.19. Detection of chemical-induced immune dysfunction

Tier I	Tier II
Immunopathology	Immunopathology (extended)
Haematology	Host resistance
Organ weights	Cell-mediated immunity (extended)
Histology	Humoral immunity (extended)
Cell-mediated immunity	Macrophage function
Lymphocyte blastogenesis	Granulocyte function
NK cell activity	Bone marrow cell quantitation
Humoral immunity	

Cardiovascular system (W. M. Haschek)

Introduction

Cardiovascular diseases are the major cause of death in the USA with major risk factors being cigarette smoking, diabetes, obesity, hypertension, hyperlipidaemia, and genetic factors (Benowitz, 1992). Although many chemicals have been shown experimentally to be potentially cardiotoxic, the role of low-level chronic exposure to chemicals in the workplace in the aetiology of chronic cardiovascular disease in humans is largely unknown.

The cardiovascular system can be a primary target for chemicals or may be affected secondarily by damage to other organs such as the nervous system and the kidney. Susceptibility to injury is due to factors such as exposure to chemicals at maximal concentrations, often for prolonged periods; presence of low concentrations of protective/detoxification enzymes in the heart; and extreme sensitivity of the heart to hypoxia due to its high metabolic rate. Some chemicals produce solely functional changes, such as cardiac arrhythmias. Nevertheless, these can have serious, and often lethal consequences. Other chemicals produce primary structural changes with secondary functional alterations that can have results that are just as serious.

Structure and function of the cardiovascular system

The cardiovascular system consists of the heart, which pumps blood by rhythmic contraction of its chambers; the arteries, muscular vessels that carry oxygenated blood away from the heart to the tissues; the capillaries, tiny vessels that transport oxygen and nutrients from blood to the tissues, and collect carbon dioxide and waste products from the tissues; and the veins, large, thin walled vessels that carry blood from the capillaries back to the heart, and then to the lung for reoxygenation. The entire circulatory system is lined by a single cell layer called the 'endothelium'. Veins and arteries have a subendothelial layer consisting of connective tissue (the intima). Beneath this layer lies smooth muscle (the media), which is well developed and highly elastic in the larger arteries, and an outer layer of loose connective tissue (the adventitia). The most common vascular disease, atherosclerosis, is characterised by plaque formation due to intimal degeneration and lipid deposition. This can result in partial to complete occlusion of the vascular lumen. Contraction of the smooth muscle in the media can result in vasospasm or vasoconstriction.

The heart muscle or myocardium consists of cardiac muscle cells, whose main functions are (1) electrical impulse generation and conduction, and (2) contraction. These cells cannot regenerate; therefore injury leading to cell death (necrosis) can result in significant problems. Both the sympathetic and parasympathetic divisions of the autonomic nervous system innervate the heart. Blood supply to the myocardium is through the coronary arteries. Because of the high energy demand of the myocardium, any interference with blood supply (such as coronary atherosclerosis) leading to hypoxia or ischaemia can have serious consequences. These can be manifested clinically as angina pectoris (severe chest pain), heart attack, or sudden death.

Classification of cardiovascular toxicity

There are many ways to classify cardiovascular toxicity. Classification can be based on the type of injury (as shown in Table 3.20), clinical manifestations, mechanism of toxicity (see Table 3.21), and organellar localisation of injury. Direct cardiovascular injury is discussed under mechanisms below.

Detection and evaluation of cardiovascular injury

Evaluation of workplace exposure as a factor in cardiovascular disease is very difficult since cardiovascular disease from other causes is very common

Table 3.20. Types of cardiovascular injury with examples

Heart
1. Disturbances in electrical impulse formation or conduction (leading to arrhythmia) e.g. halogenated hydrocarbons, organophosphates, arsine
2. Direct myocardial injury, e.g. arsenic, arsine
3. Ischaemia due to coronary vasospasm, e.g. organic nitrates
4. Asphyxia, e.g. carbon monoxide, cyanide, hydrogen sulphide

Vessels
1. Vasoconstriction (functional injury leading to hypertension), e.g. lead, carbon disulphide
2. Atherosclerosis/arteriosclerosis, e.g. carbon disulphide
3. Vasculitis, e.g. arsenic, gold, many drugs

in the general population and the clinical signs are usually non-specific as to cause. Major clinical features of acute toxicosis are electrocardiographic changes, arrhythmias, acute cardiac failure and death. Knowledge of potentially cardiotoxic chemicals and their effects on other organ systems are helpful in defining the role of chemical exposure in the cardiovascular disease of a specific patient since chemical exposure may aggravate pre-existing conditions. Evaluation of chemical-induced cardiovascular injury is identical to that for other causes of cardiovascular disease.

Mechanisms of cardiovascular toxicity

Cardiovascular toxicity may be due to direct or indirect injury or due to an interaction with exogenous or endogenous chemicals as shown in Table 3.21. Pharmacological or functional effects arise from alteration of electrical or contractile properties of the heart, without detectable structural injury. This type of toxic effect is frequently manifested as arrhythmia and sometimes as sudden death. Effects such as these have been reported following short term occupational exposure to high concentrations of organic solvents or fluorocarbons (Benowitz, 1992). At lower levels of exposure, these solvents sensitize the heart to the effects of endogenous catecholamines, which cause increased contractility, accelerated heart rate and even arrhythmias leading to hypoxia. Endogenous catecholamines may be released due to central nervous stimulation induced by the solvents themselves, or due to physiological responses such as those following exercise or excitement (Benowitz, 1992).

Table 3.21. Mechanisms of direct cardiotoxicity

Pharmacological (functional)
Cardiotonic agents increase the force of myocardial contraction by:
    Inhibiting Na^+/K^+ ATPase, e.g. digitalis
    Increasing Na^+ influx, e.g. ciguatoxin

Table 3.21. (*Contd.*)

Increasing Ca^{2+} influx, e.g. catecholamines, F^-
Myocardial depressants acting by:
  Decreasing Na^+ permeability, e.g. polyethylene glycol, higher
  alcohols
  Replacing sarcolemmal Ca^{2+} and increasing Ca^{2+} influx,
  e.g. cadmium
  Interaction with exogenous or endogenous chemicals,
  e.g. organic solvents

Direct cellular injury
Reaction with functionally or structurally important molecules,
e.g. cobalt
Reactive metabolite binding to macromolecules, e.g. allylamine
Reactive oxygen radical formation, e.g. adriamycin

Hypersensitivity responses
  To, for example, penicillin

Aggravation of pre-existing disease

Reaction with functionally or structurally important molecules by a chemical or its metabolite can cause a direct effect on the heart, frequently resulting in degeneration and necrosis of cardiac muscle, sometimes accompanied by inflammation. Allylamine, an industrial chemical, is metabolised by amine oxidase to acrolein which conjugates to and depletes glutathione. This puts cardiac muscle at risk of damage due to free radicals. Chemotherapeutic agents such as the anthracyclines (e.g. adriamycin) form reactive oxygen radicals which can directly injure cardiac muscle. Immune mediated hypersensitivity reactions can also affect the cardiovascular system. These are not dose related, are primarily induced by drugs, and are characterised by inflammation, especially vasculitis.

Several chemicals have been found to aggravate pre-existing cardiovascular disease. Carbon disulphide, combustion products, and arsenic irreversibly accelerate coronary heart disease (Benowitz, 1992). Carbon monoxide and nitroglycerin may also aggravate coronary artery disease, but the association is not as strong. Carbon monoxide can lead to decreased oxygen availability (myocardial asphyxiation) manifesting as increased heart rate (tachycardia) and other electrocardiographic changes suggestive of hypoxia. Nitroglycerin and other organic nitrates can cause vasospasm of the coronary artery and thus lead to ischaemic heart disease, even in the absence of atherosclerosis (Benowitz, 1992).

Examples of cardiovascular injury from workplace exposure

Many chemicals are known to be potentially cardiotoxic; however, few have been shown to be of unequivocal importance in the workplace. Those workplace chemicals which have been identified as significant include: substituted aliphatic hydrocarbons, such as chloroform, fluorocarbons, and propylene glycol; heavy metals such as cadmium, lead, and nickel; and carbon monoxide (CO) and carbon disulphide. Table 3.22 lists those workplace chemicals that are accepted, on the basis of epidemiological studies, to have a role in cardiovascular disease; also listed is the type of injury produced (Kristensen, 1989; Benowitz, 1992).

Table 3.22. Workplace exposures implicated in cardiovascular disease*

Disease	Cause	
	Definite	Probable
Atherosclerotic ischaemic heart disease	Carbon disulphide	Tobacco smoke
Nonatheromatous ischaemic heart disease	Organic nitrates	
Myocardial asphyxiant	Carbon monoxide Cyanide Hydrogen sulphide	
Direct myocardial injury	Arsenic Arsine	Antimony
Arrhythmias	Halogenated hydrocarbons Organophosphates Arsine Hypertension	Antimony Arsenic Lead Carbon disulphide
Peripheral arterial occlusive disease	Arsenic Lead Carbon disulphide	

*Adapted from Benowitz (1992).

Gastrointestinal system (W. M. Haschek)

Introduction

Although many industrial chemicals cause gastrointestinal symptoms and even tissue injury, little information is available regarding their specific toxic effects and even less regarding their mechanism of action. This may be due to the generally held view that the gastrointestinal tract is not an important site of action of toxic chemicals, except when exposure is to corrosive agents and carcinogens.

The gastrointestinal tract is the site of entry for ingested chemicals, for inhaled chemicals that are removed from the lung by coughing or expectoration and then swallowed, and those excreted in the bile. Gastrointestinal toxicity may occur from ingested chemicals themselves, or secondarily by chemicals reaching the tract through the circulation or from the bile. Susceptibility of the gastrointestinal tract to injury is due to its barrier role, allowing direct contact with ingested chemicals; its marked absorptive capacity; and its high mucosal proliferative and metabolic rate. Protective mechanisms against chemicals include the low pH in the stomach, the mucus surface layer, and presence of biotransforming enzymes. These enzymes are present both within the lining epithelium and within endogenous lumenal bacteria; they may metabolise chemicals to either reactive or less toxic intermediates. Reactive metabolites may be directly toxic to the gastrointestinal tract or may be absorbed into the circulation to reach other target organs. The intestines also contain large amounts of inert binding materials that can act as protective adsorbents.

Structure and function of the gastrointestinal tract

The gastrointestinal tract is a tubular organ whose wall consists of a mucosa, a submucosa, smooth muscle, and serosa. The mucosa is the primary site of chemical-induced injury. It consists of an epithelial lining, a lamina propria of vascularised connective tissue, and the muscularis mucosae, a thin layer of muscle that delineates the mucosal boundary. The epithelium that covers the lumenal surface of the mucosa functions as a selectively permeable barrier to substances within the lumen, and facilitates the transport and digestion of food, as well as the absorption of water and digestive products. Abundant lymphoid tissue is also present in the mucosa and submucosa; protection against infection is primarily through IgA production.

In the stomach, the mucosa is folded into rugae. The major types of epithelial cells are the mucous, parietal, and chief cells, which secrete large amounts of mucus, hydrochloric acid, and pepsinogen and lipase, respectively. The mucous protects the surface from the secreted acid as well as from ingesta. In the small intestine, the mucosa is folded into villi with crypts present at the base. The crypt epithelial cells are the progenitor cells with high mitotic rates. They differentiate as they move up the villus into non-dividing absorptive cells which line the lumenal surface. The renewal rate for the mucosal epithelium is less than 5 days in humans. The crypt epithelial cells are very sensitive to compounds that interfere with cell division such as radiation and chemotherapeutic agents. Damage to these cells ultimately decreases the availability of absorptive cells, resulting in malabsorption as well as diarrhoea. The absorptive cells are rich in biotransforming enzymes, similar to those present in the liver, and therefore can metabolise chemicals. Resident bacteria can also metabolise ingested chemicals. The large intestine does not have villi, only crypts, with many mucous cells. It is the major site for water absorption from the intestinal contents and for mucous production.

Chemicals that enter the digestive tract may: pass straight through and be excreted unchanged in the faeces; be directly toxic to the mucosa; be absorbed, primarily by passive diffusion, into the epithelial cells; or be metabolised by bacteria in the lumen. Once within the cell, a chemical may be: directly toxic to the cell; metabolised to reactive or less toxic intermediates; or may be bound to protein before passing into the lymphatics or capillary bed. After passing through the liver, the absorbed chemical can then be excreted in the urine or the bile. Enterohepatic circulation occurs when the chemical excreted in the bile is absorbed from the intestines, re-enters the circulation, and is once more excreted by the liver into the bile. This process may be repeated several times resulting in concentration of the chemical and increased toxicity.

Classification of gastrointestinal toxicity

Classification of gastrointestinal toxicity can be based on the type of injury (as shown in Table 3.23), or on the pathophysiological or clinical response (as shown in Table 3.24). There are four major types of tissue response to injury: ulceration; necrosis and inflammation (which often occur together); and proliferation, including cancer. (For additional information, see the section below on mechanisms.)

Table 3.23. Classification of gastrointestinal toxicity based on tissue response

Ulceration
Necrosis
Inflammation
Proliferation

Table 3.24. Clinical manifestations of chemical-induced gastrointestinal injury

Clinical sign	Example
Diarrhoea	Mercury, solvents
Vomiting	Arsenic
Constipation	Lead
Change in motility	Lead, organophosphorus compounds
Abdominal pain	Arsine, lead, bromochloromethane

Classification based on pathophysiological responses (see Table 3.24) is useful in the detection of injury, as discussed below. Diarrhoea is the most common presenting sign associated with toxicity and can result from increased mucosal permeability and exudation, hypersecretion, malabsorption, or abnormal motility of the gastrointestinal tract (Bertram, 1991). The consequences include dehydration from loss of water, acidosis from loss of bicarbonate and electrolyte imbalance. Vomiting can result from direct gastric irritation, an effect on the central nervous system, or liver damage. Constipation can sometimes be present as a result of functional abnormalities, including neurological effects, or a result of structural changes, such as the presence of a tumour. Changes in motility due to chemicals can result in spasms, diarrhoea or constipation. These can be due to neurological effects, either regional or central, as well as direct toxicity.

Detection and evaluation of gastrointestinal injury

Gastrointestinal symptoms, especially nausea and vomiting, are very widespread after exposure to chemicals. Most of the time these effects are regarded as secondary, with the intestine not considered a target organ. However, it is probable that more visible injury to other organs, such as liver (e.g. chloroform-induced hepatotoxicity), overshadows intestinal toxicity. Gastrointestinal injury can be detected based on clinical signs, as shown in Table 3.24; however, determination of a role for chemical exposure in the clinical disease syndrome relies on an accurate history of exposure and exclusion of other possible causes. Evaluation of chemical-induced gastrointestinal injury is similar to that used to diagnose gastrointestinal disease from other causes. Endoscopic examination, radiography, and biopsy may be useful. Measures of the rate of absorption and propulsive activity can also be obtained.

Mechanisms of gastrointestinal toxicity

The mechanisms of chemical-induced gastrointestinal injury are listed in Table 3.25. Carbamate and organophosphorus compounds exhibit a pharmacological effect by inhibiting cholinesterase. Muscarinic actions are the predominant effects exhibited. These include anorexia, nausea, vomiting, abdominal cramps and diarrhoea. These chemicals may also increase motility and tone, and induce vomiting due to central neurogenic effects (Scheufler and Rozman, 1986). Other chemicals can alter absorptive functions resulting in malabsorption. Abnormal absorption can occur due to alteration in epithelial transport mechanisms, reduction of surface area, or binding of chemicals to unabsorbed intestinal contents (Bertram, 1991). Decreased blood supply and resultant hypoxia, such as occurs in shock and hypotension, increases the susceptibility of the mucosa to injury and is frequently manifested as ulceration. Alteration of the local protective mechanisms is important in gastric ulceration induced by steroidal and non-steroidal anti-inflammatory drugs.

Table 3.25. Mechanisms of chemical-induced gastrointestinal injury

Pharmacological effects

Alteration of absorptive functions

Decreased blood supply or hypoxia

Indirect damage to the mucosa

Direct cytotoxicity
  Parent compound
  Reactive metabolite (binding to macromolecules)

Hypersensitivity reactions

DNA damage

Direct toxicity to epithelial cells by the parent chemical or its metabolite can result in necrosis and inflammation (gastritis, enteritis, colitis) with subsequent malabsorption and maldigestion. Crypt epithelial cells are highly susceptible to cytostatic chemicals such as epoxides, which are DNA alkylating agents, and radiation which also damages DNA. Absorptive cells on the other hand are frequently injured by corrosive chemicals, due to direct contact, or chemicals that require metabolic activation for toxicity. Aldehydes, for example, are potent local irritants and phenols are highly corrosive agents on ingestion. Arsenic is cytotoxic to the vasculature and results in increased capillary permeability. Immune-mediated hypersensitivity reactions, characterised by an inflammatory process, may also occur. DNA damage, such as that induced by some nitrosamines, can lead to cancer. Since colon cancer is the second most common cancer in humans, the contribution of chemicals to this process is under active investigation.

Examples of gastrointestinal injury from workplace exposure

A large number of chemicals are corrosive and their ingestion typically causes severe gastrointestinal damage. However, workplace exposure to chemicals more commonly occurs by inhalation and dermal exposure routes. Table 3.26 lists chemicals known to cause gastrointestinal injury. Epidemiological studies show that workers in plants producing polyvinyl chloride and those exposed to asbestos have a higher incidence of intestinal cancers than control populations (Pfeiffer, 1985). Lead poisoning can cause gastric ulcers and gastric hypoacidity, while chronic mercury poisoning has been associated with diarrhoea and recurrent bouts of abdominal pain (Pfeiffer, 1985).

Table 3.26. Examples of gastrointestinal injury from workplace exposure

Asbestos

Corrosive chemicals

Halogenated aromatic hydrocarbons
    Chlorobenzene
    Hexachlorobenzene

Metals
    Lead
    Mercury
    Arsenic
    Cadmium

Polyvinyl chloride manufacture

Solvents

References

Alden, C. L. and Frith, C. H., 1991, Urinary system, in Haschek, W. M. and Rousseaux, C. G. (Eds) *Handbook of Toxicologic Pathology*, pp. 315–87. San Diego: Academic Press.

Amdur, M. O., Doull, J. and Klaassen, C. D. (Eds), 1991, *Casarett and Doull's Toxicology. The Basic Science of Poisons*, 4th Ed. New York: Pergamon Press.

Arias, I. M., Jakoby, W. B., Popper, H., Schachter, D. and Shafritz, D. A. (Eds), 1988, *The Liver—Biology and Pathobiology*, 2nd Edn. New York: Raven Press.

Bai, C., Canfield, P. J. and Stacey, N. H., 1992, Individual serum bile acids as early indicators of carbon tetrachloride- and chloroform-induced liver injury, *Toxicology*, **75**, 221–34.

Benowitz, N. L., 1992, Cardiac toxicology, in Sullivan, J. B. and Krieger, G. R. (Eds) *Hazardous Materials Toxicology. Clinical Principles of Environmental Health*, pp. 168–78. Baltimore: Williams & Wilkins.

Bernard, A. M. and Lauwerys, R. R., 1992, Renal toxicity from hazardous chemicals, in Sullivan, J. B. and Krieger, G. R. (Eds) *Hazardous Materials Toxicology. Clinical Principles of Environmental Health*, pp. 163–7. Baltimore: Williams & Wilkins.

Bertram, T. A., 1991, Gastrointestinal tract, in Haschek, W. M. and Rousseaux, C. G. (Eds) *Handbook of Toxicologic Pathology*, pp. 195–251. San Diego: Academic Press.

Dean, J. H. and Murray, M. J., 1991, Toxic responses of the immune system, in Amdur, M. O., Doull, J. and Klaassen, C. D. (Eds) *Casarett and Doull's Toxicology. The Basic Science of Poisons*, 4th Edn, pp. 282–333. New York: Pergamon Press.

Dixon, R. L. (Ed.), 1981–, *Target Organ Toxicology Series*. New York: Raven Press.

Dossing, M. and Skinhoj, P., 1985, Occupational liver injury. Present state of knowledge and future perspective, *Int. Arch. Occ. Environ. Health*, **56**, 1–21.

Haschek, W. M. and Rousseaux, C. G. (Eds), 1991, *Handbook of Toxicologic Pathology*. San Diego: Academic Press.

Hewitt, W. R., Goldstein, R. S. and Hook, J. B., 1991, Toxic responses of the kidney, in Amdur, M. O., Doull, J. and Klaassen, C. D. (Eds) *Casarett and Doull's Toxicology. The Basic Science of Poisons*, 4th Edn, pp. 354–82. New York: Pergamon Press.

Irons, R. D., 1991, Blood and bone marrow, in Haschek, W. M. and Rousseaux, C. G. (Eds) *Handbook of Toxicologic Pathology*, pp. 389–420. San Diego: Academic Press.

Irons, R. D., 1992, Benzene and other hematotoxins, in Sullivan, J. B. and Krieger, G. R. (Eds) *Hazardous Materials Toxicology. Clinical Principles of Environmental Health*, pp. 718–31. Baltimore: Williams & Wilkins.

Kristensen, T. F., 1989, Cardiovascular disease and the work environment. A critical review of the epidemiologic literature on chemical factors. *Scand. J. Work Environ. Health* **15**, 245–64.

Landrigan, P. J., Goyer, R. A., Clarkson, T. W., Sandler, D. P., Smith, J. H., Thun, M. J. and Wedeen, R. P., 1984, The work-relatedness of renal disease, *Arch. Environ. Health*, **39**, 225–30.

Pfeiffer, C. J., 1985, Gastrointestinal tract, in Mottet, N. K. (Ed.) *Environmental Pathology*, pp. 230–47. New York: Oxford University Press.

Rappaport, A. M., 1980, Hepatic blood flow: morphologic aspects and physiologic regulation, *Int. Rev. Physiol.*, **21**, 1–63.

Scheufler, E. and Rozman, K., 1986, Industrial and environmental chemicals, in Rozman, K. and Hanninen, O. (Eds) *Gastrointestinal Toxicology*, pp. 397–415. Amsterdam: Elsevier.
Smith, R. P., 1991, Toxic responses of the blood, in Amdur, M. O., Doull, J. and Klaassen, C. D. (Eds) *Casarett and Doull's Toxicology. The Basic Science of Poisons*, 4th Edn, pp. 257–81. New York: Pergamon Press.
Zimmerman, H. J., 1978, *Hepatotoxicity*, New York: Appleton Century Crofts.
Zimmerman, H. J., 1982, Chemical hepatic injury and its detection, in Plaa, G. L. and Hewitt, W. R., (Eds) *Toxicology of the Liver*. New York: Raven Press.

Bibliography

Kidney

Bach, P. E. and Lock, E. A. (Eds), 1987, *Nephrotoxicity in the Experimental and Clinical Situation*. Lancaster: Martinus Nijhoff.
Brenner, B. M. and Rector, F. C. (Eds), 1986, *The Kidney*. Philadelphia: W. B. Saunders.
Hook, J. B. (Ed.), 1981, *Toxicology of the Kidney*. New York: Raven Press.
Hook, J. B. and Ford, S. M., 1983, Mechanisms of nephrotoxicity, *J. Toxicol. Sci.*, **8**, 1–14.
Rush, G. F., Smith, J. H., Newton, J. F. and Hook, J. B., 1984, Chemically induced nephrotoxicity: role of metabolic activation, *CRC Crit. Rev. Toxicol.*, **13**, 99–160.
Wedeen, R. P., 1984, Occupational renal disease, *Am. J. Kidney Dis.*, **4**, 241–57.

Nervous system

Ellenhorn, M. J. and Barceloux, D. G., 1988, *Medical Toxicology: Diagnosis and Treatment of Human Poisoning*. New York: Elsevier.
EPA, 1990, *Indoor Air Health: Neurotoxic Effects of a Controlled Exposure to a Complex Mixture of Volatile Organic Compounds*. Research Triangle Park North Carolina. US Environmental Protection Agency.
Doull, J., Klaassen, C. D., and Amdur, M. O. (Eds), 1986, *Cassarett and Doull's Toxicology. The Basic Science of Poisons*, 3rd Edn. New York: Macmillan.
Friberg, L., Nordberg, G. F. and Vouk, V. B. (Eds), 1979, *Handbook on the Toxicology of Metals*. Amsterdam: Elsevier/North Holland.
Hayes, W. J., 1982, *Toxicology of Pesticides*. Baltimore: Waverly Press.
Rosenstock, L. and Cullen, M. R., 1986, *Clinical Occupational Medicine*. Philadelphia: W. B. Saunders.
WHO, 1985, *Organic Solvents and the Central Nervous System. Environmental Health 5*. Copenhagen: World Health Organisation.
WHO, 1986, *Early Detection of Occupational Diseases*. Geneva: World Health Organisation.
Worksafe, 1990, *Industrial Organic Solvents*. Canberra: Worksafe Australia/AGPS.

Haematopoietic system

Irons, R. D. (Ed.), 1985, *Toxicology of the Blood and Bone Marrow*. New York: Raven Press.
Leventhal, B. G. and Khan, A. B., 1985, Hematopoietic system, in Mottet, N. K. (Ed.) *Environmental Pathology*, pp. 344–55. New York: Oxford University Press.

Rosner, F. and Grunwald, H. W., 1990, Chemicals and leukemia, in Henderson, E. S. and Lister, T. A. (Eds) *Leukemia*, pp. 271–87. Philadelphia: W. B. Saunders.

Testa, N. G. and Gale, R. P. (Eds), 1988, *Hematopoiesis*. New York: Marcel Dekker.

Young, N. S., 1988, Drugs and chemicals as agents of bone marrow failure, in Testa, N. G. and Gale, R. P. (Eds) *Hematopoiesis*, pp. 131–57, New York: Marcel Dekker.

Cardiovascular system

Balazs, T. (Ed.), 1981, *Cardiac Toxicology*. Boca Raton, FL: CRC Press.

Balazs, T. and Ferrans, V. J., 1978, Cardiac lesions induced by chemicals, *Environ. Health Persp.* **26**, 181–91.

Hanig, J. P. and Herman, E. H., 1991, Toxic responses of the heart and vascular systems, in Amdur, M. O., Doull, J. and Klaassen, C. D. (Eds) *Casarett and Doull's Toxicology. The Basic Science of Poisons*, 4th Edn, pp. 430–62. New York: Pergamon Press.

Magos, L., 1981, The effects of industrial chemicals on the heart, in Balazs, T., *Cardiac Toxicology*, Vol. II, pp. 203–11. Boca Raton, FL: CRC Press.

Van Steen, E. W. (Ed.), 1982, *Cardiovascular Toxicology*. New York: Raven Press.

Van Vleet, J. F., Ferrans, V. J. and Herman, E., 1991, Cardiovascular and skeletal muscle systems, in Haschek, W. M. and Rousseaux, C. G. (Eds) *Handbook of Toxicologic Pathology*, pp. 540–624. San Diego: Academic Press.

Gastrointestinal tract

Banwell, J. G., 1979, Environmental contaminants and intestinal function, *Environ. Health Perspec.*, **33**, 61–9.

Klaassen, C. D. and Rozman, K., 1991, Absorption, distribution, and excretion of toxicants, in Amdur, M. O., Doull, J. and Klaassen, C. D. (Eds) *Casarett and Doull's Toxicology. The Basic Science of Poisons*, 4th Edn, pp. 50–87. New York: Pergamon Press.

Rozman, K. and Hanninen, O. (Eds), 1986, *Gastrointestinal Toxicology*. Amsterdam: Elsevier.

Schiller, C. M., 1979, Chemical exposure and intestinal function. *Environ. Health Perspec.*, **33**, 91–100.

General

WHO, 1986, *Early Detection of Occupational Diseases*. Geneva: WHO.

Chapter 4

Respiratory Toxicology

G. Baker

Introduction

The respiratory system is both a route of entry and an exit from the human body for toxicants, as well as a target organ for chemical effects. The study of the inhalation route as a portal of entry and excretion has developed into the subspeciality of inhalational toxicology. However, the emphasis in this chapter is on the respiratory system as the target organ; that is, respiratory toxicology. The respiratory system may be the site where a critical dose of toxicant is achieved at the cellular level and results in a pathophysiological process. Although the lung contains over 40 different cell types organised with regional, anatomical and functional diversity, the responses of the lung are relatively few.

There are two special issues that are important in human pulmonary toxicology. The human lung comes into contact with approximately 20 kg of air each day and the attendant suspended chemical and microbial load. Although the inhaled chemical load of the home environment may be quite different from the work environment, the respiratory system is the same. The potential for interactive health effects between chemicals is great, for instance between tobacco smoke and workplace chemicals. To cope with this massive environment, the lung has developed a sophisticated defence system. The pulmonary health effects of chemicals are a consequence of both the toxicant effects and the response of the lungs. Individuals have varying degrees of susceptibility, which often are based on the lungs' ability to respond to the environmental chemical load. Susceptibility can be different depending on inherited traits, or due to acquired diseases. Thus it is necessary to consider potential chemical interactions and make allowances for variation in susceptibilites.

Occupational pulmonary toxicology has a special emphasis. It is concerned with preventing adverse pulmonary health effects from workplace exposures. Frequently, the question asked is: How can one work with this substance safely? The answer is based on an assessment on the potential adverse health effects. The health-risk assessment provides the basis for the development of appropriate control measures for exposure and health monitoring/surveillance.

A particularly useful approach to toxicological risk assessment of respiratory tract hazards is the mechanistic approach, as outlined in Table 4.1. Here, 'mechanism' refers to the critical biological factors that regulate the occurrence of a particular process and the nature of the interrelationship between these factors. It is important to define the level of the biological response in which there is an interest. One could be interested in the molecular, the cellular, the pulmonary, the individual or the population level. At each level of biological organisation, the mechanisms responsible for the effects can be considered. The focus here is on the mechanisms with respect to the human individual. However, to understand those effects, attention will also be paid to the biochemical, cellular and tissue effects.

Table 4.1. Mechanistic approach

Tissue dose of chemical
- Dosimetry
- Clearance
- Toxicokinetics

Chemical effect

Pathophysiological response
- Biochemical
- Cellular
- Pulmonary
- Clinical

The respiratory tract can be divided into four major compartments with different functional, dosimetric, and pathophysiological characteristics.

There are a number of advantages in adopting this approach to pulmonary toxicology, as opposed to a more descriptive approach. In particular, information from animal studies and cell culture studies as well as clinical and epidemiological studies can be integrated. The potential for predicting new effects or interactive effects, for example, is greatly enhanced. Such an approach to assessing the risk can incorporate concerns about interactions and susceptibility, and has the potential to become more accurate as more information is gathered.

In conducting a risk assessment for a pulmonary toxicant it is useful to consider the sequence of events that the toxicant undergoes (see Table 4.1). The three important questions encompassed by this approach are;

1. What is the tissue dose of the toxicant?
2. What are the chemical effects on the cells?
3. What is the pathophysiological response?

Answers to these questions will provide the basis for directing controls, exposure monitoring, and health surveillance in the occupational setting.

Structure and function

Anatomy

The lung has marked regional differences. A useful approach is to consider the respiratory system as having four compartments (Figure 4.1). There is the nasal pharyngeal compartment, which is from the nares to the vocal cords; the tracheobronchial compartment, from the vocal cords down to the respiratory bronchioles; the parenchymal compartment from the respiratory bronchioles to the alveoli; and, finally, the pleural space. Each of these compartments has particular epithelial cells, special interstitium and particular protective responses. The nasopharyngeal compartment filters, humidifies and warms the air.

The tracheobronchial compartment is concerned primarily with conducting gases to the alveolar region. The surface area is approximately 0.25–0.5 m^2. This surface area can receive the full load of inhaled toxicants. However, the tracheobronchial compartment has a very active protective response.

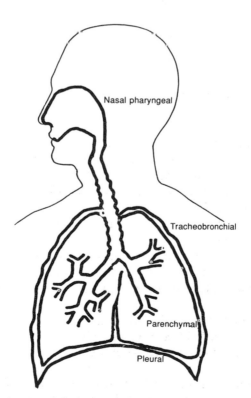

Figure 4.1. The respiratory tract can be divided into four major compartments with different functional, dosimetric, and pathophysiological characteristics.

In order to achieve optimal gas exchange the lung provides a vast air/blood interface. The surface epithelium has an intimate interaction with the vascular, nervous and immune systems within this tissue. Like the skin, the lung epithelium comes into contact with the outside world. However, there are major differences between the environmental contact of the lung and the skin. Firstly, the surface area of the lung is approximately 140 m^2 compared with 2–3 m^2 of the skin. The actual thickness of the barrier between the environment and the vascular compartment is approximately three orders of magnitude less in the lung being of the order of 10^{-6} m in the alveolus compared with skin thickness of 10^{-3} m.

Physiology

This specialised anatomy of the pulmonary system has particular functions relevant to toxicants (Table 4.2). The chief function of the lungs is to ensure efficient and effective gas exchange of oxygen and carbon dioxide. The system is organised to protect this function as a priority. The respiratory system also functions as a barrier between foreign chemicals and the body. Furthermore, the lung has biotransformation capabilities. The lung is able to maintain these functions through a well developed system of pulmonary defences.

Table 4.2. Functions of lung

Gas exchange
Barrier to foreign chemicals
Metabolic function

Pulmonary defences

An outline of some of the pulmonary defences is shown in Table 4.3. An important early defence is the detection of chemical odour. This can induce a behavioural response, such as the avoidance of entering into a space which has odour. Some chemicals can elicit a bronchoconstrictive response which does not require any previous sensitisation. This direct effect results in decreased breathing and hence entry of air containing the chemical into the body. The lung is lined with fluid which provides another defence mechanism. In the upper two compartments of the respiratory tract this is mainly mucous, whereas in the lung parenchyma this is a lipid based surfactant fluid. This fluid barrier contains enzymes, proteases and antibodies. The aqueous or lipid matrix of the fluid dissolves particles and gases and there are biochemical defences which can inactivate chemicals in the fluid itself. The lung is very active in clearing material. An early response to chemicals being deposited in the particular regions is increased secretions of mucous and surfactant, as relevant to the region. The cilia in the bronchial and upper respiratory tract epithelium move the secretions out of the airway where it is either swallowed or coughed up. A cough is a mechanism to remove bulk fluid. The lower respiratory tract contains alveolar macrophages which can phagocytose material and carry it either into the mucociliary escalator or into the interstitial space and to lymph nodes. If a substance remains in the lung there are mechanisms that enable containment of the material. The connective tissue matrix of the lung can wall off sections of the lung containing chemical material. A good example of this is seen with silicosis.

Table 4.3. Pulmonary defences

Avoid inhaled toxicants
● Smell
● Bronchoconstriction

Deactivate toxicants
● Secretion
● Antibodies, antioxidants, antiproteases

Clear toxicants
● Cough
● Mucocilary escalator
● Phagocytosis

Contain toxicants
● Phagocytosis
● Connective tissue

In workers exposed to a pulmonary toxicant, evidence of operating pulmonary defence mechanisms is often observed before overt toxicity occurs. The observed clinical effect of a toxicant is usually a combination of the effects of the chemical and the pulmonary defence mechanism.

Determinants of tissue dose

Exposure

The two scenarios normally considered for workplace exposures are acute high exposure and chronic low exposure. These can be regarded as ends of a spectrum. Exposure standards for chemicals may be peak values or time weighted average; some chemicals have both. Actual exposures probably consist of a combination of episodic acute high exposures and continual very low exposure.

Deposition

When considering where the toxicant is deposited there are a number of important questions to be addressed. Firstly, what is the physical form of the toxicant? Table 4.4 shows a useful classification which separates gases and vapours from particulates. For gases the important determinant for tissue dose is the water and lipid solubility. Water soluble gases tend to be deposited in the upper respiratory tract because of the mucous lining this tissue. In contrast, lipid soluble materials tend to be more soluble in the lower respiratory tract. For particles, size and shape are important. The larger size particles are deposited in the upper respiratory tract and only the smaller particles get to the lower respiratory tract. Fibrous shapes collect at bifurcation points which is important because some small local areas may receive very high doses relative to cells nearby.

Table 4.4. Dosimetry

Gases	*Deposition site*
Solubility	
Water	Upper tract
Lipid	Lower tract
Particles	
Size	
Large	Upper tract
Small	Lower tract
Shape	
Fibrous	Bifurcations
Spherical	

Clearance

The clearance of the two upper compartments of the respiratory tract is different from the lower compartment and the pleural space. The upper two compartments rely on secretion and ciliary movement while the parenchyma relies on phagocytosis as does the pleural space.

The clearance rate is very important because often clearance depends upon cellular function, which itself can be compromised by the toxicant; for instance, ciliary function in the airways or phagocytosis in the lower respiratory tract. An important concept that requires consideration is the saturation of clearance mechanisms by high doses. This is particularly relevant when considering the heterogeneous nature of deposition, and the fact that local area defences may be overwhelmed.

Biotransformation

The lung epithelium has an active cytochrome P450 mixed function oxidase enzyme system, which can metabolise and activate chemicals.

Modifiers

People can have anatomical variations or deficiencies in some of these clearances mechanisms. This may modify the tissue dose of toxicants. For

instance, people with ciliary abnormalities, or abnormalities in phagocytosis, or obstructed airways will have different dosimetry profiles from
people without such changes.

Classification, nature, mechanism and detection of chemical-induced effects

Classification

The important chemical effects are outlined in Table 4.5. Chemicals may
have direct cellular toxicity which may be first observed in the epithelium
cells lining the respiratory tract. Initially there may be abnormal function
of these cells while at higher doses the toxicity may be due to direct
necrosis of these cells. Many of these effects become evident as irritation.
Another important effect is sensitisation which is due in part to the high
levels of immune activity in the lung. Chemicals, by acting as haptens, can
elicit an allergic response. The mechanism of these effects is not well
understood partly because of the difficulty in creating animal models. The
third type of response is that of carcinogenesis. Chemicals have been
reported to act as initiators or promoters in the respiratory tract This is an
area of active research because of the ability to model *in vitro* the effects of
chemicals and cells.

Table 4.5. Biochemical interactions
between chemicals and tissues

Cellular toxicity
Sensitisation
Carcinogenesis

The effects of chemicals may be enhanced or reduced by the presence
of other chemicals. Toxicant interaction can be very important in occupational respiratory toxicology. For instance, there appears to be a synergism
between tobacco smoke and asbestos. Cellular mechanisms also exist which
could modify these effects. Examples include anti-oxidant levels, suppressor
genes and DNA repair mechanisms.

Nature and mechanism

There are six major pathological processes that can occur from toxicants in
the lung (Table 4.6): asphyxiation, irritation, infection, allergy, structural
changes, and neoplasia.

Table 4.6. Pulmonary pathological processes

Asphyxiation
Irritation
Infective
Immunological
Structural
Neoplasia

Asphyxiation refers to the failure of gas exchange at the tissue level. This may result from failure of the respiratory system or from systemic effects such as the failure of central nervous system control due to poisoning of oxidative phosphorylation at the cellular level. Symptoms can range from behavioural change and headaches to death. *Irritation* refers to a cluster of symptoms involving pain, hypersecretion, and acute breakdown of the epithelial barrier. *Infections* can be a sign of toxicant inhalant because of the disturbance of the normal pulmonary defence system and the normal micro-organism barrier. A relatively common respiratory effect is one of *allergic* reactions, which requires the development of sensitisation and leads to symptoms at very low exposures to the toxicants. *Structural changes* can occur in any of the compartments and may involve obstruction such as blockage of airways or destruction of the parenchymal tissue which may lead to emphysema. Finally, *neoplasia* can occur as a result of carcinogenic actions of toxicants. Most of these pathophysiological reactions can occur in any of the four compartments of the respiratory system.

Detection

The approaches for measuring and detecting pathophysiological effects in the four compartments differ (Table 4.7). Toxic effects in the naso-pharyngeal compartment, and to a lesser extent in the tracheobronchial compartment, can often be identified by structured questionnaires, which elicit information on symptoms. Many of these symptoms are features of an activated pulmonary defence system. Standardised spirometry which measures lung volume and rate of volume change, such as the force expiratory volume in one second, are very useful for detecting disease in the tracheobronchial compartment. In addition, lung volume measurements can detect disease in the lung parenchyma or pleural space. Parenchymal disease can be assessed by gas exchange tests. The simplest is exercise performance which can be evaluated from a person's work or exercise performance or quantified on laboratory/exercise tests situation. Finally, disease of the pleural compartment and the lung parenchyma can be detected by the chest radiograph. These methods of detecting respiratory disease of questionnaire, spirometry, exercise and chest radiographs have been developed to the stage where they can often be used as surveillance tools to detect disease resulting from inhaled toxicants.

Table 4.7. Methods for detecting respiratory disease

Method	Compartment			
	Naso-pharyngeal	Tracheobronchial	Parenchyma	Pleura
Questionnaire	+++	++	+	
Spirometry		+++	++	+
Exercise		++	+++	+
Chest radiograph		+	++	+++

The clinical methods for measuring respiratory pathophysiology have different
usefulness in the different respiratory compartments.
+ some   ++ reasonable   +++ most

Conclusion

It is important to consider each of the aspects discussed above in assessing
respiratory toxicological risk. The consideration of the tissue dose may help
to identify critical sites within the respiratory tract. Consideration of the
chemical/biological actions helps to identify the types of pathophysiological
effects that might be anticipated. Knowledge of the pathophysiological consequences allows appropriate end-points to be recognised and measured.
The consideration of the three together allow an assessment, which can
result in a recommendation for an acceptable level of exposure. Furthermore, it can identify appropriate exposure monitoring and health surveillance protocols.

An increasingly important concept in the development of safe exposures
to respiratory toxicants is the recognition of the role of the pulmonary
protective mechanisms. It appears that if a toxicant exposure results in a
tissue dose which does not overwhelm the protective response, then it is
unlikely to cause adverse pathophysiological effects. If, however, these
processes are overwhelmed then disease can develop.

Example—crystalline silica

Description

Silicon oxide (or silicon dioxide) is a mineral which is a major component
of the Earth's crust. It can occur basically in a crystalline form where the
silicon and oxygen atoms are arranged in a definite regular tetrahedral
pattern throughout the crystal or in an amorphous form where the silicon
oxide has no definite regular pattern. There are also intermediary forms.
Crystalline silica dust is often produced when working with minerals or
rocks. It is one of the oldest known respiratory toxicants. It will be
considered using a mechanistic approach.

What is the chemical dose?

Exposure

Exposure to crystalline silica may be to high concentrations of dust for short periods of time or, as more commonly occurs, to lower doses over a long period of time.

Deposition

Crystalline silica consists of particles which can vary in size from large particles down to the respirable, range 0.1–100 μm. The silica particles are deposited on the epithelium throughout the whole respiratory tract.

Clearance

The clearance rate is different in the different respiratory regions and it depends on the dose. There is some evidence that the silica deposited in the airways can penetrate into the basement membrane and similarly silica can be found underneath the alveolar epithelium. The material that reaches the tissue appears to have a very long half-life.

Biotransformation

It is uncertain whether silica is actually changed.

Chemical effects

In vitro evidence suggests that crystalline silica can result in the production of oxygen radicals, particularly in the presence of metal ions. In addition, the silicon itself can be internalised by cells. *In vitro* studies also indicate that silicon oxide in the crystalline form can act as a genotoxic agent. This profile of activity has some similarities to other common respiratory toxicants such as tobacco smoke.

Pathophysiological effects

Acute

Acute high level exposures cause acute irritant effects to the airways (bronchitis) or the lung parenchyma (pulmonary alveolar proteinosis). In this latter condition there is an outpouring of surfactant secretion (up to 100-fold), which fills the alveolar space, and causes respiratory failure.

Chronic

In low dose chronic exposure structural changes develop in the airways (chronic bronchitis), in the terminal airways (emphysema) and in the parenchyma (fibrosis). There is some evidence for cancer.

Systemic effects

There is some suggestion of scleroderma and renal disease.

Conclusion

Consideration of crystalline silica as a respiratory toxicant from a mechanistic perspective has highlighted a number of aspects of a historically well-known toxicant. In particular, disease may occur in any respiratory compartment, and may involve obstructive and neoplastic pathophysiology, as well as pneumoconiosis. The mechanistic approach is useful for identifying interactions.

Bibliography

Dungworth, D., Kimmerle, G., Lewkowski, J., McClellan, R., and Stober, W. (Eds), 1988, *Inhalation Toxicology. The Design and Interpretation of Inhalation Studies and Their Use in Risk Assessment*. New York: Springer-Verlag.

Frank, R., O'Neill, J. J., Utell, M. J., Hackney, J. D., Van Ryzin, J. and Brubaker, P. E. (Eds), 1985, *Inhalation Toxicology of Air Pollution: Clinical Research Considerations*. Philadelphia: ATSM.

Gardner, D. E., Crapo, J. D. and Massaro, E. J. (Eds), 1988, *Toxicology of the Lung*. New York: Raven Press.

International Agency for Research on Cancer (IARC), 1986, Tobacco smoking, *IARC Vol. 38*. IARC: Lyon. France.

Klaassen, C. D., Amdur, M. O. and Doull, J. (Eds), 1986, *Casarett and Doull's Toxicology. The Basic Science of Poisons*. 3rd Edn. New York: MacMillan.

Methods in pulmonary toxicology. *Environ. Health Perspect.*, 1984, **56**, 1–183.

Miller, F. J. and Menzel, D. B. (Eds), *Fundamentals of Extrapolation Modelling of Inhaled Toxicants: Ozone and Nitrogen Dioxide*. Washington, DC: Hemisphere Publishing Corporation.

Monograph on pulmonary toxicology. *Environ. Health Perspect.* 1984, 55.

Morgan, W. K. C. and Seaton, A., 1984, *Occupational Lung Diseases*. 2nd Edn. Philadelphia: W. B. Saunders.

Phalen, R. F., 1984, *Inhalation Studies: Foundation and Techniques*. Boca Raton, FL: CRC Press.

Samet, J. M., Marbury, M. C. and Spengler, J. D., 1987, Health effects and sources of indoor air pollution. Part I, *Am. Rev. Respir. Dis.*, **136**, 1486–508.

Samet, J. M., Marbury, M. C. and Spengler, J. D., 1988, Health effects and sources of indoor air pollution. Part II, *Am. Rev. Respir. Dis.*, **137**, 221–42.

The Health Consequences of Smoking. Cancer and Chronic Lung Disease in the Workplace. A Report of the Surgeon General, 1985. Rockville, Maryland: US Dept of Health and Human Services.

Chapter 5

Occupational Skin Disease

E. A. Emmett

The skin is a major site for the effects of occupational skin disease as a result of contact with toxic substances and/or electromagnetic radiation. It is also one of the most important routes for absorption of toxic substances into the body as a result of industrial exposure.

Structure and function

Structure of the skin

The skin is one of the major organs which interfaces with the environment. Accordingly, it provides a barrier not only against chemicals but also against micro-organisms, heat, cold, trauma, electric current and ionising and non-ionising radiation. Conversely, it is a protective covering which keeps the constituents of the body's fluids intact. Damage to the skin may both lower the resistance of the barrier to external agents of injury and lead to potentially severe or even fatal loss of fluids.

The skin is a layered organ. The two major layers are the epidermis and the dermis. The epidermis is the outer layer. The most numerous cell type is the keratinocyte. The epidermis is generally considered to consist of several zones or layers depending on the behaviour of the keratinocytes. The innermost basal layer consists of rapidly dividing, metabolically active, keratinocytes. The keratinocytes migrate towards the surface through the spinous or prickle cell layer and then the granular cell layer. As they migrate they become less metabolically active and undergo the process of keratinisation. By the time they reach the outermost layer, the stratum corneum, the cells are dead and cornified (consist of horny material). The stratum corneum is the major barrier for the passage of water, electrolytes and most chemicals. In the stratum corneum the remains of the keratinocytes are filled with a filamentous network of keratin proteins, embedded in a matrix containing mucous and lipids surrounded by a thickened, highly chemically resistant cell envelope. Between the 'cornified' cells is an intercellular material containing lipid ceramides the properties of which also contribute to the barrier function. Depending on the presence of moisture or the humidity at the outer surface of the skin, the water content of the

89

stratum corneum varies from around 10% to 70%. The higher the water content the more soft and supple the epidermis and the more permeable the stratum corneum barrier to water soluble substances.

The epidermis also contains specialised cell types including melanocytes and Langerhans cells. The melanocytes are dendritic cells derived from the neural crest; they synthesise specialised organelles, the melanosomes in which melanin is synthesised. When mature the melanosomes are transferred to keratinocytes where they are aggregated and destroyed. The major function of the melanin system is to provide protection against ultraviolet (UV) radiation. There are substantial racial differences in the behaviour of melanocytes and melanosomes. In black-skinned individuals melanosomes are larger, more numerous, contain more melanin and are less easily destroyed in keratinocytes and thus provide much more UV protection than in white-skinned individuals.

The Langerhans cell is another dendritic cell, which forms a network in the lower layers of the epidermis. Langerhans cells have a critical function in the immune reactions of the skin since they are responsible for antigen recognition and processing

The keratinocyte population of the epidermis is continually renewing itself. In the human, under normal conditions, it takes a cell about 12–14 days following its formation in the basal layer to move up through the living cell layers to the stratum corneum and about another 14 days to reach the outer surface of the stratum corneum and to be lost as an imperceptible scale. These turnover times are shortened after injury and in certain skin diseases. These times are longer than in most of the species used for experimental toxicological studies such as mice and rats, which have a much thinner epidermis than humans.

The epidermis is separated from and attached to the dermis by a basal lamina. Over most of the body this junction is ridged. In contrast to the epidermis, the dermis consists mainly of strong, flexible but loose connective tissue, containing collagen, reticulin and elastic fibres and glycosaminoglycan ground substance. This dermal connective tissue provides a slow diffusion medium for tissue fluids and chemical substances in general. There are scattered cells in the dermis including macrophages, mast cells and lymphocytes which are involved in various toxicologic reactions as well as fibroblasts which produce the dermal fibres and tissue.

Whereas the epidermis is avascular, the dermis has substantial plexuses of blood vessels and has a rich supply of lymphatics which drain to the regional lymph nodes. The dermal blood supply is potentially greatly in excess of that required for metabolic activity; vasodilation of these vessels is important in regulation of heat loss from the body. In contrast to the epidermis, the dermis generally provides little barrier against the passage of toxic substances.

Other important structural features of the skin are the hair follicles, sebaceous glands, nails, eccrine sweat glands and apocrine sweat glands. All are modified epidermal structures and consist of specialised epidermal tissue.

Percutaneous absorption

Absorption across the skin and absorption from the respiratory route have long been recognised as the major primary routes of entry of toxic agents into the body from occupational exposures. Generally much more attention has been paid to airborne exposures and entry via the respiratory tract; more recently it has been recognised that the cutaneous route of entry is very important for many toxic substances in industry. However, percutaneous absorption is complex, variable and affected by a variety of factors and still defies simple measurement in workplace situations. For this reason it is frequently not given the attention it deserves. Percutaneous absorption occurs through a process of passive transfer. The rate of penetration of different substances varies markedly by at least four orders of magnitude. Generally lipophilic compounds penetrate more rapidly than hydrophilic compounds, from hydrophilic solutions. This may not be true if the applied solution is lipophilic. Water is lost from the surface of the skin, in the absence of sweating, as insensible perspiration.

The sequence of passage of a chemical passing through the skin following application to the outer surface is as follows: absorption at the surface of the stratum corneum, passage through the dead horny layers of the stratum corneum, then through the living layers of the epidermis. Here it may be biotransformed or photochemically altered (see next section). The substance will then pass through the connective tissue of the dermis before reaching a blood capillary. The stratum corneum presents the greatest barrier and penetration through the stratum corneum may be very slow. Some compounds such as certain organic solvents may severely damage the epidermis. Since such damage may impair the barrier function more rapid absorption may occur subsequently.

In addition to penetration through normal epidermis for very lipophilic and large molecules there may be some penetration through hair follicles and sweat glands. Physicochemical studies have shown that Ficks law of diffusion gives a reasonable approximation of the absorption of a number of agents across the skin.

According to Ficks law, the steady-state penetration flux J is given by:

$$J = k_p C$$

where k_p is the permeability constant, and C is the concentration difference of the solute across the membrane.
Furthermore,

$$k_p = \frac{K_M D_M}{\delta_M}$$

where K_M is the partition coefficient between the stratum corneum membrane and the vehicle, D_M is the diffusion constant, and δ_M is the thickness of the membrane.

The partition coefficient will depend on the relative solubilities of the substance in the vehicle and the stratum corneum and, since this will vary depending on the vehicle involved, the penetration of a substance from different mixtures is not a constant but depends on the particular solvent or vehicle in which it is dissolved.

Mathematical modelling of skin penetration is possible but complicated; particular difficulties are posed by the several layers in the skin (especially if the substance does not readily pass through the layers beyond the stratum corneum) and biotransformation occurs.

Measurement of percutaneous absorption

Percutaneous absorption may be measured *in vitro* or *in vivo* under laboratory or carefully controlled circumstances. There are no measurements particularly suitable for routine occupational use, although if percutaneous absorption is the only or main method of ingress of a substance, biological monitoring will primarily measure the amount crossing the skin.

In vitro studies generally use excised skin or stratum corneum. The tissue can be placed in an experimental cell with the applied solution on one side and a perfused physiological solution on the other, so that the passage across the membrane can be measured. Human skin samples may be used for this purpose.

In vivo studies may be performed by topically applying substances to the intact skin of whole animals. Radiolabelled tracers are commonly used for this purpose. The selection of species is critical since rodents generally have higher permeability than man because of their thinner epidermis. Pigs and monkeys are more similar to humans.

Some *in vivo* human data have been obtained by application of fluids or solutions to the skin of volunteers and later measurement of compounds in the blood and urine. The results can be compared with those obtained following a known injected dose or airborne exposure. This comparison allows computation of the percutaneous absorption.

It has previously been indicated that percutaneous absorption is variable and complex in occupational circumstances. By understanding the sources of this variability we may develop an appreciation of the factors which are important in determining whether or not there is likely to be a hazard from absorption across the skin in any particular occupational setting. Sources of variability are the type of penetrant, the vehicle or solution and the skin and/or the method of application. These factors will be briefly considered in turn.

TYPE OF PENETRANT
Simple polar compounds such as alcohols penetrate the skin reasonably well, at about the same rate as water. Electrolytes penetrate poorly, the ionisation of a weak electrolyte markedly reducing its permeability.

Small molecules with both hydrophilic and lipophilic properties penetrate well.

Organic liquids penetrate well, some organic solvents such as acetone and hexane additionally damage the barrier which can then produce a fairly porous non-selective membrane. True gases penetrate the skin reasonably well. Molecules with a molecular weight of greater than 500 are poorly absorbed through skin.

VEHICLE OR SOLVENT

The vehicle, by altering the partition coefficient, may make a profound difference to penetration. For example *N*-nitrosodiethanolamine, a hydrophilic substance, penetrates the skin 200 times faster from olive oil than water. The vehicle may also influence absorption in other ways; through its pH, as non-ionised compounds generally penetrate faster; by damaging the skin barrier in the case of some solvents; or through the presence of surfactants which increase the permeability of water and other polar substances.

SKIN AND METHOD OF APPLICATION

The amount absorbed will depend on the applied amount, the time before washing or removal, the concentration and the surface area of application. Hair may interfere with contact with the stratum corneum, vigorous sweating may wash material from the surface or may help dissolve or leach substances from solid objects. If the stratum corneum is damaged, abraded or removed, absorption is accelerated. Skin diseases which involve the epidermis may reduce the barrier function and enhance penetration. There is quite profound regional variation in the barrier function. The scrotum, forehead and angle of jaw show much more rapid penetration, for example, than the palm, forearm, soles of the feet or ankles.

The regional variation in absorption helps account for the distribution of toxic reactions on the skin. For example, the first recognised occupational cancer was scrotal cancer in chimney sweeps, the prime occurrence on the scrotum reflecting the ease of absorption of carcinogenic polycyclic aromatic hydrocarbons at that site.

Increased hydration of the stratum corneum will increase the penetration of hydrophilic substances. Occlusion of a site of contact by an impermeable barrier, such as polyethylene plastic sheeting or gloves will increase percutaneous absorption by ensuring good contact, increasing hydration and increasing the surface temperature.

Transformation of chemicals in the skin

Chemicals may be transformed within the skin in two important ways, by biotransformation and photochemical reaction. Transformation may be important in increasing or decreasing the toxicological effects.

The inner viable layers of the epidermis may significantly biotransform foreign substances. One of the more studied examples in the skin is that of aryl hydrocarbon hydroxylase (AHH) activity. The conversion of a number of polycyclic aromatic hydrocarbons to active epoxides by this microsomal enzyme activity in the skin is considered responsible for their carcinogenicity. Epidermal enzyme activity may also detoxify some compounds, for example some dermally applied organophosphates may be detoxified in passing through the skin.

Ultraviolet (UV) radiation penetrates the epidermis and, to a lesser extent, the dermis and is able to produce photochemical reactions with a number of substances and is thereby able to produce phototoxic and photoallergic reactions described later in this chapter. This type of transformation is generally confined to the skin and the eye, since the photochemically active UV rays do not generally penetrate to deeper structures.

Excretion from the skin

Although not usually the major source of loss from the body, a number of potentially toxic substances are lost from the skin in desquamated cells, hair or nails, or secretions such as tears or sweat.

Quantitatively significant amounts of some metals are excreted in sweat particularly under hot conditions or with heavy work rates. In these circumstances excretion in sweat of lead, cadmium and nickel may exceed that in urine. Water soluble drugs are excreted in sweat, sometimes in significant amounts.

The loss in hair rarely, if ever, approaches these amounts, however analysis of hair may be helpful in establishing the timing of exposure to metals such as arsenic, cadmium and lead which are incorporated into the matrix of growing hairs and remain in the hair tissue until it is lost. Thus, analysing segments of hair may give an indication of the period of exposure.

Major patterns of toxic skin reaction

Contact dermatitis

The most frequent toxic skin reaction is contact dermatitis. Contact dermatitis is an inflammatory reaction of the skin, more or less confined to the areas contacted by the inciting agent. Clinical signs in affected human subjects may include one or more of erythema (reddening), oedema, vesiculation, scaling and thickening, and may be accompanied by itch or a burning sensation. In experimental animals contact dermatitis is usually manifest by erythema and oedema.

Contact dermatitis may occur from irritation or from an allergic reaction. Photosensitivity may also cause contact dermatitis which will be described separately. Irritant reactions are more frequent than allergic, accounting for about 60–80% of cases of contact dermatitis referred to dermatologists. Minor degrees of irritant dermatitis are particularly common.

Irritant reactions

Cutaneous irritants are agents which produce a local cutaneous inflammatory response (dermatitis) by direct action on the skin; that is, not mediated through an immunological reaction.

There is a spectrum of degrees of severity of irritant reactions. The severity depends both on the potency of the irritant, the circumstances of contact and the skin site affected. Since irritation depends on damage to the lower, living layers of the epidermis, those factors which enhance penetration of a substance will generally increase the severity of the irritant response it produces. The distribution of the dermatitis on the skin will involve sites of contact; but the pattern may be modified in that sites with a stronger barrier (e.g. palms and soles) may show little or no dermatitis when other areas are markedly affected.

Irritant responses may be considered as encompassing corrosion, acute irritation and cumulative irritation. *Corrosion* occurs from direct chemical action on skin which results in its disintegration and irreversible alteration at the site of contact, there is ulceration and necrosis with subsequent scar formation. Corrosive changes in humans are sometimes colloquially referred to as 'chemical burns'. *Acute irritation* is a local reversible inflammatory response, generally resulting from a single contact with an irritant substance. *Cumulative irritation* results from repeated or continuous exposure to milder irritants which may not be sufficiently potent to cause dermatitis on a single contact. The dermatitis produced by cumulative irritation is described as 'cumulative insult dermatitis', and the substances which produce this type of reaction are termed 'marginal irritants'.

Irritant reactions are produced by a wide variety of substances and by a variety of chemical mechanisms, most of which are poorly understood. There are, accordingly, minor differences between the responses caused by different agents.

Examples of strong irritants are sodium hydroxide, triphenylphosphate and other strong alkalies, sulphuric acid, hydrofluoric acid, tin tetrachloride and many others. Greater exposure to strong irritants will often result in corrosion rather than acute irritation. Some agents present special hazards, for example phenolics produce local anaesthesia so that warning symptoms may be less noticeable. Nitrogen mustard and organotin compounds characteristically produce severe reactions, but only after a delay of some hours.

Marginal irritants include soaps, detergents and a wide variety of industrial products.

The standard tests for predicting irritation potential are based on the test described by Draize and colleagues in 1944. Because of the large numbers of laboratory animals sacrificed and ethical concerns about such testing, substantial efforts are being made to find alternative ways of determining irritant potential, but none are yet universally accepted.

In Draize-type tests, substances are applied under gauze patches, immobilised under an impervious covering, to abraded and intact skin of albino rabbits which has been clipped free of hair. The patches are removed after 24 h of exposure, the reactions are scored against standard criteria (redness, swelling, etc.) immediately, and once again 72 h after application. Irritancy is classified on the basis of the score obtained. Since the rabbit is generally more sensitive than humans to irritants and the testing is carried out under occlusive conditions, the test will satisfactorily predict strong irritants, although comparative studies have revealed substantial interlaboratory variation in the results.

A major deficiency is the failure to identify marginal irritants which might produce cumulative insult dermatitis with product use. This hazard is better predicted by cumulative irritation patch testing where the substance is repeatedly applied to the same skin site for up to 21 days. Such testing may be performed in rabbits or human volunteers.

Allergic contact reactions

Allergic contact dermatitis occurs as a result of allergy to one or more specific substances (antigens) as a result of cell-mediated immunity. Such reactions can be provoked by very small amounts of the allergen in some sensitised persons.

There are two main phases in cell-mediated immunity: the sensitisation phase (in which the person becomes 'allergic' to the antigen) and the elicitation phase. The induction of sensitisation usually takes 10–21 days. Once sensitisation has been induced and the individual is re-exposed to the antigen, a reaction is obvious after a characteristic delay of about 12–48 h; hence the name 'delayed hypersensitivity' for this type of cell-mediated immunity.

The first step in the biological process of sensitisation is absorption of the antigen (hapten) into the skin and covalent binding to a carrier protein. This bound complex is termed a 'complete antigen'. The antigen is then bound to the cell surface of Langerhans cells in the epidermis or to macrophages. The complete antigen is processed in these cells by altering the configurational arrangement. Processed antigen is held at the cell surface where it interacts with T-lymphocytes. Antigen-bearing T-lymphocytes undergo clonal proliferation in the regional lymph node to produce two populations of sensitised lymphocytes, effector T-lymphocytes which are distributed to the skin surface via the blood stream and memory cells which will proliferate to form new populations of sensitised lymphocytes on recontact with the antigen.

In the elicitation phase, contact with the hapten and formation of complete antigen results in activation of effector T-lymphocytes. Activated lymphocytes and other skin cells then synthesise a variety of substances called 'cytokines', which mediate the inflammatory response.

Strong allergens usually have a molecular weight of less than 500 (RMW) and are quite reactive with protein. Amongst the most important allergens currently in industry are rubber additives including: mercaptobenzthiazole, thiurams and *p*-phenylenediamine; epoxy oligomer; methacrylate and other acrylic monomers; formaldehyde; nickel and chromium salts; and various substances in plant species. The number of potent allergens is fairly small, but several thousand substances have been reported to have caused sensitisation in one or a few individuals.

Cross-sensitisation may occur when two or more substances share similar chemical groups. For example, aromatic substances sharing *p*-amino groups may cross-react. Thus a person sensitised to one of these substances may react to another, even though they have had no prior contact with the second, chemically related, compound.

Predictive patch testing to identify the sensitisation potential of chemicals is usually performed in guinea-pigs or in panels of human volunteers. Repeated applications (or sometimes injections in the case of guinea-pigs) are made, usually three times a week for 3 weeks. After a rest period of a few weeks, the individual is re-exposed to the substance at a concentration which is non-irritating. If there is a reaction, sensitisation is considered to have occurred. Such tests are generally able to identify strong sensitisers but are less effective in detecting weaker sensitisers.

Allergic contact dermatitis is diagnosed in affected individuals by the use of diagnostic patch testing. In these tests a non-irritating concentration of the suspect substance is applied to the normal skin on the back under occlusion for 48 h. Readings are generally made 24–96 h after removal of the patch. If the person is sensitised a contact dermatitis reaction will be seen at the site of the test. *In vitro* tests using lymphocytes from blood (such as the lymphocyte transformation test) are also available, but have not yet been sufficiently validated for routine use.

Photosensitisation

Photosensitisation is an abnormal adverse reaction to ultraviolet and/or visible radiation. Photosensitisation may be produced by a number of substances. There is an action spectrum for each of these responses. The action spectrum is the relative response to different wavelengths of radiation. The action spectrum usually approximates the absorption spectrum of the chemical. Most photosensitisation reactions have an action spectrum which is strongest in the mid-ultraviolet range.

The two most important types of chemical photosensitivity, phototoxicity and photoallergy, are broadly analogous to irritant and allergic reactions, respectively.

Phototoxicity refers to chemically induced increased skin reactivity on a non-immunolgical basis. Phototoxic agents include 8-methoxypsoralen, various polycyclic aromatic hydrocarbons, some dyes and other substances. The intensity of a phototoxic reaction depends on the concentration of the chemical in the skin, and the amount of radiation of the appropriate wavelengths to which the skin is exposed. Pigmentation may provide some partial protection against phototoxic reactions. Phototoxic reactions are usually characterised by erythema and swelling and hyperpigmentation may be induced. With some phototoxic agents there is sharp pain at the affected sites during exposure to sun. Phototoxicity may be detected in a range of tests including *in vitro* tests where cells are exposed to chemicals and subsequently to radiation, or by tests where human or animal skin is so exposed.

Photoallergic reactions are less common than phototoxic ones. In these reactions a substance which absorbs ultraviolet radiation is photochemically converts an absorbing substance into a photoproduct which is a sensitiser or which is bound with a skin protein in such a manner that it becomes a complete antigen. The process appears to resemble that of usual contact allergy except for the additional role of ultraviolet radiation in producing the complete antigen. Photoallergic dermatitis is usually confined to sun exposed areas of skin, but where there is extreme photosensitivity the amount of ultraviolet radiation which penetrates clothing may cause reactions on apparently unexposed skin. Photoallergens include halogenated salicylanilides, phenothiazides and certain coumarin derivatives. A serious complication of photoallergy from some agents is the development of a persistent light reaction in which marked sensitivity to ultraviolet persists for years, despite the apparent removal of exposure to the photoallergen.

Urticarial reactions

Urticarial reactions (weal and flare responses) as a result of contact with external substances may be produced in the skin in two major ways: as direct reactions or as a result of immediate hypersensitivity. The reactions usually occur within 30–60 min of contact with the offending agent.

A number of substances directly release histamine and other vasoactive agents. These include biogenic polymers released from plant species and animals (caterpillars, jellyfish). Other substances produce urticaria as a result of allergic sensitisation with the production of specific immunoglobulin E (IgE). Because the reactions occur shortly after exposure this type of immunological reaction is called 'immediate hypersensitivity'. Severe reactions may involve other organs, including angioedema with swelling of distant tissues, bronchial asthma, anaphylactoid reactions and gastrointestinal dysfunction, and even death from respiratory obstruction.

Urticaria may also occur as a component of an immediate hypersensitivity reaction to an airborne occupational allergens such as phthalic anhydride.

The causes of immediate hypersensitivity reactions may be confirmed by cutaneous prick tests or a radioallergosorbent test (RAST) confirming the presence of the specific IgE.

Acne

Greases, oils, coal-tar pitch and creosote exacerbate acne vulgaris, (the usual form of juvenile acne) and may produce the typical lesions of acne, namely comedones (blackheads) and inflammatory folicullitis on susceptible areas of the body.

Certain halogenated aromatic compounds produce a more specific type of acne, i.e. chloracne. In this condition the predominant lesions are small, straw coloured cysts and comedones and inflamed follicles. The most sensitive areas of skin, which may be the only ones involved, are below and to the outer side of the eye and behind the ear. Chloracne may occur after the exposure has ceased, possibly because of release from body stores and may persist for years. 2,3,7,8-Tetrachlorodibenzo-*p*-dioxin (TCDD) is the most potent chloracnegen; other structurally related substances causing this condition include polyhalogenated dibenzofurans, 3,4,3′,4′-tetrachloroazoxybenzene and 3,3′,4,4′-tetrachlorazobenzene.

Other toxic skin reactions

Other possible toxic reactions on the skin, which will not be described here in detail, include skin cancer, increases or loss of pigmentation, granuloma and nail or hair change or loss.

The investigation of occupational skin disease

Toxicological understanding is often essential in investigating actual or suspected occupational skin disease. As with other occupational conditions, the relationship of potential causal exposures to the clinical disease is key.

The goal should be a precise aetiological diagnosis identifying single or multiple causal agents since this is needed for the management and rehabilitation of the affected patient, prevention of further cases, and for the determination of compensation and/or other liability claims.

The investigation of an occupational dermatosis may involve consideration of one or more of: the nature of the exposure, the toxic potential of the substances contacted, the clinical nature of the condition, and the epidemiology of the skin disease. Each of these is considered briefly below.

Nature of the exposure(s)

The nature of the exposure may be established through the history of the patient, direct observation (e.g. by a walk-through survey), and measurement of exposures to the skin. Some of the details of a patient's history of particular interest to toxicologists are indicated in Table 5.1.

Table 5.1. Selected historical details important in investigating occupational skin disease

Work history
Occupation—present and past
Exposure to substances and processes
Method of handling substances
Use of protective measures
Skin cleansing methods
Environmental conditions (temperature, humidity, etc.)
Modifications, changes to job
Second job?

Skin disease
When and where did it start
Appearance
How did it progress
Recurrences, periodicity
Effect of weekends, vacations, sick leave
Exacerbation by specific work activities

Past skin disease/history of atopy

Other exposures and influencing factors
Home
Hobbies
Cosmetics, etc.

Direct observation by a walk-through survey of the workplace is a standard occupational hygiene technique. When the objective is the investigation or a risk assessment related to occupational skin disease, emphasis must be given to the potential for skin contact. Items to be noted include:

● The particular processes and tasks (especially with respect to opportunities for skin contact).

● General housekeeping and cleanliness of surfaces.

● Ambient environment including temperature, humidity.

● Use or potential for use of protective clothing.

● Hygienic facilities, washing facilities, showers, emergency showers, cleaning agents used.

● Identity of substances used.

The measurement of actual dermal exposure is difficult and not well standardised. Wipe sampling of environmental surfaces may be used to assess surface contamination, but it does not relate the mass of contaminant on a surface to the mass transferred to a worker's skin. The quantity of chemical contaminants deposited directly on the skin may be assessed more directly by: the use of 'exposure pads' where a sampling material is attached to the skin or clothing; measurement of substances deposited in clothing; measurement of substances found by swabbing or rinsing the skin; or, by surface measurement of radioactive labels or fluorescent traces added to or as part of a mixture. Although such measurements indicate the exposure of the skin, they do not tell us the amount absorbed. Biological monitoring will measure substances which pass through the skin, but also absorption from other routes. None of these methods is ideal and all must be interpreted with caution.

Toxic potential of contactants

The composition of materials contacted in occupational settings is generally available on Material Safety Data Sheets (MSDS). The hazards to the skin should also be described in the MSDS. The adequacy of this information varies, in part depending on resources available to the person preparing the MSDS. The MSDS is generally a reliable guide for corrosive and strong irritant properties but the following points should be borne in mind:

● Despite legal obligations, some suppliers appear reluctant to disclose the sensitising properties of ingredients in their products.

● The potential for producing cumulative irritation may not be apparent from standard Draize-type tests, thus substances considered to be non-irritating by the manufacturer may produce cumulative insult dermatitis.

Accordingly, in cases of doubt, an independent search of appropriate literature is warranted.

Nature of the clinical condition(s)

As described earlier in this chapter, there are numerous different occupational dermatoses, each of which have individual diagnostic features. Nevertheless, some general diagnostic criteria can be applied in determining whether a particular hazardous exposure or toxic substance has caused a particular condition.

● The physical appearance and type of reaction and its distribution on the surface of the body is consistent with disease due to the suspected agent.

- There is an appropriate history of exposure at the workplace to the agent or an appropriate combination of agents.

- There is a logical time relationship between exposure and the onset or exacerbation of the condition. For example, it would be illogical for cancer to have followed 7–10 days after an exposure started, or for dermatitis from a severe corrosive material to have taken this long to develop, whereas this would be a sensible time for the development of new allergic contact dermatitis.

- Removal from the suspected causal agent leads to improvement in the illness.

- Possible non-occupational causes have been ruled out or appear unlikely.

- In certain types of disorder, diagnostic tests may show a specific possible causal relationship. For example, patch testing in allergic contact dermatitis, and the presence of glass fibre filaments on adhesive tape stripping of skin in glass fibre dermatitis.

None of the above criteria is absolute, but consideration of these factors should lead to an appropriate judgement.

Epidemiological studies

Epidemiological studies may sometimes be helpful in establishing causal relationships with occupational skin diseases. Epidemiology is particularly useful in occupational skin cancer. For some other conditions, observations on individuals are quite powerful, particularly where there is a clear relationship between the nature of the exposure, and the site of the dermatitis on the skin and the timing of episodes of dermatitis, so that more complex epidemological studies on groups are not necessary to confirm a relationship.

Prevention of toxic skin reactions

In order to prevent toxic reactions of the skin and/or ill effects from percutaneous absorption under workplace conditions, a toxicological evaluation and assessment of risk should be performed, followed as appropriate by substitution, training and the institution of control measures. It may also be necessary to identify individuals who may be at particular risk, and/or appropriate monitoring procedures.

Toxicological assessment of risk

In order to assess whether there is a risk at the workplace a review should be made of the toxic properties of the various agents used with respect to both their ability to damage the skin and to produce systemic toxic effects following percutaneous absorption. The latter may be apparent from consideration of the physicochemical properties of the compound or published experimental studies, field investigations or case reports of ill effects after skin penetration. Information on toxic properties is available from MSDS and the scientific literature.

A site visit may help identify opportunities for skin exposure. Other factors to be taken into account in the risk assessment include: the ambient working environment, including heat, humidity and the likelihood of abrasion; education level; standard of general housekeeping; level of personal hygiene of workers; opportunities for spills and upset conditions; and possibilities for interactions or additive toxic effects of multiple agents. As a result of this assessment hazards should be identified, hazardous substances appropriately labelled and education and control measurements should be instituted as necessary.

Substitution

Less hazardous agents may be substituted for more hazardous or the hazard may be reduced, for example by encapsulation. In the case of potent allergens, allergen replacement by substances of low allergenicity is desirable.

Reactive monomers may be replaced by less reactive substances of higher molecular weight. For example, allergic contact dermatitis from epoxies has been greatly reduced by the use of epoxy preparations which exclude the highly allergenic monomer with a molecular weight of 340 (RMW).

Dermatitis from chromates in cement has been reduced in Denmark by adding ferrous sulphate to cement with the subsequent reduction in the amount of available hexavalent chromium.

Education and training

Potentially exposed individuals need training to understand and identify hazards to the skin, the means by which contact and subsequent effects may be prevented, how to remove materials from the skin and when to report spills and untoward occurrences.

Engineering and hygiene controls

Engineering and hygiene controls are designed to prevent contact of toxic substances with workers' skin. Closed or isolated operations may achieve this, devices such as splash shields may help. Particular attention needs to be given to operations where dusts or liquids are transferred from one container to another, and spraying operations including the spraying of agricultural chemicals.

Protective clothing

Protective clothing may be necessary when contact with hazardous substances cannot be avoided. Such clothing may range from full body suits to gloves, aprons and impervious covers for shoes. Sometimes, very localised protection may be sufficient such as an impervious fingercot over one finger.

Whereas the effectiveness of appropriate protective clothing has been demonstrated in a number of studies, several conditions are necessary to achieve satisfactory results. There are also dramatic examples of the failure of some personal protection, for example, contact dermatitis from methylmethacrylate in surgeons despite the use of surgical gloves. Protective clothing must be impervious to the chemicals against which protection is desired. The American Society of Testing and Materials (ASTM) has developed testing methods to determine the effectiveness of protective clothing against different substances. Accordingly manufacturers are now sometimes able to provide information on appropriate protection. Temperature, humidity and of course physical damage will affect the quality of the barrier. Some chemicals will affect the physical properties of the materials resulting in variability in durability. Breakthrough times are now available for some chemical/glove combinations.

Protective clothing may have its own hazards. Heat stress will be promoted by extensive coverage of the body with occlusive material. Contact dermatitis can occur from protective clothing, especially from additives to rubber. If the inner surface of protective gloves is contaminated, the gloves should be immediately discarded since percutaneous absorption of the contaminant may be enhanced under the occlusive conditions. Protective clothing caught in machinery may lead to mechanical injury.

Barrier creams

Despite substantial commercial claims, there is little proof that barrier creams other than sunscreens are particularly effective. Reasons include the difficulty of maintaining an even film on the skin. Different barrier creams are used against water-soluble or hydrophobic solutions. Barrier creams are likely to be most effective where minimal, temporary, protection is required.

Individuals at particular risk

Certain individuals may be identified as at increased risk from particular hazards. Persons with prior sensitisation will need to avoid particular allergens or cross-reacting substances. Atopic persons may have difficulties with a wide range of irritants and may be at particular risk in certain occupations, for example hairdressing. In order to minimise the potential for discriminatory practices, at-risk individuals should be counselled as early as possible (e.g. for atopic persons this should preferably be done before they have made a final choice of careers) and subsequently work-place protection should be designed to eliminate risk as far as possible to those who are particularly susceptible.

Monitoring and surveillance

Occupational hygiene monitoring procedures for skin exposures are less well established than those for airborne exposures. Surface wipe proced-ures, use of fluorescent tracers or detection of fluorescent compounds by the use of long-wavelength UV 'backlights' may be considered. The occur-rence of skin disease or symptoms may be detected through reports of illness and results of periodic examinations or specific surveys. Biological monitoring may be used to monitor percutaneous absorption of some substances.

Removal of contaminants from the skin

Prompt removal of toxic substances from the skin is essential and facilities should be provided to make this possible. Contaminated clothing should also be removed.

Bibliography

Adams, R. M., 1990, *Occupational Skin Disease*, 2nd Edn. Philadelphia: W. B. Saunders.
Bronaugh, R. L. and Maibach, M. I., 1985, *Percutaneous Absorption*. New York: Marcel Dekker.
Emmett, E. A. and Tindall, J. P., 1987, Occupational dermatoses in Fitzpatrick, T. B. (Ed.) *Dermatology in General Medicine*, 3rd Edn. New York: McGraw Hill.
GrandJean, P., 1990, *Skin Penetration: Hazardous Chemicals at Work*. London: Taylor & Francis.
McArthur, B., 1992, Dermal measurement and wipe sampling methods: a review, *Appl. Occup. Environ. Hyg.*, 7, 599–606.

Chapter 6

Reproduction, Development and Occupational Health

C. Winder

Introduction

A number of hazardous agents have been associated to varying degrees with impairment of reproductive function and the health of the developing embryo. These agents include:

- Aspects of lifestyle (e.g. tobacco, alcohol or drug use).

- Ionising radiation.

- Non-ionising radiation.

- Hot or cold environments.

- Hyperbaric/hypobaric environments.

- Noise.

- Vibration.

- Infectious agents.

- Overexertion and stress.

- Some pharmaceuticals.

- Some chemicals, including occupational exposures.

The focus of this chapter, however, is on the reproductive effects of hazardous chemicals encountered in the work environment.

General aspects of reproduction and development

Background considerations

The complexity of the continuum called 'reproduction' is masked by a tendency to focus on discrete components of the process, such as sperm or egg cell

107

or the embryo. However, reproductive capacity also encompasses pregnancy, embryonic and fetal development, lactation, child health, development and growth, puberty, behavioural development, reproductive senescence and the integration of reproductive functions with the overall health of the individual.

Fertility

Approximately 7–10% of couples in which the female partner is of child-bearing age (15–44 years) are unintentionally infertile. This may be temporary. The causes of infertility are multifactorial:

- Heritable, such as genetic malformations.
- Nutritional.
- Ethnic.
- Age related.
- Iatrogenic (medication induced).
- Pathological, including infectious diseases.
- Environmental, including pollution.
- Sociobehavioural, including alcohol, tobacco, exercise, stress.
- Work related.

Analysis of these factors reveals large gaps in scientific knowledge, and even sparse information on possible interactions with these and other (for example, occupational) factors.

Embryonic loss

Embryonic loss is a normal part of the reproductive process. Only about one-quarter to one-third of all embryos that are conceived (zygotes) develop to become live born infants. Embryonic loss is higher at the earlier stages of pregnancy, often before a diagnosis of pregnancy is made.

Fetal malformations

The study of birth defects is called 'teratology', from the Greek word *teras*, meaning 'monster'. Fetal malformations (more generally called 'birth defects') are usually thought of as structural or anatomical changes in neonatal and postnatal organisms. In recent years, the term has also come to include physiological, functional or behavioural defects as well. Therefore, the current meaning of the word 'teratogen' includes any agent which induces structural malformations, metabolic or physiological dysfunction, or psychological or behavioural deficits in offspring, either at birth or in a defined postnatal period.

The background developmental abnormality rate in the community is between 2% and 3%. This means that of every 100 babies born, two or three will be malformed for no obvious reason. Figures for the incidence of congenital defects are often underestimated because a number of congenital disorders (mental reproduction, defects of the sense organs, enzyme disorders, abnormal sexual development) are not detectable during early postnatal life. Approximately one-half of the total number of birth defects are apparent at birth, the remainder become apparent over the first few years of life. The most common malformations involve the cardiovascular system and the male urogenital system.

Indeed, the detection rate of overall incidence of congenital defects may not be useful in detecting specific causal factors, as slight increases in some malformations may be masked by background incidence. The causes of the majority of birth defects are unknown, but best estimates are provided in Table 6.1.

Table 6.1. Causes of malformations in humans

Cause	%
Known genetic transmission	20
Chromosomal aberration	3–5
Environmental causes	
Radiation	< 1
Infections	2–3
Maternal metabolic imbalance	1–2
Drugs and environmental chemicals	4–6
Unknown	65–70
Potentiating interactions	?

It has been estimated that there are approximately 70 000 chemicals in commercial use (in the USA). Of these, approximately 2800 chemicals have been tested for teratogenicity. Of these:

- 180 are clearly positive in two or more species, representing about 6% of the total tested.

- Just over 600 (21%) are probably positive (based on limited testing or positive in the majority of species tested).

- 291 (10%) are possibly teratogenic (equivocal or variable reaction, and/or less than obvious response).

- The remaining 62% of tested chemicals are probably not teratogenic.

It is also possible to establish that about 50 of these are human teratogens. As this is based on a sample size of 2800 of a total sample of 70 000, it is possible to estimate that there are 1200 human teratogens that have not as yet been identified.

Occupational health and safety issues

The reproductive and developmental effects of industrial chemicals are a relatively new concern in occupational health and safety. This has been due in part to the emphasis of research and study in other areas, such as occupational injury or carcinogenicity as well as the increasing number of women present in the workforce. As a sequel to this phenomenon, interest in male reproductive capacity has also increased.

Table 6.2. Range of possible effects on reproduction

Prior to conception	Conception/pregnancy	After delivery
Altered libido	Effects on implantation	Effects on labour, (abnormal, prolonged) parturition
Genetic material (mutation)		
	Effects on the mother	
		Low birth weight
Effects on gamete Production (ovulation and spermatogenesis)	Spontaneous abortion	Low APGAR* score
	Congenital malformation	Effects on the mother
Abnormal sperm production/transport		Effects on lactation
Ejaculatory disorders and impotency	Effects on embyrogenesis	Postnatal abnormalities leading to developmental disabilities
	Effects on pregnancy	
Ovulatory disorders abnormal menses		Effects on postnatal development
	Altered/prolonged gestation	
Infertility		Neonatal or childhood death
Reversible or irreversible sterility	Hypertension of pregnancy	
	Pre-eclampsia	Altered reproductive capacity (duration of menses, impairment of spermatogenesis)
	Fetal death	
	Transplacental carcinogenesis	

* APGAR, A numerical expression of the condition of a new born infant usually determined 60 seconds after birth being the sum of points gained on assessment of heart rate, respiratory effect, muscle tone, reflex irritability and colour. Named after Virginia Apgar, American Anaesthesiologist (1909–1974).

There is little information available and considerable uncertainty regarding the potential for reproductive and developmental toxicity of industrial chemicals. Reproduction is a complex and dynamic sequence of events, which are critically timed and under strict hormonal control. This process can be impaired at many points through a variety of mechanisms. The range of possible reproductive effects is outlined in Table 6.2.

The four principal manifestations of impairment of the developmental process are:

- Death of the conceptus (fetal death).

- Structural abnormality.

- Altered growth.

- Functional deficit.

In some cases, these manifestations can be correlated to different developmental stages:

- Preimplantation—embryolethality.

- Organogenesis—embryolethality, birth defects.

- Fetal—growth retardation.

- Functional deficits—fetal death, transplacental carcinogenesis.

- Neonatal—growth retardation, functional alterations of nervous, immune and endocrine systems, childhood cancer.

Estimating reproductive function

Reproductive function in adults can be assessed by relatively simple means, including a detailed patient history, physical examination and analysis of blood and urine samples.

The sort of information required in a reproductive history should include:

- Identification (name, sex, age).

- Familial health (medical conditions, diseases and conditions in relatives).

- Lifestyle characteristics (smoking, alcohol, social drugs, domestic exposures).

- Medical history (injuries, medical conditions/diseases, surgical procedures, medication).

- Reproductive history (previous and present exposures).

- Reproductive history (past reproductive outcomes, reproductive difficulties or disorders).

In men, it is also possible to collect a semen sample, which can be subjected to analysis for:

- Ejaculate appearance, pH and volume.

- Sperm density, counts, motility, vitality and morphology.

The correlation of changes in these parameters with exposure is not easy, especially as the significance of a number of functional changes is not clear. However, there is some evidence to suggest that sperm counts and morphology (presence of increased numbers of spermatozoa) may be sensitive to exogenous factors.

Demonstrating impaired reproductive function

The demonstration of occupational causes of infertility can be made through the following steps.

- Non-occupational causes must be excluded:
  (a) prior ovarian, uterine, cervical or testicular injury;
  (b) surgery on the organs of reproduction, such as hysterectomy, tubal ligation, vasectomy, etc.;
  (c) mumps;
  (d) primary endocrinopathy;
  (e) gonadotoxic exposures, e.g. to cytotoxic drugs, such as dibromo-chloropropane (DBCP); and
  (f) urological abnormalities, such as ductal obstruction, retrograde ejaculation, variocele.

- A gonadal dysfunction should be demonstrated, through reproductive history, clinical and biochemical measures or by analysis of semen.

- Demonstration of exposure to an established or suspect agent sufficient to cause reproductive dysfunction.

- In many cases, deficits in reproductive performance (with the possible exception of azoospermia) are likely to be reversible. Therefore, improvement on removal from exposure can be supportive in providing evidence of diagnosis.

Occupational reproductive and developmental toxicology

The study of occupational reproductive and developmental toxicology involves the experimental, clinical and epidemiological sciences. The evolution of developmental and reproductive toxicity studies in experimental animals has produced non-standardised protocols, and the strategies employed in such testing tend to be selected on the basis of regulatory requirements, rather than design. The study of human reproductive capacity and function involves case studies and prospective and retrospective epidemiology studies, but they generally lack statistical power because of unsure end-points and small sample sizes. Most investigations have involved female exposures, with male aspects having received only limited attention. This is an area that is beginning to receive closer attention.

It is important to make the distinction between reproduction toxicity and developmental toxicity, as they represent distinct concepts. *Reproductive toxicity* is the effect of a toxic agent on the process of reproduction. Examples of toxic effects include those on specific reproductive parameters, such as:

- Gametogenesis,

- Fertility,

- Lactation, or

- Delayed or impaired growth.

Other biological systems that can indirectly affect reproductive capacity may also be involved. These include effects such as impaired metabolic capabilities, a damaged or reduced immune system, or compromised liver function. If there is likely to be an effect on reproductive capacity, it tends to be produced by long-term exposure to chemicals and often it is difficult to detect causal relationships between a non-clinical reproductive effect and exposure to a chemical (for example, a non-specific infertility).

Experimentally, reproductive toxicity is determined in multigeneration (usually 2–3 generations) reproduction studies (sometimes incorporating a teratology component) using long-term exposure to the chemical. Such studies are required for all new food additives, pesticides and therapeutic substances.

Developmental toxicity is the effect of a toxic agent on the process of development, that is, within the maternal/fetal unit. The main effect is teratogenesis, the production of physical defects on the developing embryo, including death from lethal defects. Exposure to the teratogenic agent must occur during critical developmental periods and will generally occur at doses that do not cause observable maternal toxicity. Exposures that cause severe effects on the embryo or neonate may have no effect on the mother. Also, exposures that cause maternal illness do not necessarily affect development. Signs of maternal toxicity are not normally considered to be developmental effects. Note that fetal death can be from either reproductive (for example, impairment in nutrient transfer to the fetus) or developmental (a lethal abnormality) effects.

The principles of teratology

There are three main principles, which can be best illustrated by the axiom: a teratogenic response depends on the administration of a specific treatment of a particular dose to a genetically susceptible species when the embryo(s) are in a critically susceptible stage of development.

Dose dependency. Teratogenicity is governed by dose–effect relationships, though the dose–effect curve is generally quite steep. While the duration of exposure or treatment is an important factor, single or acute exposure at the critical stage is the major concern to the developing embryo. Moreover, every teratogen that has been realistically tested has been shown to have a no observable effect level. It is probable that developmental abnormality and death are simply degrees of reaction to the same stimuli.

Susceptible species. Not all species are equally susceptible or sensitive to teratogenic influences. The susceptibility of developing processes to insult is likely to vary among species. There is a number of factors which contribute to this susceptibility, including metabolic capacity of the maternal or embryonic organism, placenta type and the length of gestation. Animal data should be applied to humans with caution. In the case of thalidomide (almost a prototype teratogen) the human is probably the most susceptible species.

Susceptible stages of development. The timing of exposure is an important determinant of effect. During the predifferentiation period, the conceptus is generally resistant to the induction of birth defects, though embryonic death or resorption (in some species) may occur. During embryonic differentiation (organogenesis), the embryo is highly susceptible to teratogenic insult, and because organ development is continual, a greater specificity of effects is observed as the embryo develops. Following differentiation, the fetus becomes progressively less susceptible to teratogenic stimuli. Therefore, for an exposure of an agent to have a teratogenic effect, it must occur during the period of organogenesis. The importance of this principle can again be illustrated with thalidomide, where time of treatment was shown to be the critical factor in failure to predict its teratogenic properties.

Effects on reproductive and developmental processes may also arise even if exposure occurred before conception. Reasons for this include:

● Hazardous agents or metabolites may be retained or persist in the body for long periods of time (for example polychlorinated biphenyls (PCBs) in fat or lead in bone).

● Prior damage to germ cells which is irreversible or has not been repaired:
   (a) sperm toxicity is usually repaired by cell turnover in several months, while
   (b) ovarian damage may persist for years.

However, the key point remains: damage arises when delivery of an insult to the critical process occurs at the critical time.

Teratology testing

A teratology test should be able to answer three questions:

- Can the agent induce developmental defects (teratogenic potential)?

- What are the effective doses (teratogenic potency)?

- Are the effective doses below adult toxic doses (teratogenic hazard)?

Experimentally, developmental toxicity is determined through classic animal teratology studies following appropriate exposure of pregnant animals (usually rabbits or small rodents) to the agent.

A quantitative evaluation of the predictive value of teratogenicity tests is lacking, though arguments have been presented on qualitative grounds. The accuracy (and therefore the validity) of such testing is impaired by:

- Different observed lesions in humans and animals.

- Human exposure data are often poorly estimated.

- Dose response data in humans are largely inaccurate, unsatisfactory or absent.

- Animal studies are often inconsistent, even between studies using the same species and doses.

The predictive ability of animal results to known human teratogens varies on the species used, and there is no *a priori* basis for selecting a certain species as a suitable model for predicting teratogenic hazard in humans. Indeed, no one species has been demonstrated to be the one of choice, although the rabbit and rat are the species most often used.

Epidemiological and clinical studies

Descriptive and analytical epidemiological studies are also employed to study reproductive or developmental impairment. These studies often suffer from methodological problems because sample sizes of worker populations may be too small to significantly demonstrate effects on reproductive or developmental end-points whose frequency is low in the general population (such as congenital malformation). Many reproductive end-points (for example, spontaneous abortion, depressed libido) are difficult to measure. Some study designs do not adequately control for the possibility of paternally, rather than maternally, mediated effects. Exposure is nearly always difficult to estimate and characteristics of lifestyle (such as use of alcohol, tobacco or drugs) can confound study results.

All these factors tend to contribute to the problems inherent in interpreting the results and conclusions of epidemiological studies. However, criteria exist for the recognition of a new teratogenic agent in humans. These have been used to identify the teratogenic agent in two teratological catastrophes, namely those caused by rubella (German measles) and thalidomide. These criteria are:

● An abrupt increase in the frequency of a particular defect or association of defects (syndrome).

● coincidence of this increase with a known change in exposure conditions, such as sudden exposure to a chemical or widespread use of a drug.

● Absence of factors common to all pregnancies yielding infants with characteristic defects.

For the criteria to work, they need the presence of a distinctive defect or pattern of defects, and sufficient number of cases. In the case where the defect is rare, fewer cases are needed.

Using such criteria, some 18 or so therapeutic drugs, one social drug (alcohol) and one chemical (methylmercury) have been identified as teratogens to humans.

Effects of chemicals

The structures and biological activities of chemicals with confirmed or suspected adverse effects on reproduction range broadly.

For some chemicals, there is scientific evidence regarding a cause and effect association with exposure and dysfunction in humans. This is based on:

● The number of studies that have reported toxicity;

● Insufficient occupational evidence is supported by the results of animal studies; or

● The effect of the chemical is predictable based on known biological activity.

Exposures to classes of chemicals, such as pesticides, oral contraceptives, or organic solvents and industries or processes where several chemicals are used, such as the rubber industry, or laboratory work, should also be included as producing evidence of reproductive or developmental dysfunction in occupationally exposed individuals.

Data are also available from animal studies alone. While such information should always be evaluated carefully with particular regard to mechanisms of toxicity and likely occupational exposures, it does often serve as a useful pointer to potential problems.

Health effects by occupation

There are many difficulties in establishing causal relationships between workplace exposures and reproductive outcomes. There are three main reasons for this:

- Limited parameters evaluated:
  (a) sperm analysis and its relationship with fertility;
  (b) availability of other measures of fertility, especially in women;
  (c) significance of fetal outcome; and
  (d) unavailability of histopathological assessment (except in animal studies).

- Limited data resources.

- Absence of systematic structure–activity studies.

However, a small number of occupations have been identified as having an increased risk, or an association with effects on reproductive function, as shown in Table 6.3.

Table 6.3. Occupations and reported effects on reproduction

Occupation	Reported effect(s)
Dental technicians	Increased spontaneous abortion
Factory workers	Decreased viability at birth; low birth weight; CNS and musculoskeletal malformations
Construction workers	CNS and musculoskeletal malformations
Transportation/communications workers	Oral clefts
Food industry workers	Musculoskeletal malformations
Laboratory technicians	Increased abortion and birth defects; chromosomal damage; increased perinatal death rate
Plastics industry workers	CNS defects
Printers	Gastroschisis
Teachers	Oral clefts
Telephone operators	Oral clefts

Table 6.3. (*Contd.*)

Occupation	Reported effect(s)
Operating theatre	Decreased fertility; increased personnel spontaneous abortion; low birth rate; possible birth defects
Registered nurses	Increased birth defects, especially cleft lip
Pulp and paper industry workers	Pregnancy complications
Lead production (males)	Reduced libido, lowered sperm counts, increased rate of miscarriage in partners

Health effects in female workers

For many years, the study of the interaction between occupational health and reproduction has focused on the female, especially with the recent increase in numbers of women joining the workforce. In many industries, this has caused a change in the way that hazards are controlled and workers are exposed. For example, policies such as exclusion of women and fetal protection are being re-examined and in many cases, discarded.

There is a number of older and now emerging hazards on reproduction and development in the females, as shown in Table 6.4.

Table 6.4. Effects reported in female workers

Adverse outcome	Agent
Menstrual and other gynaecological disorders	Aniline, benzene, chloroprene, formaldehyde, inorganic mercury, PCBs, styrene, toluene
Abortion or infertility	Anaesthetic gases, aniline, arsenic, benzene, cytotoxic drugs, ethylene oxide, formaldehyde, lead, 2,4-trichlorophenol
Decreased fetal growth, low birth weight or poor survival	Carbon monoxide, formaldehyde, PCBs, toluene, vinyl chloride
Prematurity	Lead, thermal stress
Teratogenic effects	Hexachloroprene, radiation, organic mercury, vinyl chloride
Maternal death related to pregnancy	Beryllium, benzene
Cancer	Diethylstilboestrol, hepatitis B

PCBs, polychlorinated biphenyls.

Health effects in male workers

One important outcome of the increased study of reproductive hazards in women has been an increase in attention on reproductive effects in men.

Effects of other agents on reproduction and development in the male (particularly male workers) are shown in Table 6.5.

Table 6.5. Effects reported in male workers

Adverse outcome	Agent
Decreased libido and impotence	Chloroprene, manganese, inorganic and organic lead, inorganic mercury, toluene diisocyanate, vinyl chloride
Testicular damage or infertility	Chloroprene, kepone, dibromochloropropane, inorganic and organic lead
Spermatoxicity	Carbaryl, carbon disulphide, cytotoxic drugs, dibromochloropropane, lead, radiation, thermal stress, toluenediamine/dinitrotoluene mixture

The archetypical male reproductive hazard is dibromochloropropane (DBCP) a nematocide previously used on pineapples and other crops. Initial indications of long-term (some argue permanent) azoospermia in a small cohort of production workers only came to light in circumstances whereby the workers themselves realised that they shared a common problem.

Toxicological effects in experimental animals

Data are also available from animal studies alone. While such information should always be evaluated carefully with particular regard to mechanisms of toxicity and likely occupational exposures, it does often serve as a useful pointer to potential problems.

Table 6.6. Chemical-induced effects reported in animals (but not humans)

Adverse outcome	Agent
Testicular damage or reduced male fertility	Benzene, benzo[a]pyrene, boron, cadmium, epichlorohydrin, ethylene dibromide, PBBs
Spermatoxicity	Arsenic, chloroprene, ethylene glycol ethers, ethylene oxide, halothane, kepone, mercury, nitrous oxide, trichloroethylene, triethyleneamine
Embryolethal or fetotoxic effects	Chloroform, dichloromethane, ethylene dichloride, ethylene dioxide, inorganic mercury, nitrogen dioxide, PBBs, selenium, tetrachloroethylene, thallium, trichloroethylene, vinylidine chloride
Teratogenic effects	Arsenic, benzo[a]pyrene, chlorodifluoromethane, chloroprene, monomethyl formamide, acrylonitrile, methyl ethyl ketone, tellurium, vinyl chloride
Transplacental carcinogenesis	Arsenic, benzo[a]pyrene, vinyl chloride

PBBs, polybrominated biphenyls.

With regard to occupational exposures, very few of these reported effects were from studies in which the amount of chemical was in the order of that found at the workplace.

Summary

There are many possible adverse health effects that may result from exposure to hazardous chemicals. Exposure of both males and females to such chemicals during the reproductive cycle can also have adverse outcomes on development of the embryo, fetus and infant. Such effects manifest themselves through fetal death, malformation, retarded growth, organ dysfunction, and so on. Knowledge concerning these health effects, including the interaction of a host of factors (familial, lifestyle, medical, etc.) is limited.

These unknowns indicate that the central issue in the protection of reproductive health and procreative capacity of working men and women is the management of uncertainty. Options for control of reproductive hazards are presently limited in scope and application. Nevertheless, while policy makers and employers may never have complete information regarding the full extent of reproductive dysfunction and its causes, the provisions of occupational health and safety legislation are that employers must provide as safe a working environment as is reasonably practicable. It becomes axiomatic that a cautious preventive approach should be taken to limit worker exposure to chemicals to a level as low as reasonably practicable.

Further research efforts should be intensified. These should concentrate on better and more efficient methods of identification (both experimental and epidemiological), increasing the precision of risk assessment processes (including its assumptions, methodologies and research needs), and optimising the usefulness of preventive strategies for exposed populations.

Bibliography

Barlow, S. M. and Sullivan, F. M., 1982, *Reproductive Hazards of Industrial Chemicals.* London: Academic Press.

Chamberlain, G. (Ed.), 1984 *Pregnant Women at Work.* London: Royal Society of Medicine/Macmillan.

Christian, M. S., Galbraith, W. M., Voytek, P. and Mehlman, M. A. (Eds), 1989, *Assessment of Reproductive and Teratogenic Hazards. Advances in Modern Environmental Toxicology III.* Princeton, NJ: Princeton Scientific Publishers.

Dixon, R. L. (Ed.), 1985, *Reproductive Toxicology (Target Organ Toxicology Series).* New York: Raven Press.

Dixon, R. L. and Hall, J. L., 1982, Reproductive toxicology, in Hayes, A. W. (Ed.) *Principles and Methods of Toxicology*, student edition, Chap. 4, pp. 107–40. New York: Raven Press.

Hemminki, K., 1987, Pregnancy outcome and occupation. Keynote Address to 22nd International Congress on Occupational Health, Sydney, September 1987.

Hemminki, K. and Vineis, P., 1985, Extrapolation of the evidence on teratogenicity of chemical between humans and experimental animals: chemicals other than drugs, *Terat. Carcin. Mutagen*, **5**, 251–318.

Khera, K. S., 1987, Maternal toxicity in humans and animals: effects on fetal development and criteria for detection, *Terat. Carcin. Mutagen*, **7**, 287–95.

Kirsch-Volders, M., 1981, *Mutagenicity, Carcinogenicity and Teratogenicity of Industrial Pollutants*. New York: Plenum Press.

Lemasters, G. K. and Selevan, S. G., 1984, Use of exposure data in occupational reproductive studies, *Scand. J. Work Environ. Health*, **10**, 1–6.

MacDonald, A. D. and MacDonald, J. C., 1988, Fetal death and work in pregnancy, *Br. J. Ind. Med.*, **45**, 148–57.

Manson, J. M. and Wise, L. D., 1991, Teratogens, in Amdur, M. O., Doull, J. and Klaassen, C. D. (Eds) *Casarett and Doull's Toxicology. The Basic Science of Poisons*, 4th Edn., Chap. 7. New York: Pergamon Press.

Manson, J. M., Zenick, H. and Costlow, R. D., 1982, Teratology test methods for laboratory animals, in Hayes, A. W. (Ed.) *Principles and Methods of Toxicology*, student edition, Chap. 5, pp. 141–85. New York: Raven Press.

Mattinson, D. R., 1983, The mechanisms of action of reproductive toxins, *Am. J. Indust. Med.*, **4**, 65–79.

Meyers, V. K. (Ed.), 1988, *Teratogens: Chemicals Which Cause Birth Defects (Studies in Environmental Science 31)*. Amsterdam: Elsevier.

OTA, 1985, *Reproductive Hazards in the Workplace*. Washington, DC: Office of Technology Assessment, US Government Printing Office.

Schrag, S. D. and Dixon, R. L., 1985, Occupational exposures associated with male reproductive dysfunction, *Ann Rev. Pharmacol. Toxicol.*, **25**, 567–92.

Schardien, J. L., 1985, *Chemically Induced Birth Defects (Drug and Chemical Toxicology 2)*. New York: Marcel Dekker.

Shepard, T. H. (Ed.), 1986, *Catalog of Teratogenic Agents*, 5th Edn. Baltimore: Johns Hopkins University Press.

Thomas, J. A., 1991, Toxic responses of the reproductive system, in Amdur, M. O., Doull, J. and Klaassen, C. D. (Eds) *Casarett and Doull's Toxicology. The Basic Science of Poisons*, 4th Edn., Chap. 16. New York: Pergamon Press.

Wilson, J. G., 1973, *Environment and Birth Defects*. New York: Academic Press.

Wilson, J. G., 1977, Teratogenic effects of environmental chemicals, *Fed. Proc.*, **36**, 1698–703.

Chapter 7

Genetic Toxicology

A. D. Mitchell

Introduction

Genetic toxicology involves the identification of agents that interact with nucleic acids to alter the hereditary material of living organisms; agents that produce such alterations are termed 'genotoxic'. Genetic toxicology is both an investigative science and an applied science which incorporates principles from the fields of genetics, microbiology, cell biology, molecular biology, biochemistry, and toxicology to develop and utilise tests that are predictive of mutagenesis and carcinogenesis. Thus, an understanding of these disciplines, and especially the basic genetic processes that may be influenced by genotoxicants, is necessary not only for the development and appropriate use of assay systems that measure the effects of potentially genotoxic agents, but also to interpret the significance of results that are obtained.

During the relatively short time that the field of genetic toxicology has been recognised, extensive efforts have been devoted to defining and evaluating the utility of numerous testing approaches for predicting heritable genetic effects and cancer. Today, because genetic toxicology tests are well defined, assess effects directly related to those observed in humans, and are relatively efficient and economical, they are mandated as an initial step for regulatory assessments. To provide an introduction to genetic toxicology, the rapid development of the field is summarised, some of the more extensively used tests, as well as the current application of genetic toxicology approaches for human monitoring and for product registration, are described, and references to suggested reading are provided for those who may wish to pursue this topic further.

Development of genetic toxicology

In comparison with toxicology, the science of poisons, the origins of which can be traced to antiquity (Casarett and Bruce, 1980), the origin of genetics dates only to the rediscovery of the works of Gregor Mendel, shortly after the turn of the century. Genetic toxicology is an even newer discipline; the first published study on radiation-induced mutations in *Drosophila* was that by H. J. Muller in the late 1920s; not until after World War II was the first

123

work on chemically-induced mutations (by mustard gas) published by Charlotte Auerbach (Wassom, 1989).

At least another decade elapsed before geneticists recommended that tests for mutagenicity be developed as a routine component of toxicology testing because of concerns that some chemical products of benefit to industrialised society may adversely affect human health and the environment. During the 1960s, several laboratories focused on developing methods suitable for testing chemicals for mutagenicity, and by the end of the decade, the first *in vivo* tests to assess heritable effects had been defined.

The identification of the field as 'genetic toxicology' and its exponential growth occurred during the 1970s when numerous methods for evaluating the genotoxic effects of chemicals were developed and published. Of great importance to many of these approaches was the development of *in vitro* metabolic activation systems (Malling, 1971) that permitted *in vitro* tests to reflect more closely *in vivo* metabolism. Also during this time, substantial efforts were made to enhance awareness of the public and governmental agencies to the potential threat of chemicals to the human gene pool, which resulted in the promulgation of regulations mandating that industry evaluate the potential genotoxic hazards of their products.

Objectives of genetic toxicology

Genetic toxicology testing has two objectives: (a) the identification of agents capable of inducing heritable effects, the initial goal; and (b) the prediction of carcinogenicity, a goal that gained momentum in the mid-1970s following the publication of test results which suggested that carcinogens are mutagens (McCann *et al.*, 1975a,b; Bridges, 1976; Sugimura *et al.*, 1976; Ames, 1979). Indeed, when most of the currently available genetic toxicology approaches were developed, their efficacy was first demonstrated by testing a group of classical mutagens that are also carcinogens.

Mutagenesis

Essentially all basic genetic toxicology test systems measure the induction of DNA damage and/or resulting mutations in DNA which, with the exception of some RNA viruses, is the molecule containing hereditary information for all living organisms. If DNA is damaged, it may: (a) be correctly repaired with no genetic consequences; (b) lead to cell death, again with no genetic consequences; or (c) be replicated with the damage misrepaired. Only the latter leads to mutations, defined as DNA alterations that are propagated through subsequent generations of cells or individuals. Mutations do occur spontaneously, but any increase in the rate of mutation induction is the consequence of unusual circumstances. While biological diversity may be considered to be a result of the accumulation of beneficial mutations over time, it is generally accepted that most mutations are deleterious, and it is the concern of many genetic toxicologists that the human genome received from our ancestors be none the worse when it is passed on to future generations.

Carcinogenesis

Carcinogenesis is known to proceed through a number of steps, and the first step, initiation, is generally believed to involve mutation in somatic cells. As described above, a somatic cell mutation would be of no consequence if it resulted in death of the cell or if the mutated cell failed to divide, but it would be of consequence if it occurred in a dividing cell or if a second mutation, e.g. in an oncogene, resulted in resumption of cell division of an otherwise non-dividing mutated cell. Support of the role of mutagenesis in carcinogenesis includes the clonal origin of tumours, the association of specific chromosomal abnormalities with certain cancers, information about genetically determined cancer-prone conditions, and the number of carcinogens that have been shown to be mutagens. However, some carcinogens, including hormones and inert materials have not been shown to be mutagenic, and it is thought that they may act through non-genotoxic, 'epigenetic' mechanisms such as alterations in cell regulatory mechanisms, including the induction of proliferation in otherwise non-dividing cells.

A significant number of carcinogens are mutagens, but correlations between carcinogenicity and mutagenicity are not complete, as was predicted by Malling and Chu (1974). The degree of correlation observed between these two end-points is highly dependent upon the test system used, the precision of testing, the class of chemicals tested, and the methods used to evaluate the results. For example, a number of rodent carcinogens that have yielded 'negative' results in *in vitro* genetic toxicology tests (Tennant *et al.*, 1987) are insoluble *in vitro*. However, because resources are insufficient for testing more than a small percentage of commercially important chemicals in long-term *in vivo* cancer bioassays, and because a reduction in the requirements for testing in animals is a generally accepted goal, over 200 short-term relatively inexpensive genetic toxicology tests have now been developed to assess the genetic hazards of chemicals and to assist in predicting the results of long-term testing.

Genetic toxicology testing for product registration

Genetic toxicology tests that have been proposed for product registration will be described. For various reasons, many regulatory requirements for genotoxicity testing evolved independently within different governmental agencies and in various geographical areas. Initially, these regulatory requirements were often based as much on theoretical considerations as on the actual performance of the tests. However, with increasing use and evaluation of the test systems, it has been found that only a few of the tests are appropriate for routine use. Many have been inadequately evaluated, and some have been found to be insensitive to important classes of chemicals, while others appear to yield too many 'false positive' results, and still others are too time consuming and/or costly. Thus, today, relatively few genetic toxicology tests are routinely used for initial assessments of genetic effects, with the selection of protocols often based on published regulatory guidelines and the experience of industry. To assist companies wishing to market chemicals and pharmaceuticals in diverse geographical areas, concerted efforts are being made by regulatory agencies to reach agreement on which genetic toxicology testing protocols should be universally required for regulatory submissions.

Many testing schemes utilise a battery of tests which usually fall into three tiers, as shown in Table 7.1. When currently proposed changes in regulations are implemented, it is probable that the basic, initial tier of tests recommended by various agencies will be limited to tests for (a) gene mutations in bacteria; (b) gene mutations in mammalian cells; (c) chromosomal mutations *in vitro*; and (d) chromosomal mutations *in vivo*. There is less agreement on which tests should be used after the initial tier. Tests that have been recommended and used in a second tier include unscheduled DNA synthesis (UDS), the dominant lethal test, the sex-linked recessive lethal test in *Drosophila*, *in vivo* chromosomal aberrations, and mammalian cell transformation. Assessments of genomic mutations predominate in the third tier of tests but, in general, tests for genomic mutations use large numbers of animals, are labour intensive and, hence, expensive, and the number of laboratories proficient in these tests is limited. Furthermore, as discussed by Prival and Dellarco (1989), the development of pharmaceuticals and industrial chemicals is often discontinued when initial test results indicate mutagenicity. Although regulatory agencies have used positive results in initial mutagenicity tests to justify requests for additional information on the mutagenicity and/or carcinogenicity of chemicals, because of the time and expense involved in this additional testing, a request for additional information may preclude a new product from being marketed.

Table 7.1. Example battery of genetic toxicology tests

Tier 1 Simple and rapid tests for:
Gene mutations in bacteria
Gene and chromosomal mutations in mammalian cells
Chromosomal mutations *in vivo*

Tier 2 Intermediate tests for:
Mutations in *Drosophila*
Dominant-lethal in mice
Repair of DNA damage

Tier 3 Long-term tests in animals:
Visible or biochemical specific locus test in mice
Heritable translocation test in mice

To establish that a test chemical is negative, *in vitro* tests must be conducted in the absence and presence of exogenous metabolic activation, and positive and negative controls must be within historical ranges. The latter is also applicable to *in vivo* tests, and, in addition, animals must be maintained under conditions that minimize the influence of environmental variables, and bioavailability must be considered when selecting the route of administration of a test material. Some current testing guidelines specify that the results obtained should be demonstrably reproducible in independent experiments. However, many scientists believe that it is not necessary to repeat appropriately conducted assays that are clearly positive or negative, particularly for *in vivo* tests, as this is contrary to the objective of minimising the use of animals. Also, replication for its own sake (i.e. an exact repeat of the first assay) may not be informative; instead, repeat assays should be designed to correct any deficiencies of the first assay. If one assay results in a negative response and the other in a positive response, and if there is no reason to give greater weight to either one of them, the overall evaluation must be equivocal, and the assay should be repeated again.

Applicability of genetic toxicology for human population monitoring

As described by Albertini and Robinson (1991), human population monitoring involves quantitating and characterising genotoxicant exposures and genetic effects *in vivo* in humans for human health risk assessments. Many of the laboratory assays used for monitoring are similar or identical to those that will be described for traditional genetic toxicology. However, traditional genetic toxicology deals with the identification of potential genetic hazards and is important for interpreting the results of population monitoring, while human population monitoring deals with another level of risk, i.e. the identification of effects that may have occurred in humans. Population monitoring is also related to two other activities concerned with human populations—human genetic screening, which defines genetic susceptibilities within populations; and epidemiology, which is the topic of another chapter in this text.

Measures of human genotoxicant exposure related to the tests described below include: the use of *Salmonella* mutagenesis to detect mutagens or their metabolites in urine concentrates; assessing UDS in human tissues (e.g. blood) shortly after chemical exposure to measure genotoxicant interactions with DNA; evaluating chromosome damage in peripheral blood lymphocytes as an index of irreversible genotoxic effects; assessing *hprt* mutations in human blood cells as a measure of human somatic cell gene mutations; and using markers of both chromosomal- and gene-level genetic effects which are detectable in human sperm. These and other approaches are described in Albertini and Robinson (1991), and it is anticipated that with the current rapid developments in the field of molecular biology, additional measures of human exposure will be used in the future.

The spectrum of genetic toxicology tests

The virtual universality of DNA as the genetic material and the observation that chemicals that induce genetic effects in one species or test system frequently induce similar effects in other species or test systems provides the basis for a diversity of test systems—bacteria, yeast and fungi; plants; submammalian animal species, e.g. *Drosophila*; mammalian cells in culture; and rodents—for assessing the mutagenic activity of chemicals. Mutations can range from a single nucleotide change to changes in chromosome number. Thus, they may be classified according to complexity or the extent of the genetic alteration, as gene mutations, chromosomal mutations, or genomic mutations.

A wealth of literature is available for those who wish to pursue further the development and use of specific test systems, including texts on genetic toxicology (Brusick, 1980; Li and Heflich, 1991), the series *Chemical Mutagens* by Hollaender and de Serres (1971–1983), and a number of established journals in the field, including *Environmental and Molecular Mutagenesis* (Wiley-Liss), *Mutagenesis* (IRL Press), and *Mutation Research* (Elsevier). In the latter may be found the series of US Environmental Protection Agency Gene-Tox reviews of specific test systems.

To illustrate the diversity of test systems available, representative examples are briefly described below. Descriptions of other test systems that have been developed but that are not widely used for initial regulatory submissions at this time may be found in the texts by Brusick (1980) and Li and Heflich (1991) and include: tests in yeast, fungi (e.g. *Neurospora*), and plants; measurements of DNA adducts (DNA binding); and the use of host-mediated assays. The tests that are summarised in this chapter are also detailed in those references.

Tests for gene mutations

A gene is the simplest functional unit in a DNA molecule, and gene (or point) mutations are changes in the nucleotide sequence at one or a few coding segments. Base pair, or base substitution, mutations occur when one nucleotide base is replaced with another. Frameshift mutations occur through the addition or deletion of one or more bases, which alters the sequences of bases in DNA, and hence the reading frame in RNA. These changes may occur at the site of the original mutation or at a second site on the chromosome. Missense mutations are gene mutations that specify the insertion of an 'incorrect' amino acid into a polypeptide and usually result in impaired function of the affected cell or organism. Nonsense mutations introduce terminator codons into the DNA, resulting in the premature cessation of polypeptide synthesis, which is usually associated with complete loss of function of the altered gene. Forward mutations lead to loss of normal function of a gene product; reverse, or back, mutations restore the normal function of the gene.

Using molecular biology techniques, an increasing number of gene mutations are being identified in the human population, and molecular genetic techniques have now become sufficiently powerful to allow the routine identification of the specific DNA sequence changes responsible for mutant phenotypes. However, as yet, these techniques are, for the most part, used to enhance our understanding of molecular genetic mechanisms rather than as genetic toxicology test systems. Tests for gene mutations use phenotypic changes in nutritional requirements or drug resistance to indicate that genotypic changes have occurred (at the nucleotide level) in large numbers of cells or organisms in order to demonstrate statistically and/or biologically significant increases over spontaneous mutation frequencies.

Gene mutations are tested most frequently in bacteria, insects, and mammalian cells. Although extensive literature exists on mutagenesis testing in yeast (*Saccharomyces cerevisiae*) and mould (*Neurospora crassa*), the use of these organisms has declined because of problems associated with chemical permeability and the presence of endogenous target cell metabolism (Brusick, 1980). Currently, there are no well-established *in vivo* gene mutation assays. However, various laboratories have used host-mediated assays, in which bacteria or mammalian cells are implanted in the peritoneal cavity of animals, the animals are exposed to the test material, and the cells then removed for continuation of the test *in vitro*. Also, a number of laboratories are currently evaluating gene mutation assays in transgenic mice, e.g. mice carrying a bacterial gene that, following *in vivo* exposure, is 'rescued' and re-inserted into bacteria, which are then cloned to assess mutagenesis. Because the transgenic mouse mutagenesis assays can assess mutations in the DNA from essentially any tissue, which cannot be done with the host-mediated assay, it is anticipated that one or more of the transgenic mouse gene mutation assays, when sufficiently developed and evaluated, will meet the critical need for an *in vivo* point mutation assay.

Tests for gene mutations in bacteria

The most extensive testing for gene mutations is in bacteria, particularly using reverse mutation assays in *Salmonella typhimurium* and *Escherichia coli*. Bacterial tests present the advantages of relative ease of performance, economy and efficiency, and the ability to identify specific DNA damage that is induced, e.g. frameshift or base pair mutations. Bacterial tests can also provide information on the mode of action of the test chemical, as the bacterial strains used vary in their responsiveness to different chemical classes.

The *S. typhimurium*/microsome reverse mutation assay (the Ames test) and the *E. coli* reverse mutation assay are among the most economical and rapid genetic toxicology assays. The Ames test, which is the most widely used and considered by many to be the cornerstone of genetic toxicology testing, features unique strains of histidine dependent *S. typhimurium* designed for sensitivity in detecting gene mutations, specifically frameshift mutations and base pair substitutions, which revert the bacteria to histidine independence. The *Salmonella* strains are histidine auxotrophs by virtue of mutations in the histidine operon: when these histidine-dependent cells are grown on minimal medium agar plates containing a trace of histidine, only those cells that revert to histidine independence are able to form colonies. The small amount of histidine allows all the plated bacteria to undergo a few divisions; in many cases, this growth is essential for mutagenesis to occur, and the histidine revertants are easily visible as colonies against a slight lawn of background growth. The spontaneous reversion rate of each strain is relatively constant (McCann *et al.*, 1975a; Maron and Ames, 1983), although these rates may vary with different solvents, and when the bacteria are exposed to mutagens, the mutation rates are increased, usually in a dose-related manner.

In addition to the histidine operon, most of the indicator strains carry a deletion that covers genes involved in the synthesis of the vitamin biotin (*bio*), and all carry the *rfa* mutation that leads to a defective lipopolysac-charide coat and makes the strains more permeable to many large mole-cules. All strains also carry the *uvrB* mutation which results in impaired repair of ultraviolet (UV) induced DNA damage and renders the bacteria unable to use accurate excision repair to remove certain chemically or physically damaged DNA, thereby enhancing the strains' sensitivity to some mutagenic agents. Additional strains contain the resistance transfer factor, plasmid pKM101, which is believed to cause an additional increase in error-prone DNA repair, leading to even greater sensitivity to most mutagens (McCann *et al.*, 1975b; Maron and Ames, 1983). Plasmid pKM101 also confers resistance to the antibiotic ampicillin, which is a convenient marker for detecting its presence in the strains.

In Ames testing, one strain is used for a preliminary concentration range-finding assay, then mutagenesis assays are conducted with four or five strains. For example, some protocols use five well established strains: TA1535, TA1537, TA1538, TA98 and TA100. Other protocols may use the four strains recommended by Maron and Ames (1983): TA97a (formerly TA97), TA98, TA100 and TA102. Strains TA1535 and TA100 are reverted to histidine independence by base pair mutagens; strains TA1537, TA1538, TA97a and TA98 are reverted by frameshift mutagens; and strain TA102 detects a variety of oxidants and cross-linking agents that are not detected by the other strains (Levin *et al.*, 1982a, b, 1984).

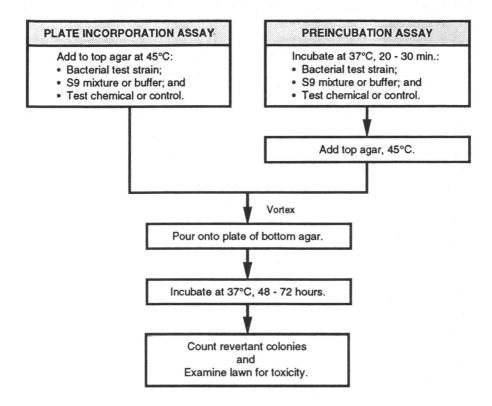

Figure 7.1. Comparison of representative plate incorporation and preincubation assays for reverse mutation in bacteria. For each strain and dilution of the test material or positive control, three sterile 13 × 100-mm test tubes are placed in a heating block; six test tubes are used for each negative (solvent) control. In the plate incorporation assay, the heating block is maintained at 45°C, and the following are added for each sample: (a) 2.0 ml of molten top agar containing histidine for *Salmonella* or tryptophan for *E. coli*, NaCl, Vogel–Bonner medium E, and glucose; (b) 0.5 ml of the metabolic activation mixture or buffer; (c) a dilution of the test material or the positive or negative control; and (d) 0.1 ml of the tester strain (about 10^8 bacteria) from an overnight culture. This mixture is then mixed and poured on a previously prepared plate containing about 25 or 30 ml of bottom agar (minimal agar with glucose). After the top agar sets (about 15 min), the plates are inverted and incubated for 48–72 h for growth of mutant colonies. Preincubation assays differ in that top agar (at 45°C) is not added until the bacteria have been incubated, at 37°C, with the chemical and the metabolic activation mixture or buffer for 20–30 min. Because the top agar contains a trace of histidine or tryptophan, which is soon depleted, the bacteria form a background lawn, but only those bacteria which have reverted to histidine- or tryptophan-auxotrophy can continue to grow and form colonies. A reduction in the background lawn indicates toxicity.

E. coli strain WP2 *uvrA* (pKM101) is a tryptophan auxotroph by virtue of a base pair substitution mutation in the tryptophan operon. The *uvrA* mutation renders it deficient in the repair of some physically or chemically induced DNA damage, and the presence of plasmid pKM101 enhances

sensitivity to most mutagens, as was described, above. Prior to the development of the *S. typhimurium* strains TA100 and TA98, the *E. coli* WP2 assay
was strongly recommended to complement the Ames test; its use has continued, particularly in conjunction with the *Salmonella* strains, to address
international regulatory requirements based on the finding that some chemicals that are negative in *Salmonella* are detected by *E. coli*.

Basic microbial mutagenesis protocols use the plate incorporation approach or a preincubation modification of this approach (Maron and Ames,
1983). They are outlined in Figure 7.1. In the standard plate incorporation
protocol, the test material, bacteria, and either a metabolic activation
mixture (S9) or buffer are added to liquid top agar which is then mixed, and
the mixture is immediately poured on a plate of bottom agar. After the agar
gels, the bacteria are incubated, at 37°C, for 48–72 h; then, the resulting
colonies are counted. The preincubation modification is used for materials,
including volatile and water-soluble compounds, that may be poorly detected in the plate incorporation assay. In this protocol, the test material,
bacteria, and S9 mixture (if used) are incubated for 20–30 min at 37°C
before top agar is added, mixed, and the mixture poured on a plate of
bottom agar. Increased activity with preincubation in comparison with
plate incorporation is attributed to the fact that the test compound,
bacteria, and S9 are incubated at higher concentrations (without agar
present) than in the standard plate incorporation test (Prival *et al.*, 1979).
Other modifications of the assays provide for exposing the bacteria to
measured concentrations of gases in closed containers and/or the use of
metabolic activation systems from a variety of species.

Tests for gene and chromosomal mutations in mammalian cells

Although measurements of mutagenesis in mammalian cells are more time
consuming and expensive than bacterial assays, the test results obtained
reflect the greater complexity of mammalian cells and chromosomes in
comparison with those of prokaryotes, and thus they more closely approximate the genetic effects of chemicals in rodent species and humans. In
contrast to bacteria, mammalian cells are essentialy diploid (2*n*, with two
copies of each chromosome), and their chromosomes are located within the
nucleus of the cell and contain non-functional and non-coding, as well as
functional, coding sequences. In addition, whereas in bacterial cells all
genes are usually expressed, in diploid cells, there are usually two copies of
each gene (one on each chromosome), and one dominant form of the gene
may be expressed while the other recessive gene remains unexpressed, unless
both copies are recessive. If both copies of the gene are the same the cell or
organism is homozygous for that trait; a heterozygous condition exists if
the copies are different; and, if only one chromosome is present to carry the
trait, the condition is hemizygous. Hemizygous traits are found on the X

chromosome in mammals because males have only one X chromosome and, in female cells, only one X chromosome is expressed.

In mammalian cell mutagenesis assays, the chemical exposure step must be followed by an expression period, during which mutant (and non-mutant) cells increase in number and the non-mutant protein (enzyme) present in the mutated cells and the RNA coding for that protein are depleted. Then a selective agent is added which permits only the mutated cells to grow and form colonies. The most extensively used mammalian cell mutagenesis tests employ established cell lines from mice and Chinese hamsters. Three such well-characterised protocols are shown in Table 7.2. The AS52/*xprt* mutation assay in Chinese hamster cells is a fourth, newer protocol.

Table 7.2. Examples of tests for mammalian cell mutagenesis

Chinese hamster ovary (CHO) *hprt* gene mutation assay
V79 (Chinese hamster lung fibroblast) *hprt* gene mutation assay
L5178Y/*tk*$^{+/-}$ mouse lymphoma cell mutation assay (with colony sizing)

The L5178Y/*tk*$^{+/-}$ and AS52/*xprt* assays measure mutations at heterozygous, rather than hemizygous, loci; therefore, cells with chromosomal mutations, as well as cells with less extensive damage (gene mutations), survive and are enumerated. These protocols are used to determine whether a test material will induce chromosomal effects as well as gene mutations *in vitro*. In contrast, the CHO and V79/*hprt* assays measure mutagenesis at a hemizygous locus; thus, cells with more extensive (chromosomal) damage do not survive and cannot be enumerated. For a number of years these *hprt* mutation assays were used at least as extensively as the L5178Y mouse lymphoma cell mutagenesis assay; then, in many laboratories, the *hprt* assays were favoured because some publications suggested that the L5178Y assay was too sensitive, i.e yielded too many 'false positive' results. However, it has been found that the L5178Y assay is not overly sensitive when the appropriate protocols and evaluation criteria are used, and its use in comparison to that of the *hprt* assays is now increasing because the latter necessitates the parallel use of an *in vitro* chromosomal aberration assay.

THE CHO/*hprt* AND V79/*hprt* GENE MUTATION ASSAYS
The *hprt* gene is located on the X chromosome; therefore, mutations at this locus are measurable in virtually all diploid or near-diploid mammalian cell lines. The CHO and V79 target cells have a rapid growth rate (a 12–14 h cell doubling time), may be grown as monolayer cultures or in suspension, have a high cloning efficiency, a relatively low spontaneous mutation frequency, and may be used for cytogenetic studies (described below). CHO and V79 cells have two X chromosomes, but only one of them is actively transcribed and used in cellular processes. Thus, there are two possible

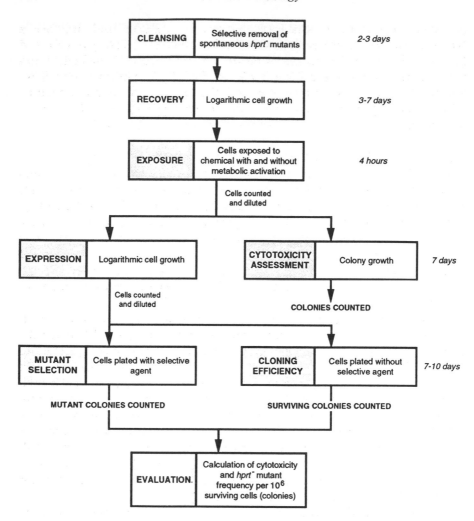

Figure 7.2. Representative CHO or V79 mammalian cell mutagenesis assay. Before each assay, spontaneous *hprt⁻* mutants are removed by maintaining a monolayer culture of cells for 2–3 days in medium containing thymidine, hypoxanthine, methotrexate and glycine (THMG). The cells are then allowed to recover from cleansing for 1 day in medium containing THG (no methotrexate); then they are grown for another 2–6 days, with subculturing every 2–3 days, before establishing the cultures to be exposed. Each culture of cells is exposed to a dilution of the test material, the negative (solvent) control, or the positive control, in the absence and presence of metabolic activation, for 4 h at 37°C. Following exposure, the cells are rinsed, detached with trypsin, centrifuged, resuspended, and counted. Then 200 cells are plated in each of three dishes and grown without subculturing for 7 days before staining and counting colonies to assess cytotoxicity, and two cultures of 1.5×10^6 cells are grown, with subculturing every 2–3 days, for expression. After expression, the two cultures are pooled and counted; 2×10^5 cells are plated in medium containing 6-thioguanine (the selective agent) in each of 12 dishes for growth of mutant colonies, and three dishes of 200 cells are plated (without the selective agent) to determine cloning efficiency of each culture. After growth of colonies (without subculturing) for 7–10 days, the colonies are stained and counted to determine the number of *hprt⁻* mutants per 10^6 cells that were cloned.

genotypes: (1) *hprt*⁺, in which the enzyme is produced and provides a 'salvage' pathway to use hypoxanthine and guanine for DNA synthesis; and (2) *hprt*⁻, in which the enzyme is either not produced or is defective, and the cell cannot use the salvage pathway for DNA synthesis. For these assays, after a 6–8 day expression period, the cells are plated in thioguanine (TG) containing medium, and *hprt*-deficient mutants are detected as surviving colonies. An outline of the procedure is shown in Figure 7.2.

THE L5178Y/*tk*⁺/⁻ GENE AND CHROMOSOMAL MUTATION ASSAY

The L5178Y mouse lymphoma assay measures gene and chromosomal forward mutations at the thymidine kinase locus, $tk^{+/-} \rightarrow tk^{-/-}$, and it yields high concordances with carcinogenicity test results. When trifluorothymidine (TFT) is used as the selective agent, many mutagens yield a biphasic curve of colony sizes which is resolved into small (σ) colonies of slowly growing mutant cells and large (λ) colonies of more rapidly growing mutants. It has been shown that most σ colony mutants have chromosomal mutations, as well as gene mutations, and that most λ colony mutants have only gene mutations (Clive and Moore-Brown, 1979).

L5178Y mouse lymphoma cells, specifically clone 3.7.2C, grow in suspension culture with a relatively short cell doubling time (9–10 h). After the expression period, the cells are cloned in culture dishes in medium containing sufficient agar to immobilise the cells to measure mutagenesis (with TFT present in the cloning medium) and survival. An approximately 2 week incubation period is required before colonies can be counted, because with shorter times the small colonies may not grow to a sufficient size to be visualised. Colony counting and sizing are conducted using colony counters that can discriminate between size ranges of the objects (colonies) counted. Both σ and λ colony mutation frequencies, as well as total mutation frequencies, should be reported for positive and negative controls and for treated cultures that yield a positive response.

At least two modifications of the L5178Y mouse lymphoma cell mutagenesis assay have been used for testing chemicals. In the first, the cells are cloned in microtitre plates in the absence of agar. In the second, an *in situ* variant, the cells are cloned in soft agar cloning medium after the exposure step, and TFT in liquid medium is added two days later, following the expression period. Because the presence of agar can retard colony growth, the microtitre approach yields more accurate measures of mutation frequencies and survival than when cells are cloned in agar; however, it is more time consuming than cloning in soft agar, and, to date, colony sizing must be accomplished subjectively, with visual (microscopic) observation of the colonies. The *in situ* approach also yields a more accurate measure of mutation frequencies, as the more slowly growing mutants are not lost by dilution during the expression period. With this approach, spontaneous and induced mutation frequencies (particularly σ colony mutation frequencies) are several times higher than with the standard approach, but to date, no chemical has been found positive with the *in situ* approach that was not also positive in the standard assay. Therefore, its future use may be for research purposes rather than for testing.

THE AS52/*xprt* GENE AND CHROMOSOMAL MUTATION ASSAY

The AS52/*xprt* cell mutation assay, a more recently developed mammalian cell assay (Tindall *et al.*, 1986), provides many features of the L5178Y cell mutagenesis assay, but CHO cells are used, with essentially the same procedures as for the CHO/*hprt* assay. The AS52 cell line carries a single functional copy of the bacterial *gpt* gene integrated into the CHO genome at a site that allows the recovery of chromosomal mutations. Although, as yet, the AS52/*xprt* assay has been successfully used in only a few laboratories, it is anticipated that, with greater availability and more extensive evaluation of its performance, this system may become more widely used in the future.

The Drosophila sex-linked recessive lethal test

The sex-linked recessive lethal (SLRL) test in the fruit fly, *Drosophila melanogaster*, is a forward mutation assay that detects the occurrence of both point mutations and small deletions in germ cells, and it is capable of screening for mutations at about 800 loci on the X chromosome (hence, sex-linked mutations). The *Drosophila* SLRL test is of historical importance because the first demonstration of mutagenesis was in *Drosophila* (Muller, 1927). In the six-plus decades that have elapsed since then, *Drosophila* have been extensively characterised genetically, hundreds of chemicals have been tested in this species, and the SLRL has been found to be responsive to mutagens from different chemical classes.

In this assay, wild-type males (3–5 days old) are treated with the test material and mated to an excess of virgin females from the Basc or Muller-5 stock, with specially marked and arranged chromosomes. The females are replaced with fresh virgins every two to three days to cover the entire germ cell cycle. Heterozygous female offspring (F_1) are mated individually to their brothers (also F_1), and the progeny (F_2) from each of these crosses are scored for phenotypically wild-type males. Absence of these males indicates that a sex-linked recessive lethal mutation has occurred in a germ cell of the parental male.

Advantages of this assay include the presence of a xenobiotic metabolic system in insects and significant economies of time and resources over similar tests in mammals. However, the SLRL is not used as an initial test for mutagenesis because of concerns that insect metabolism may be too far removed from human metabolic responses. Even though the test is more economical and rapid than tests in mammals, the assay is still labour intensive in comparison with many testing approaches because of the time required to examine thousands of progeny. At this time the SLRL is used primarily in research laboratories.

Tests for chromosomal mutations

Chromosomal abnormalities are associated with:

- Spontaneous abortion.
- Congenital malformation.
- Neoplasia.
- Infertility.

They occur in approximately 0.6% of live births in humans. It has been estimated that up to 40% of spontaneous abortuses have chromosomal defects. The rationale for measuring chromosomal effects includes: the increasing evidence that specific chromosomal defects in somatic cells are associated with most neoplasias and evidence that chromosomal rearrangement may play a role in oncogene activation; the relevance of chromosomal mutation to inheritance of genetic defects in germ cells; and the observation that substances which produce chromosomal structural changes also produce point mutations and that few gene mutagens produce no aberrations.

An understanding of mitosis and the stages of the somatic cell cycle, and their derangements, is important in the design and interpretation of results for several genetic toxicology test systems including, most particularly, cytogenetic assays. Initially it was thought that the cell cycle was composed of only two stages, mitosis or cell division, and interphase (the interval between mitoses), but interphase, which is a period of intense biochemical activity, is divided into at least three distinct stages: G_1, S and G_2 (first gap, synthesis, and second gap, respectively). During G_1, which follows mitosis, the chromosomes are greatly extended, and the cell undergoes enzymatic synthesis of proteins and nucleotides, the precursors of the DNA molecule. During S, the stage generally most sensitive to mutagens, nucleotides are incorporated during DNA synthesis and replication of the whole genome occurs. After the completion of DNA synthesis, each chromosome consists of two daughter chromatids, and the cell enters G_2, preparatory to mitosis. In normal cells, after a certain number of divisions, some may leave the cycle and become non-dividing, terminally differentiated cells in an extended G_1 phase, termed G_0. For most *in vitro* mammalian cell mutagenesis and cytogenetics tests, however, continuous cell cultures, without a G_0 stage, are used. And for tests using human lymphocytes, mitogenic stimulation is used to induce G_0 cells to re-enter the cell cycle and, after a lengthy G_1 stage, to resume the process of cell replication.

Mitosis is divided into four stages, as shown in Table 7.3.

Table 7.3. Stages of mitosis

Prophase	Chromatin begins to condense into visible chromosomes and the nuclear membrane disappears
Metaphase	The condensed, replicated chromosome is visible as two chromatids connected at the centromere, the point of spindle attachment
Anaphase	The chromatids separate and the cytoplasm begins to constrict to form two daughter cells
Telophase	Nuclear membranes reform around each set of chromosomes and cytokinesis, cell division, is completed

To visualise chromosomes, cells are arrested in metaphase, treated with a hypotonic solution to swell the chromosomes, fixed, transferred to microscope slides, and stained. The first metaphase (M) following chemical exposure (M_1) is the time when the greatest number of chromosomally damaged cells may be observed because many cells with extensively damaged chromosomes are incapable of progressing through additional cell cycles. The progression of severely damaged cells through the cell cycle to mitosis is retarded in direct relation to the extent of damage, a phenomenon that must be considered in the design of cytogenetic tests.

Chromosome breakage, which is necessary for chromosomal rearrangements (Hsu, 1979), is the classical end-point in chromosomal aberration assays designed to assess the potential health hazards of chemicals. Agents that break chromosomes are termed 'clastogens'. Following exposure to a clastogen, the number of cells with chromosome breakage and rearrangements increases in M_1 cells in a dose-related manner, but declines rapidly after M_1 because of the greatly extended cell cycle times of some cytogenetically damaged cells. A chromosomal exchange results when the broken ends of the same or different chromosomes rejoin in an aberrant manner. An inversion results from two breaks in one chromosome with the broken piece turned 180° before rejoining and cannot be visualised without special chromosome staining techniques to reveal chromosome bands. A translocation results from an interchange between different non-homologous chromosomes.

Chromosomal mutations (structural aberrations) are morphological alterations in the structure of eukaryotic chromosomes and, hence, they may affect the expression of numerous genes, with gross effects, or be lethal to affected cells. To assess chromosomal damage, test systems are used that provide for exposures *in vitro* and *in vivo*. While the L5178Y/$tk^{+/-}$ and AS52/*xprt* cell mutation assays indicate chromosomal, as well as gene, mutations, they do not provide for direct observations of broken and aberrant chromosomes or indicate possible cell-cycle specificity of test materials. Tests for chromosomal mutagenesis include *in vitro* and *in vivo* tests for chromosome aberrations, the micronucleus test, tests for dominant lethal mutations, the heritable translocation test, and mammalian germ cell cytogenetics.

In vitro chromosome aberrations

Two types of cell are routinely used for *in vitro* chromosome aberration assays, which are conducted in the absence and presence of exogenous metabolic activation, CHO cells and human lymphocytes stimulated to divide *in vitro*. Mitotic cells in the first metaphase (M_1) following chemical exposure are evaluated for the presence of chromosome and chromatid breakage and aberrations. Preliminary concentration range-finding assays are conducted with mitotic index determinations and/or assessments of cell growth (generation times) in culture to select concentrations for testing in which there will be sufficient numbers of mitotic cells for analyses.

Because some chemicals induce a delay in cellular progression to mitosis, some protocols specify use of a second, delayed, harvest time, and, if delayed harvest times are used, both the preliminary assay and the cytogenetic assay should include an analysis of whether the mitotic cells are in the first division (M_1) following exposure. This is accomplished by growing the cells in the presence of bromodeoxyuridine (BrdUrd) and then staining the chromosomes of the harvested cells using the fluorescence plus giemsa (FPG) technique, as described later for sister chromatid exchanges. When this is done, only M_1 cells will contain uniformly darkly stained chromosomes; the chromosomes of M_2 cells will have one darkly stained and one lightly stained chromatid, and M_3 cells will have a mixture of chromosomes with differentially stained and lightly stained chromatids.

The *in vitro* chromosome aberration assay in human lymphocytes is used to enhance the relevance of the effects studied to humans. To visualise chromosomes, freshly drawn blood from healthy human donors is diluted with cell culture medium containing phytohaemaglutinin (PHA), which stimulates the lymphocytes to divide *in vitro*. After a prolonged G_1 stage, the cells enter the S phase, which should be the time of addition of the test chemical to the cells. For a typical protocol, chemical exposure is initiated at 48 h, colcemid (a mitotic spindle inhibitor) is added at 70.5 h, and metaphases are harvested at 72 h. The cells are then treated with a hypotonic solution to swell the chromosomes, fixed, and dropped onto slides. The chromosomes are stained and coverslips are attached before microscopic analysis.

In vitro chromosome aberration assays in CHO cells present several advantages: Chinese hamster cells have a low chromosome number ($2n = 22$), a short generation time, and no donor-to-donor variability, as could potentially influence the results of studies with human lymphocytes. Also, because the CHO cells grow as attached monolayers, metaphase-rich populations can be obtained using mitotic shake-off procedures, which reduces the time required for microscopic analysis (although mitotic index determinations are not informative with this approach). In spite of the suggestion that the analysis of aberrations in CHO cells lacks sensitivity (Tennant *et al.*, 1987), a number of laboratories have found the assessment of aberrations in CHO cells, but not in human lymphocytes, to be overly sensitive (yielding 'false positive' results), particularly when a delayed harvest time is used. As with other assays, it is probable that such difficulties will be resolved by identifying insoluble chemicals as 'not testable', and with greater attention to procedural details, such as ensuring that the population of cells analysed is in M_1.

In vivo chromosomal aberrations

Measurements of chromosome and chromatid breakage and aberrations in the rapidly dividing population of cells in rodent bone marrow, following *in vivo* exposures, are reasonably well predictive of carcinogenesis in rodents, an outcome that may be due to the fact that the target cells are exposed to chemical metabolites under physiological conditions. Preliminary dose range-finding studies are necessary, using an evaluation of mitotic indices to select a high dose in which a sufficient number of M_1 cells will be present for analysis. Experience has shown that this dose may be lower than the LD_{50} defined in acute toxicology testing.

One testing approach utilises a single exposure (of each dose) followed by three sacrifice times to allow for variations in metabolic rates and cell-cycle delay. More recently, it has been shown that this variability is negated by repeated dosing to achieve a steady state, followed by a single sacrifice time. The latter approach conserves animals and significantly reduces the time required for microscopic analysis of the cells. For either approach, it is recommended that BrdUrd incorporation (accomplished by implanting BrdUrd in the test animals) followed by FPG staining of the cells be used to insure that the chromosomes analysed are in M_1.

Micronucleus tests

Because of the need for careful microscopic analysis of a sufficient number of cells to determine statistical significance of results, chromosomal aberration assays have historically been time and labour intensive. Furthermore, the analysis of chromosomal aberrations requires a high level of training and expertise to preclude the introduction of subjective bias. However, most regulatory agencies consider the micronucleus test to meet the requirements for an assay to assess cytogenetic damage *in vivo*, and micronucleus testing has virtually replaced the use of *in vivo* chromosome aberration tests, because the micronucleus test is more rapid, considerably less expensive, and requires minimal training.

Micronuclei result when nuclear membranes form around broken pieces of chromosomes; therefore, micronucleus tests in rodents measure chromosome breakage, the process necessary for essentially all cytogenetic aberrations. Following exposure, micronuclei may be readily observed microscopically in stained preparations of (otherwise anucleate) erythrocytes from the bone marrow of rats or mice or in the peripheral blood of mice as, in mice, the spleen does not remove micronucleated cells from the blood. Bone marrow cells are a more heterogeneous population and give a more informative index of toxicity, but peripheral blood erythrocytes are evaluated more efficiently. Furthermore, because mice are less expensive than rats, most micronucleus testing is now conducted with mice. As was described, above, for *in vivo* chromosomal aberration tests, either single dosing followed by three sacrifice times or multiple dosing to achieve a steady state of exposure, followed by one sacrifice time can be used, with the latter providing economies of time and animal usage.

The dominant lethal test in rodents

The dominant lethal test in rodents has been used for over 50 years to assess the effects of mutagenic agents. A dominant lethal mutation is one that occurs in a germ cell without causing dysfunction of the gamete, but that is lethal to the fertilised egg or developing embryo. Male rats or mice are exposed to the test material then mated to untreated virgin females, and susceptibility of the various germ cell stages can be tested by the use of sequential mating intervals. After an appropriate interval, the pregnant females are sacrificed, and the contents of the uteri are examined to determine the numbers of implants and live and dead embryos. A positive response is indicated by an increase in the number of dead implants in the treated group in relation to the number observed in the untreated group, and indicates that the test substance has affected germinal tissue of the test species. Dominant lethal effects are generally considered to be the result of structural and numerical chromosomal aberrations (i.e. genomic mutations), but gene mutations and toxic effects cannot be excluded.

Because the correlation between positive results in this assay and animal carcinogenicity is poor, the dominant lethal test is not generally recommended as a predictive test for carcinogenicity. However, it has been recommended as a second-tier test for chromosomal mutations, e.g. to indicate whether chromosomal effects observed in bone marrow cells could also be observed in germinal tissues. In contrast with the tests that will be described for genomic mutations, the dominant lethal test is relatively economical and can be performed in most toxicology laboratories.

The heritable translocation test

The mouse heritable translocation test detects structural and numerical chromosome changes, specifically reciprocal translocations (between chromosomes) and, if female progeny are included, X chromosome loss in germ cells as recovered in the F_1 generation. The heritable translocation test is an important third-tier test for assessing the potential of a test material to induce heritable chromosomal mutations. However, because of the large numbers of mice that are required and the time and expense associated with this test, its current usage is limited to research, rather than testing, laboratories.

To test for heritable translocations, sexually mature male mice are administered the test material (using either single dosing or repeated dosing over several weeks), then mated with two or three virgin females each; then the females are caged individually. When the females give birth, the date, litter size and sex of the progeny are recorded; all F_1 males are weaned, and all F_1 females are discarded unless the experimental design includes assessment of X chromosome loss. F_1 males (300–500 per initial dose level) are then raised to maturity, and each is mated to approximately three virgin females to test for fertility. The presence of heritable translocations is detected by reduced fertility (litter size) of the F_2 generation, and is confirmed by cytogenetic analysis of meiotic cells from the F_1 males. XO Females are recognised by a change in the sex ratio among their progeny from 1:1 males vs. females to 1:2, and are confirmed cytogenetically by the presence of 39 (instead of 40) chromosomes in bone marrow mitoses.

Tests for genomic mutations

In germinal tissues, eukaryotic chromosomes undergo meiosis, when the diploid ($2n$) chromosome number is reduced to a haploid (n) number, ensuring that each gamete has one copy of each pair of genes. During meiosis, homologous chromosomes (one of paternal origin and one of maternal origin) are paired then assorted independently, and a high level of chromosome recombination may occur; therefore, each gamete carries a discrete complement of genetic traits. Without these processes, genetic variability would be limited to rare mutational events that survive natural selection. Interference with normal meiosis may result in genomic mutations which are changes in the number of chromosomes, or aneuploidy, and are also referred to as 'numerical aberrations'.

Genomic mutations include: monosomy, when one of a pair of chromosomes is lost; trisomy, the addition of a chromosome; and polyploidy, when the complete set of chromosomes is increased in number. Virtually all genomic mutations arise in germ cells of the previous generation and are detrimental to the health of the individual. In humans, well known genomic mutations include several trisomies such as Down's (trisomy 21) and Kleinefelter's (XXY) syndromes. At present, there is no direct evidence that specific chemicals induce inherited defects in humans and no way to measure the induction of specific mutations in human germ cells. However, the induction of mutations by physical and chemical agents in a wide variety of species suggests that humans are also susceptible to mutations by the same or similar agents.

There is some redundancy in the classification of genomic mutation tests. For example, genomic mutation tests include the *Drosophila* sex-linked recessive test (which is also a test for gene mutations), the heritable translocation test (which is also a test for chromosomal mutations), and the specific locus test in *Neurospora* (de Serres, 1992). In the design of dosing times and interpretation of test results for heritable damage, it is necessary to be aware of the time involved in cells' traversing each stage of meiosis to the formation of gametes. However, apart from research on stage-specific effects, testing protocols usually incorporate dosing over the entire meiotic sequence.

The mouse visible specific locus test, initially developed by W. L. Russell in 1951, for studying the effects of radiation and later used to study chemical mutagens, and the more recently developed biochemical specific locus test in mice (Malling and Valcovic, 1978), are generally considered to be definitive tests for heritable germ cell mutations. The mouse visible specific locus test involves the use of developed strains that differ in selected gene loci so that mutations in these loci can be visualised as a phenotypic change due to the expression of recessive genes in the F_1 generation. The biochemical specific locus test is similar, using mice from defined inbred strains, but presumptive mutants are identified by variations in the electrophoretic mobility of proteins. For each mutagenic agent that is evaluated in each specific locus test, thousands of mice are examined to assess the induced mutation frequency. For this reason, and because the number of laboratories in which they can be performed competently is limited, the specific locus tests are infrequently used as third-tier, or final, tests. Rather, their importance stems from the information they provide on basic processes of mutagenesis in mammals.

Tests for the repair of primary DNA damage

As it is thought that the incorrect repair of damage to DNA may be an early step in mutagenesis and/or carcinogenesis two short-term tests, in particular, have been used to measure the repair of primary DNA damage: tests for sister chromatid exchanges (SCEs) and tests for unscheduled DNA synthesis (UDS).

Sister chromatid exchange

The induction of DNA lesions by genotoxicants leads to the formation of sister chromatid exchanges (SCEs), which may be related to recombinational or postreplicative repair of DNA damage at the chromosomal level. SCEs are revealed by a 'harlequin' pattern of differentially stained chromatid segments in chromosomes from cells grown in the presence of BrdUrd for two rounds of DNA replication, then stained with the fluorescence-plus-Giemsa (FPG) technique so that one chromatid is more lightly stained than the other. Because SCEs can be enumerated more rapidly than chromosomal aberrations, SCE assays are more efficient and economical than aberration assays. SCEs can also be measured *in vitro*, e.g. in CHO cells or human lymphocytes, or *in vivo*, primarily in mice. For the latter, BrdUrd is implanted in mice which are then exposed to the test material.

SCE assays have been used as supplementary tests rather than as alternative assays for measuring cytogenetic damage. However, the apparently high sensitivity of SCE assays, uncertainty about the significance of SCE induction, and a lack of a close correlation with results from chromosome aberration tests, has led to a virtual discontinuation of SCE testing for regulatory submissions. Today, UDS is used for submissions to those agencies still requiring assessments of primary DNA damage and its repair.

Unscheduled DNA synthesis

Unscheduled DNA synthesis (UDS) is the incorporation of DNA precursors at times other than the scheduled, S-phase, synthesis of DNA in the cell cycle. It indicates that an active form of a chemical has damaged cellular DNA and that the cell was capable of (correctly or incorrectly) repairing the damage. UDS is evaluated *in vitro* by exposing cells to the test chemical in the presence of tritiated thymidine ([³H]TdR). Then, autoradiographic techniques are used to reveal the extent of incorporation of [³H]TdR in the nuclei of non-S-phase cells that have undergone UDS, i.e. the [³H]TdR-exposed silver grains in an autoradiographic emulsion over the cell nuclei are counted, a process that may be semi-automated. When tested with and without addition of a metabolic activation system, UDS may be examined *in vitro* in any cells blocked from entering the S phase, or *in vivo* in various tissues. Rat hepatocytes are routinely used because they are metabolically competent and normally exhibit little scheduled DNA synthesis; therefore, no S-phase inhibition or exogenous metabolic activation is required.

As UDS testing is an indirect measure of mutagenesis, regulatory agencies are discontinuing requirements for UDS testing in initial batteries of tests. Instead, UDS tests are often used in a second tier to evaluate whether the test material has interacted with DNA.

Mammalian cell transformation

Morphological transformation is sometimes used as a test for *in vitro* carcinogenesis, rather than mutagenesis, and is the process whereby mammalian cells with a limited number of generations in culture, and/or cells that proliferate with an oriented pattern on a plastic surface, are converted into cells with unlimited capacities to divide and random patterns of growth. The relevance of tests for transformation stems from their measurement of other than strictly mutagenic events leading to carcinogenesis. Hence, they extend the range of short-term test batteries.

Examples of mammalian cell transformation protocols include tests in BALB/c-3T3 cells and C3H-10T1/2 cells. The BALB/c-3T3 cell line has been studied extensively for postconfluent inhibition of cell division, when the cultures have a cobblestone-like morphology. This inhibition is reversed by various treatments including exposure to carcinogens, with and without metabolic activation, to yield transformed foci of cells. The C3H mouse prostate cell line C3H-10T1/2 is acutely sensitive to postconfluent inhibition of cell division and has been transformed with a variety of carcinogens to produce foci of cells that yield malignant fibrosarcomas when administered to irradiated recipient mice. The C3H-10T1/2 cell line has a lower rate of spontaneous transformation than BALB/c-3T3 cells, but the C3H-10T1/2 cell line is customarily used for testing only in the absence of metabolic activation. Mammalian cell transformation assays are currently used more extensively for screening antineoplastic agents for efficacy rather than as genetic toxicology tests.

The future of genetic toxicology

In the preceding text the origins and development of genetic toxicology and many of its current practices were described. During the past two decades, the use of genetic toxicology tests for product registration has gained acceptance and has matured with the more precise definition and more extensive evaluation of many of the tests. International consensus is being sought on those tests and protocols that are most predictive and useful. Thus, it is anticipated that the emphasis of applied genetic toxicology in the immediate future may be on the more extensive use of specific tests to reduce the backlog of chemicals that are as yet untested. The emphasis of investigative genetic toxicology is to draw upon developments in related disciplines to understand the basis of tests for assessing the potential risk of exposing humans to various agents. The use of molecular biology techniques has led to the definition of many human genetic diseases. Thus, the development of polymerase chain reaction (PCR) in combination with molecular techniques to identify changes in DNA, and the use of fluorescence *in situ* hybridisation (FISH), pulsed-field gel electrophoresis, restriction enzyme mapping and associated techniques for probing the larger genetic changes should also lead to the definition of new and improved approaches for probing genotoxic mechanisms. These, in turn, should bring the field closer to the goal of accurately assessing effects directly related to those observed or with the potential to occur in humans.

References

Albertini, R. J. and Robinson, S. H., 1991, Human population monitoring, in Li, A. P. and Heflich, R. H. (Eds) *Genetic Toxicology*, pp. 375–420. Boca Raton, FL: CRC Press.

Ames, B. N., 1979, Identifying environmental chemicals causing mutations and cancer. Science, **204**, 587–93.

Bridges, B., 1976, Evaluation of mutagenicity and carcinogenicity using a three-tier system, *Mutat. Res.*, **204**, 17–115.

Brusick, D., 1980, *Principles of Genetic Toxicology*. New York: Plenum Press.

Casarett, L. J. and Bruce, M. C., 1980, Origin and scope of toxicology, in Doull, J., Klaassen, C. D. and Amdur, M. O. (Eds) *Casarett and Doull's Toxicology. The Basic Science of Poisons*, pp. 3–10. New York: Macmillan.

Clive, D. and Moore-Brown, M. M., 1979, The L5178Y/TK$^{+/-}$ mutagen assay system: Mutant analysis, in Hsie, A. W., O'Neill, J. P. and McElheny V. K. (Eds) 'Banbury Report 2; Mammalian Cell Mutagenesis: The Maturation of Test Systems'. New York: Cold Spring Harbor Laboratory, pp. 421–9.

de Serres, F. J., 1992, Development of a specific-locus assay in the *ad*-3 region of two-compartment heterokaryons of *Neurospora*: a review, *Environ. Mol. Mutagen.*, **20**, 225–45.

Hollaender, A. and de Serres, F. J., 1971–1983, *Chemical Mutagens. Principles and Methods for their Detection*, Vols 1–8. New York: Plenum Press.

Hsu, T. C., 1979, Foreword. Mammalian Chromosomes Newsletter, **30**, 59–70.

Levin, D. E., Hollstein, M., Christman, M. F., Schwiers, E. A. and Ames, B. N., 1982a, A new *Salmonella* tester strain (TA102) with A.T base pairs at the site of mutation detects oxidative mutagens, *Proc. Natl. Acad. Sci. USA*, **79**, 7445–9.

Levin, D. E., Yamasaki, E. and Ames, B. N., 1982b, A new *Salmonella* tester strain, TA97, for the detection of frameshift mutagens. A run of cytosines as a mutational hot-spot, *Mutat. Res.*, **94**, 315–30.

Levin, D. E., Hollstein, M., Christman, M. F. and Ames, B. N., 1984, Detection of oxidative mutagens with a new *Salmonella* tester strain (TA102), *Methods Enzymol.*, **105**, 249–54.

Li, A. P. and Heflich, R. H., 1991, *Genetic Toxicology*. Boca Raton, FL: CRC Press.

Malling, H. V., 1971, Dimethylnitrosamine: formation of mutagenic compounds by interaction with mouse liver microsomes, *Mutat. Res.*, **13**, 425–9.

Malling, H. V. and Chu, E. H. Y., 1974, Development of mutational model systems for the study of carcinogenesis, in Ts'o, P. O. and DiPaolo, J. A. (Eds) 'Chemical Carcinogenesis,' Part B. pp. 545–63. New York: Marcel Dekker, Inc.

Malling, H. V. and Valcovic, L. R., 1978, New approaches to gene detection in mammals, in Flamm, G. and Mehlman, M. (Eds) *Advances in Modern Toxicology*, Vol. 4, pp. 149–71. New York: Hemisphere Press.

Maron, D. M. and Ames, B. N., 1983, Revised methods for the *Salmonella* mutagenicity test, *Mutat. Res.*, **113**, 173–215.

McCann, J., Choi, E., Yamasaki, E. and Ames, B. N., 1975a, Detection of carcinogens as mutagens in the *Salmonella*/microsome test: assay of 300 chemicals, *Proc. Natl. Acad. Sci. USA*, **72**, 5135–9.

McCann, J., Spingarn, N. E., Kobori, J. and Ames, B. N., 1975b, Detection of carcinogens as mutagens: bacterial tester strains with R factor plasmids, *Proc. Natl. Acad. Sci. USA*, **72**, 979–83.

Muller, H. J., 1927, Artificial transmutation of the gene, *Science*, **64**, 84–7.

Prival, M. J. and Dellarco, V. L., 1989, Evolution of social concerns and environmental policies for chemical mutagens, *Environ. Mol. Mutagen.*, **14**(S16), 46–50.

Prival, M. J., King, V. D. and Sheldon Jr, A. T., 1979, The mutagenicity of dialkyl nitrosamines in the *Salmonella* plate assay, *Environ. Mutagen.*, **1**, 95–104.

Sugimura, T., Sato, S., Nagao, M., Yahagi, T., Matsushima T., Seino, Y., Takeuchi, M. and Kawachi, T., 1976, Overlapping of carcinogens and mutagens, in Magee, P. N., Takayama, S., Sugimura, T. and Matsushima, T. (Eds) *Fundamentals in Cancer Prevention*, pp. 191–215. Baltimore, MD: University Park Press.

Tennant, R. W., Margolin, B. H., Shelby, M. D., Zeiger, E., Haseman, J. K., Spalding, J., Caspary, W., Resnick, M., Stasiewicz, S., Anderson, B. and Minor, R., 1987, Prediction of chemical carcinogenicity in rodents from *in vitro* genetic toxicity assays, *Science*, **236**, 933–41.

Tindall, K. R., Stankowski Jr, L. F., Machanoff, R. and Hsie, A. W., 1986, Analyses of mutation in pSV2gpt-transformed CHO cells, *Mutat. Res.*, **160**, 121–31.

Wassom, J. S., 1989, Origins of genetic toxicology and the Environmental Mutagen Society, *Environ. Mol. Mutagen.*, **14**(S16), 1–6.

Chapter 8

Carcinogenesis and its Prevention

H. Vainio

Introduction

The history of environmental carcinogenesis bears the strong imprint of the clinical observations that led to successful identification of aetiological factors. The story begins with the classic description of cancers of the scrotum among chimney sweeps in 1775 (Pott, 1775), then moves to the account in the late nineteenth century of bladder cancer among workers exposed to aromatic amines (Rehn, 1895) and the experimental production in rats of skin cancer after exposure to coal tar in 1915 (Yamagiwa and Ichikawa, 1915), culminating with the identification of polycyclic aromatic hydrocarbons such as benzo[a]pyrene in coal tar in 1933 (Cook *et al.*, 1933). Thus, over a 160-year period, one class of chemicals in which carcinogens occur (polynuclear aromatic hydrocarbons) was discovered, and a specific carcinogenic agent (benzo[a]pyrene) was isolated. The relative roles of epidemiology and of experiments in gathering the information relevant to the identification and prevention of the environmental causes of cancer has since been the object of much debate.

Many of the early epidemiological successes were based on observations made either in the occupational setting or in other situations of high-level exposure (e.g. to drugs and cigarette smoking). In contrast, much of today's cancer epidemiology deals with general environmental exposures (e.g. to pollutants in ambient air and in drinking water) and with personal behaviour pattern (e.g. dietary habits, use of contraception, sexual behaviour, reproduction). Such exposure situations are more difficult to study epidemiologically than some of the earlier ones.

Toxicological approaches in non-human test systems can be used to avoid many of the problems of epidemiological studies. The capacity of animal model systems to serve as the only means for evaluating potential hazards is limited, however; therefore, the two approaches have complementary roles in the identification and prevention of environmental cancer risks.

In this chapter, aspects of environmental carcinogenesis are discussed and methods of identifying carcinogens as well as means of prevention are given.

149

Cancer as a public health burden

About 20% of the people in the developed part of the world will contract cancer. There will be around 6.35 million new cases each year, divided almost equally between the developed and developing parts of the world (Parkin *et al.*, 1988), although two-thirds of the world's population lives in the latter. The six ranking sites that account for nearly 60% of the world cancer burden are listed in Table 8.1. Taking 3 years as a gross mean for the survival time of unselected cancer patients, 6 million new cases per year implies about 20 million cancer patients (excluding non-melanotic skin cancers).

Table 8.1. The most frequent cancers world-wide (Parkin *et al.*, 1988)

Men			Women		
Site	No. of cases (×1000)	% of total	Site	No. of cases (×1000)	% of total
Lung	514	16	Breast	572	18
Stomach	409	13	Cervix	466	15
Colon/rectum	286	9	Colon/rectum	286	9
Mouth/pharynx	257	8	Stomach	261	8
Prostate	236	7	Corpus	149	5
Oesophagus	202	6	Lung	147	5

Lung cancer is by far the most common malignancy in males, as breast cancer is in females; however, when the two sexes are combined, stomach is the first ranking site, although the frequency of this cancer is declining.

Diet and lifestyle are considered to be the most prevalent causes of cancer, although it is clear that this conclusion is somewhat presumptive. Cancers at two of the leading sites in males (lung and mouth/pharynx) are due largely to the effects of tobacco, whether chewed or smoked, and abuse of alcohol. Cancer of the large bowel has been linked to diet, as has that of prostate. Breast and cervix cancer, though confined to the female sex, are third and fifth in the rank order for both sexes combined. Female breast cancer, the incidence of which seems to have stabilised in several Western populations but is increasing rapidly in populations that have hitherto been at low risk (such as in Japan), is also believed to have a dietary component. Lung cancer, sixth in rank among women, is likely to become much more common because of the current smoking habits of women. By the year 2000, lung cancer will probably be the first ranking cancer in the two sexes combined. Further discussion of the cancer burden and of target sites is given by Tomatis (1990).

The process of carcinogenesis

Carcinogenesis is a complex process involving sequential genetic events which result in altered functions of the genes that control normal cellular growth, with subsequent clonal growth of the resulting 'preneoplastic' or neoplastic cells (Farber, 1984; Boyd & Barrett, 1990). Chemical carcinogens may act by inducing mutations and/or by altering gene and cellular growth control. Figure 8.1 is a simplified schematic illustration of the development of cancer.

The incidence of many human cancers rises sharply with age. For cancers of the stomach and lung, for instance, the age-specific incidence rates increase exponentially with age, with exponents of 4–7 for ages between 30 and 65 years. This time–incidence curve reflects a multistep process for carcinogenesis that requires 4–7 independent 'events' (Armitage, 1985). Because of the heritable nature of cancer, these 'events' are probably genetic changes. Tumour development in the human colon, for instance, appears to require more than one type of genetic change; these include hypomethylation, gene mutation, recombination, and chromosomal aberrations (Fearon *et al.*, 1987; Vogelstein *et al.*, 1988). Some of these changes represent DNA damage, while others are constitutive processes that regulate gene expression.

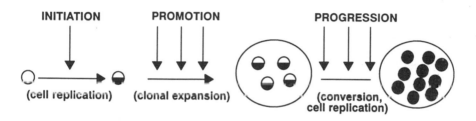

Figure 8.1. Schematic illustration of the development of cancer, depicting the stages of initiation, promotion and progression. Initiation results from the action of a chemical, physical or biological agent to alter irreversibly the information in the genetic material. Initiated cells have the potential to develop into a clone of preneoplastic cells. Promotion is characterised by alteration of genetic expression and the (reversible) clonal growth of the initiated cell population. Progression, which is the final stage of cancer development, is characterised by demonstrable changes in the number and/or arrangement of chromosomes associated with increased growth rate, invasiveness and metastasis.

Thus, the accumulated experience in the field of carcinogenesis clearly supports the concept that cancer development is a multistep process and that multiple genetic changes are required before a normal cell becomes fully neoplastic. Likewise, studies of human tumours suggest that the multistep paradigm, together with similar genetic events, is involved in the development of cancer in humans, and that the carcinogenic process is indistinguishable among mammals, from laboratory rodents to humans. This finding plus the knowledge that all chemicals known to induce cancer in humans that have been studied under adequate experimental protocols also cause cancer in laboratory animals have led most prudent investigators to the speculation that the obverse would hold true: chemicals shown unequivocally to induce cancer in laboratory animals are capable of causing cancer in humans.

As more advances are made in molecular carcinogenesis, knowledge about the mechanism of cancer induction in mammals will shed more light on the usefulness of animals as predictive surrogates for humans. The genes that control cellular growth and differentiation are likely to play a fundamental role in basic cellular function in view of the degree to which they have been conserved throughout eukaryotic evolution; for instance, the protein sequence of the H-*ras* gene, is similar in humans and rats (Barbacid, 1987).

Proto-oncogenes are cellular genes that are expressed during normal growth and development (Weinberg, 1985). The proteins coded by proto-oncogenes are involved in mitogenic regulation, including growth factors, protein kinases and signal transducers, all of which, when behaving aberrantly, may lead to uncontrolled cell proliferation. Proto-oncogenes can be activated to cancer-causing oncogenes by point mutations or by gross DNA rearrangements (chromosomal translocation or gene amplification) (Anderson and Reynolds, 1988; Bos, 1989). These lesions are especially revealing for chemicals that are apparently non-mutagenic in standard genotoxicity tests and yet cause point mutations in exposed animals (Reynolds *et al.*, 1987). Loss of specific regulatory functions (e.g. tumour suppressor genes) represents an important feature in neoplastic transformation (Weinberg, 1989). Inactivation of tumour suppressor genes, like activation of proto-oncogenes, can occur via mutations but can also result from loss of the gene or portions of the chromosome containing it. The absence of specific chromosomes in tumours frequently indicates that loss of tumour suppressor gene(s) function is associated with the aetiology of the tumour (Knudson, 1985). Hereditary inactivation of a tumour suppressor gene is the strongest risk factor for human cancer known to date—an indication of the importance of this class of genes in human carcinogenesis (Friend *et al.*, 1986; Harbour *et al.*, 1988).

In certain malignancies, such as retinoblastoma, loss of function of only a single suppressor gene is implicated. In other cancers, however, studies of restriction fragment length polymorphism studies have indicated that loss of multiple tumour suppressor genes may be necessary for progression of the full malignant condition. Examples of such malignancies include small cell lung cancer (Yokota *et al.*, 1987) and colorectal cancer (Vogelstein *et al.*, 1988).

Types of cancer risk factor

The categories of known risk factors for cancers are listed in Table 8.2; these may act individually or in combination. Individuals have some control over their behaviour, including tobacco use, diet, alcohol use, exposure to sunlight, sexual behaviour patterns and general personal hygiene. Environmental factors include occupational exposures to carcinogens, exposures during medical procedures, as well as factors that occur naturally or are man-made and contaminate water, air and soil. These factors are beyond the individual's control, and their effective control thus requires broad social action. Genetic factors are inherited at conception and their control is presently not feasible.

Table 8.2. Risk factors for cancer

Category	Example
Endogenous	
Genetic predisposition	Xeroderma pigmentosum
Hormones	Oestrogens
Exogenous	
Chemicals	Benzene
Industrial processes	Rubber industry
Hormones	Oestrogen replacement therapy
Ionising radiation	Therapeutic X-ray
Non-ionising radiation	Ultraviolet light
Viruses	Hepatitis B virus
Cultural habits	Tobacco smoking
Iatrogenic exposures	Cyclophosphamide
Diet	Excessive caloric intake
Socio-economic conditions	Less-favoured occupational class

Obstacles to the identification of specific causative factors for human cancers include:

- The long latent period between onset of exposure to causative agents and overt appearance of the disease.

- The multistage nature of carcinogenesis.

- The likelihood that most human cancers result from a complex interaction between multiple environmental and endogenous (genetic, host) factors.

Although significant progress has been made, several important questions have still not been completely resolved. These include the extent to which human cancers are due to specific causes, such as chemicals, hormones and physical and viral agents, the role of nutritional factors and the interactions of endogenous and environmental factors.

Identification of cancer risk factors

The identification of carcinogens via laboratory experiments relies on two main types of test: long-term carcinogenicity tests in rodents (mice, rats, hamsters); and short-term tests assessing the effect of an agent on a variety of genetic and related effects. These tests are valuable to the extent that such effects may reflect underlying events in the carcinogenic process. Indeed, consistent positivity in tests measuring mutations (point mutations or chromosomal mutations) is usually regarded as indicating potential for carcinogenicity of the tested agent. Results from laboratory experiments constitute useful supporting evidence when adequate epidemiological data for the carcinogenicity of an agent exist (for example, vinyl chloride) but become all the more essential when the epidemiological evidence is non-existent

Table 8.3. Established human carcinogens and their target organs

Carcinogen	Target organ (suspected target organ in humans)
Agents and groups of agents	
Aflatoxins	Liver (lung)
4-Aminobiphenyl	Bladder
Arsenic and arsenic compounds*	Lung, skin
Asbestos	Lung, pleura, peritoneum (gastrointestinal tract, larynx)
Azathioprine	Lymphatic system, mesenchyma, hepatobiliary system, skin
Benzene	Haematopoietic system
Benzidine	Bladder
N, N-bis (2-Chloroethyl)-2-naphthylamine (chlornaphazine)	Bladder
bis(Chloromethyl)ether and chloromethylmethyl ether (technical grade)	Lung
1,4-Butanediol dimethanesulfonate (Myleran)	Haematopoietic system
Chlorambucil	Haematopoietic system
1-(2-Chloroethyl)-3-(4-methylcyclohexyl)-1-nitrosourea (methyl-CCNU)	Haematopoietic system
Chromium (VI) compounds	Lung (nasal cavity)
Ciclosporin	Lymphatic system
Cyclophosphamide	Bladder, haematopoietic system
Diethylstilboestrol	Cervix/vagina, breast, testis (uterus)
Erionite	Pleura, peritoneum
Melphalan	Haematopoietic system
8-Methoxypsoralen (methoxsalen) plus UV radiation	Skin
MOPP and other combined chemotherapy including alkylating agents	Haematopoietic system
Mustard gas (sulphur mustard)	Pharynx, larynx, lung
2-Naphthylamine	Bladder (liver)
Nickel compounds	Nasal cavity, lung
Oestrogen replacement therapy	Uterus, breast
Oestrogens, non-steroidal*	Cervix/vagina, breast, testis (uterus)
Oestrogens, steroidal*	Uterus, breast
Oral contraceptives, combined†	Liver
Oral contraceptives, sequential	Uterus
Radon and its decay products	Lung
Talc containing asbestiform fibres	Lung
Thiotepa	Haematopoietic system
Treosulphan	Haematopoietic system

Table 8.3 (*Contd.*)

Carcinogen	Target organ (suspected target organ in humans)
Vinyl chloride	Liver, blood vessels (brain, lung, lymphatic system)
Alcoholic beverages	Pharynx oesophagus, liver, larynx, oral cavity (breast)
Analgesic mixtures containing phenacetin	Bladder, kidney
Betel quid with tobacco	Oral cavity, pharynx, larynx, oesophagus
Coal-tar pitches	Skin, lung, bladder (larynx, oral cavity)
Coal tars	Skin, lung (bladder)
Mineral oils, untreated and mildly treated	Skin (lung, bladder, gastrointestinal tract)
Shale-oils	Skin (gastrointestinal tract)
Soots	Skin, lung
Tobacco products, smokeless	Oral cavity, pharynx, oesophagus
Tobacco smoke	Lung, bladder, oral cavity, pharnyx, larynx, oesophagus, pancreas, kidney
Exposure circumstances	
Aluminium production	Lung, bladder (lymphatic system)
Auramine, manufacture of	Bladder (prostate)
Boot and shoe manufacture and repair	Nasal cavity, haematopoietic system (pharynx, lung, liver, gastrointestinal tract, bladder)
Coal gasification	Skin, lung, bladder
Coke production	Skin, lung, kidney
Furniture and cabinet making	Nasal cavity
Iron and steel founding	Lung (gastrointestinal tract, genitourinary system, haematopoietic system)
Isopropyl alcohol manufacture (strong-acid process)	Nasal cavity (larynx)
Magenta, manufacture of	Bladder
Painter (occupational exposure)	Lung
Rubber industry	Bladder, haematopoietic system (lung, gastrointestinal tract, skin, lymphatic system)
Underground haematite mining with exposure to radon	Lung

* This evaluation applies to the group of chemicals as a whole and not necessarily to all individual chemicals within the group.
† There is also conclusive evidence that these agents have a protective effect against cancers of the ovary and endometrium.

or inadequate in quality and/or quantity. In the latter case, although no universally accepted criteria exist to automatically translate data from long-term animal tests or short-term tests in terms of cancer risk in humans, an evaluation of the risk can be made on a judgmental basis using all available scientific evidence.

This policy has been applied by the International Agency for Research on Cancer (IARC) in a systematic programme of 'Evaluation of Carcinogenic Risks to Humans'. The IARC evaluation process is essentially qualitative, aimed at assessing the strength of evidence that an agent is or is not carcinogenic to humans (risk identification) and it does not extend to the subsequent stage of risk quantification or to risk management.

Recognised human carcinogens

For a number of chemical, physical, and biological environmental agents there is direct evidence from epidemiological studies, usually supported by experimental evidence, that they cause malignant neoplasms in humans (Doll and Peto, 1981). More than 50 agents have been shown to be causally related to human cancer (Table 8.3). The majority are chemicals to which humans have been exposed only relatively recently (Tomatis *et al.*, 1989). Most are either chemicals to which people are exposed occupationally, pharmaceutical products, or naturally occurring compounds, to which specific groups of people have been exposed, at high concentrations, for long enough so that the increased risk could be detected by the methods of epidemiology. Table 8.3 also gives the organ in which cancers have been observed; those more frequently involved are lung, urinary bladder, haematopoietic tissue and skin (see also Table 8.4).

Table 8.4. Most frequent target organs for recognised human carcinogens

Target organ	Carcinogens
Lung	Asbestos, arsenic and arsenic compounds, bis(chloromethyl)ether, chloromethylmethyl ether, chromium(VI) compounds, mustard gas, nickel compounds, talc containing asbestiform fibres
Bladder	4-Aminobiphenyl, benzidine, chlornaphazine, cyclophosphamide, tobacco smoke
Haematopoietic system	Benzene, chlorambucil, methyl-CCNU, *a* cyclophosphamide, melphalan, myleran, ionising radiation
Skin	Arsenic and arsenic compounds, coal tars, coal-tar pitches, mineral oils, soots, UV radiation, ionising radiation
Liver	Alcoholic beverages, aflatoxins, hepatitis B virus, vinyl chloride

CCNU, *a* Methyl-CCNU, 1-(2-Chloroethyl)-3(4-Methylcyclohexyl)-1-nitrosourea.

Among physical agents, ultraviolet (UV) radiation (as part of the solar spectrum) and particulate ionising radiations are clearly carcinogenic in humans.

Two parasites have been shown to be associated, probably causally, with human cancer (see Tomatis, 1990). In some areas of South-East Asia and China, infestation of bile ducts with *Chlornochis sinensis* or *Opistorchis viverrini*, two liver flukes, is followed by the development of cholangio carcinomas. In some parts of Africa, bladder cancer is one of the most common cancers and there is evidence that bilharziasis due to infestation with *Schistosoma haematobium* plays on aetiological role.

The best evidence supporting a causal evidence between a virus and a cancer, is the one linking the hepatitis B virus (HBV) to primary hepatocellular carcinoma (see Tomatis, 1990).

Diet may conceivably influence the development of cancer in a variety of ways. One mechanism is through ingestion of carcinogens formed by fungal or bacterial action during the storage of food (for example, aflatoxin B_1 produced by *Aspergillus flavus*) or through pyrolysis or pyrosynthesis during cooking of meat and fish. A second type of mechanism is by providing substrates for the formation of carcinogens in the body (for example, nitrites and nitrates) or by altering the concentration or duration of contact of carcinogens with cells in the large bowel, as may be derived through varying the quantity of fibres in the diet. Finally, being overweight, which implies overnutrition, whatever the mechanism, is associated with cancer at certain sites (such as endometrium) (National Research Council, 1982).

The knowledge derived from epidemiological and laboratory studies is unbalanced, in that we know most about the specific causal factors of cancers of the lung, urinary bladder, skin, upper aerodigestive tract and liver, and of leukaemia. We are less certain about the causes of cancers of the breast, cervix, endometrium, ovary, pancreas, stomach, colon and rectum; and we know very little about the causes of cancers of the brain and prostate and of lymphomas and sarcomas.

Potential for cancer prevention

Control of risk factors

Primary prevention of cancer implies avoidance of its occurrence, either by reducing the exposure of individuals to causative agents in the environment or by enhancing resistance to them. Prevention is clearly feasible in relation to tobacco smoking, chemicals, industrial processes, medical drugs and viruses and, to a certain extent, radiation. Another measure would be to improve socio-economic conditions. The variety of cancer risk factors of which we are aware (see Table 8.2) clearly implies that there cannot be a single approach to cancer control and prevention. An effective preventive action must therefore be focused on those factors that cause the greatest numbers of deaths and that are most easily controlled, e.g. diet, alcohol drinking, tobacco use and exposure to carcinogens in the workplace.

Diet

A high proportion of human cancers could be related directly or indirectly to dietary factors, at least if we consider cancer sites for which such a relationship is conceivable. Primary prevention of cancer through dietary intervention therefore exerts an obvious attraction, and several intervention studies are currently under-way in different parts of the world. The possibilities are rendered even more attractive by the fact that not only might we avoid exposure to carcinogens present as such in the diet or formed endogenously from what we eat, but also that certain dietary factors may protect against cancers caused by exposures to other, non-dietary factors (Vainio and Hemminki, 1989). It would be reasonable to recommend an increased intake of fresh fruit and vegetables, a reduction of animal fat, and the need to control one's weight. These recommendations will result in no harm, and the effects on cancer (and cardiovascular) risk would probably be beneficial.

Alcohol drinking

The abundant epidemiological evidence that consumption of alcoholic beverages increases the risks for certain cancers was reviewed recently by the IARC (1988). There is strong evidence that drinking alcoholic beverages increases the risks for developing cancers of the oral cavity, pharynx, larynx, oesophagus and liver. The risks are multiplied in people who also smoke. Pure ethanol has not been shown to be carcinogenic in laboratory animals, but there is no indication in humans that the carcinogenic effect is dependent on the type of beverage consumed. Thus, although the drinking of alcoholic beverages causes certain cancers, we do not know which of their constituents are responsible. The only means of prevention of those cancers, therefore, is avoidance of excessive drinking.

Tobacco use

Tobacco smoking is the major cause of cancers of the lung, larynx and bladder and an important cause of cancers of the pancreas and kidney. It is the main identified cause of cancer in industrialised countries. Risk increases with the amount smoked and with the duration of smoking.

Ambient tobacco smoke must be assumed to cause some lung cancers in non-smokers, since they are exposed in this way to the same chemicals as smokers. Tobacco smoke contains at least 40 chemicals that are carcinogenic to animals (IARC, 1985b).

Many tobacco products increase the risk for cancer: cigarettes, cigars, cigarillos, *bidis*, other tobacco products smoked in Asia, pipe tobacco and smokeless tobacco, which is chewed or snuffed. In many parts of the world, particularly in the Indian subcontinent, tobacco is chewed in a quid with areca nut and betel leaf. This habit causes cancers of the oral cavity and upper gastrointestinal tract (IARC, 1985a).

Smoking tobacco will be a factor in approximately 3 million deaths per year during the 1990s (Peto and Lopez, 1990). World-wide mortality from tobacco is still rising rapidly, particularly in less developed countries, partly because of the population growth but chiefly because of previous large increases in cigarette smoking by young adults which cause large increases in mortality rates by the time the young adults reach middle age. On the basis of current smoking habits, the date when world-wide annual mortality from tobacco will exceed 10 million has been estimated to be about 2020.

Strategies for prevention include persuading adult smokers to quit, which would have an immediate impact on incidence and mortality, and discouraging teenagers from taking up the habit. Low-tar and filter cigarettes are known to result in lower, but still substantial, risks and a switch to such brands could also markedly reduce disease.

Occupation

The main result of epidemiological studies of cancer in occupational settings has been to indicate methods for prevention, often long before the specific aetiological agents were identified and their exact relationship to human cancers elucidated. This practice is fundamental in the prevention of exposure to known or potential occupational carcinogens. Examples of carcinogens encountered in the workplace are listed in Table 8.5.

Table 8.5. Common occupational carcinogens

Agent	Organ(s) affected	Occupation
Asbestos	Lung, pleura	Insulation workers, shipyard workers, construction workers, miners
Auramine, benzidine, 2-naphthylamine, magenta, 4-aminobiphenyl	Urinary bladder	Dyestuffs manufacturers and users, rubber workers, textile dyers, paint manufacturers
Benzene	Bone marrow	Dye users, painters, shoemakers
Chromium	Nasal cavity, lung, larynx	Chromium producers, processors, welders
Coal tar, pitch, other products of coal combustion	Lung, larynx, skin, urinary bladder	Coal tar and pitch workers, coke-oven workers, gashouse workers
Nickel	Nasal sinuses, lung	Nickel smelters, mixers, roasters, electrolysis workers
Vinyl chloride	Liver	Plastics workers

Data on exposures and their association with specific cancers provide a starting point for identifying more specific problems. Firstly, although occupational carcinogens induce a wide variety of cancers, certain organs, tissues and cells have been found to be the primary targets of these agents: lung, urinary bladder, skin, lymphatic system and haematopoietic system. Secondly, there are some occupational exposures for which specific agents have been identified, but many others for which only the occupation or industrial process itself has been shown to be associated with increased cancer risk.

Furthermore, very few of the potential occupational carcinogens have been evaluated by epidemiological research. Since so few of the agents shown by the experimental methods to be potentially carcinogenic have been the subject of epidemiological investigation, it is essential that such studies continue the evaluation and explication of human risk within well-defined occupations and, where possible, in association with specific agents. An impetus for conducting studies of occupational cancer should be the immediacy of the opportunities for prevention that often arise from the findings.

Current scientific knowledge indicates two primary approaches to the prevention of cancer: avoidance of carcinogens or reduction of exposure to them. In the first instance, substances that are known or suspected human carcinogens could be removed from commercial use and replaced with materials that serve the same function. However, there is often no adequate substitute and a substitute chemical or material may not have been tested for carcinogenicity. The multiplicative interaction between cigarette smoking and many occupational carcinogens is well documented. Therefore an immediate priority is to develop strategies for smoking prevention and cessation among workers in high-risk occupations. The second approach, reduction of exposure, can be widely applied, since extensive technological advances have resulted in the development of both engineering controls that can be installed at the work-site and protective clothing and equipment that reduce or eliminate worker exposure to hazardous substances. The only limiting factors to this approach are the cost of implementing such interventions and the specificity of available data regarding those substances to which exposure should be limited.

Sunlight

Ultraviolet radiation, especially UVB, in the 320–290 nm region, appears to be related to skin cancer occurrence. The epidemiological evidence indicates that UVB is the aetiological agent of the majority of basal cell epithelioma of face and neck, of squamous cell carcinomas of the exposed surfaces, and of the cancers (Lee, 1982; Scotto *et al.*, 1982). For malignant melanoma, sunburn in childhood appears to be important, as studies of migrants from Europe to Australia have shown (Muir and Sasco, 1990).

Protection against excessive exposure to sun should reduce the burden of skin cancers substantially.

Summary

The risk for cancer in humans is increased by a variety of factors, ranging from exposure to an identified agent to a culturally determined behaviour, such as smoking, or to socio-economic conditions. Intervention is possible with regard to some of these factors, while others affect us in as yet undetermined ways. Carcinogenesis is a multievent process nearly always involving more than one aetiological agent, so complementing reduction of exposures to carcinogens in the occupational and general environment with reductions in exposures that are under the control of the individual will maximise the potential for cancer prevention. Furthermore, exciting developments in epidemiological and experimental research provide leads about factors that may reduce cancer risk. As we learn more about diet and energy intake, for instance, the potential arises for more general approaches to cancer prevention.

References

Anderson, M. W. and Reynolds, S. H., 1988, Activation of oncogenes by chemical carcinogens, in Sirica, A. E. (Ed.) *Pathology of Neoplasia*, pp. 291–301. New York: Plenum Press.

Armitage, P., 1985, Multistage models of carcinogenesis, *Environ. Health Perspect.*, **63**, 195–201.

Barbacid, M., 1987, *ras* Genes, *Ann. Rev. Biochem.*, **56**, 779–827.

Bos, J. L., 1989, *ras* Oncogenes in human cancer: a review, *Cancer Res.*, **49**, 4682–9.

Boyd, J. A. and Barrett, J. C., 1990, Genetic and cellular basis of multistep carcinogenesis, *Pharmacol. Ther.*, **46**, 469–86.

Cook, J. W., Hewett, C. L. and Higger, I., 1933, The isolation of a cancer producing hydrocarbon from coal tar, *J. Chem. Soc.*, **1**, 395–405.

Doll, R. and Peto, R., 1981, The causes of cancer, *J. Natl. Cancer Inst.*, **66**, 1197–308.

Farber, E., 1984, The multistep nature of cancer development, *Cancer Res.*, **44**, 4217–23.

Fearon, E. R., Hamilton, S. R. and Vogelstein, B., 1987, Clonal analysis of human colorectal tumors, *Science*, **238**, 193–7.

Friend, S. H., Bernards, R., Rogdej, S., Weinberg, R. A., Rapaport, J. M., Albert, D. M. and Dryja, T. P., 1986, A human DNA segment with properties of the gene that predisposes to retinoblastoma and osteosarcoma, *Nature*, **323**, 643–6.

Harbour, J. W., Lai, S.-L., Whang-Peng, J., Gazdar, A. F., Minna, J. and Kay, F. J., 1988, Abnormalities in structure and expression of the human retinoblastoma gene in SCLC, *Science*, **241**, 353–7.

IARC, 1985a, *IARC Monographs on the Evaluation of the Carcinogenic Risks of Chemicals to Humans, Vol. 37, Tobacco Habits Other than Smoking; Betel-quid and Areca-nut Chewing; and Some Related Nitrosamines.* Lyon: IARC.

IARC, 1985b, *IARC Monographs on the Evaluation of the Carcinogenic Risks of Chemicals to Humans, Vol. 38, Tobacco Smoking*. Lyon: IARC.

IARC, 1988, *IARC Monographs on the Evaluation of Carcinogenic Risks to Humans, Vol. 44, Alcohol Drinking*. Lyon: IARC.

Knudson, A. G., 1985, Hereditary cancer, oncogenes and antioncogenes, *Cancer Res.*, **45**, 1437–43.

Lee, J. A. H., 1982, Melanoma and exposure to sunlight, *Epid. Rev.*, **4**, 110–36.

Muir, C. S. and Sasco, A. J., 1990, Prospects for cancer control in the 1990s, *Ann. Rev. Public Health*, **11**, 143–63.

National Research Council, 1982, *Diet, Nutrition, and Cancer*, Washington DC, National Academy Press, Committee on Diet, Nutrition and Cancer.

Parkin, D. M., Läärä, E. and Muir, C. S., 1988, Estimates of the worldwide frequency of sixteen major cancers in 1980, *Int. J. Cancer*, **41**, 184–97.

Peto, R. and Lopez, A. D., 1990, The future worldwide health effects of current smoking patterns: 3 million deaths/year in the 1990s, but over 10 million/year eventually, *7th World Conference on Tobacco and Health*, Perth, Western Australia, 3 April 1990.

Pott, P., 1775, *Chirurgical Observations Relative to Cataract, the Polypus of Nose, the Cancer of Scrotum, the Different Kinds of Ruptures, and the Mortification of the Toes and Feet*, pp. 63–5. London: Hawes, Clarke & Collins.

Rehn, L., 1895, Blasengeschwülste bei Fuchsin-Arbeitern, *Arch. Klin. Chir.*, **50**, 588–600.

Reynolds, S. H., Stowers, S. J., Patterson, R. M., Maronpot, R. R., Aaronson, S. A. and Anderson, M. W., 1987, Activated oncogenes in B6C3F1 mouse liver tumors: implications for risk assessment, *Science*, **237**, 1309–16.

Scotto, J., Fears, T. R. and Fraumeni, J. F., 1982, Solar radiation, in Schottenfield, D. and Fraumeni, J. F. (Eds) *Cancer Epidemiology and Prevention*, p. 254–76. Philadelphia: W. B. Saunders.

Tomatis, L. (Ed.) 1990, Cancer: causes, occurrence and control, *IARC Scientific Publication No. 100*. Lyon: International Agency for Research on Cancer.

Tomatis, L., Aitio, A., Wilbourn, J. and Shuker, L., 1989, Human carcinogens so far identified, *Jpn. J. Cancer Res.*, **80**, 795–807.

Vainio, H. and Hemminki, K., 1989, Multistage process and prevention of cancer, in *Occupational Cancer in the Chemical Industry*, pp. 78–97, Copenhagen: World Health Organization, Regional Office for Europe.

Vogelstein, B., Fearon, E. R., Hamilton, S. R., Kern, S. E., Preisinger, A. C., Leppert, M., Nakamura, Y., White, R., Smits, A. M. M. and Bos, J. L., 1988, Genetic alterations during colorectal tumour development, *New Engl. J. Med.*, **319**, 525–32.

Weinberg, R. A., 1985, The action of oncogenes in the cytoplasm and nucleus, *Science*, **230**, 770–6.

Weinberg, R. A., 1989, Oncogenes, antioncogenes, and the molecular basis of multistep carcinogenesis, *Cancer Res.*, **49**, 3713–21.

Yamagiwa, K. and Ichikawa, K., 1915, Uber die künstliche Erzeugung von Papillom, *Verk. Jpn. Pathol. Ges.*, **5**, 142–8.

Yokota, J., Wada, M., Shimosato, Y., Terada, M. and Sugimura, T., 1987, Loss of heterozygocity on chromosomes 3, 13 and 17 in small-cell carcinoma and on chromosome 3 in adenocarcinoma of the lung, *Proc. Natl. Acad. Sci. USA*, **84**, 9252–6.

Toxicity by Group of Chemical

Chapter 9

Toxicity of Metals

C. Winder

Introduction

Exposure to metals and metal-containing compounds is common to many industrial workplaces. Absorption of metals can have many effects on the body. Not all of these are adverse, and it must be remembered that some metals are essential for the normal function of the body. Examples include cobalt, copper, iron, magnesium, manganese, selenium, zinc. However, many of these, when exposure occurs in excess amounts, will result in toxicological effects. Examples of metals that have primarily toxic properties are cadmium, mercury and lead.

Before a discussion of the toxicity of metals, it is necessary to consider some general properties which have a bearing on health effects.

- Metals seldom interact with biological systems in the elemental form, and are usually active in the ionic form.

- Availability of metal ions to biological processes is often dependent on solubility. Soluble salts of metals readily dissociate in the aqueous environment of biological membranes, making transport into the body easy, whereas insoluble salts are poorly absorbed (for example, reduction of chromium (VI) to the less soluble chromium (III) will decrease its absorption).

- Absorption of soluble salts may be modified by the formation of insoluble compounds in biological materials (for example, high dietary levels of phosphate will reduce absorption of lead because of the formation of insoluble lead phosphate).

- Some metals are produced as alkyl compounds. These are often very lipid soluble, and pass readily across the lipid phase of biological membranes (examples include methyl mercury and organotin compounds).

- Strong attractions between metal ions and organic compounds will influence the disposition of metals and their rate of excretion. Most of the toxicologically important metals bind strongly to tissues, are only

165

slowly excreted, and therefore tend to accumulate with continuing exposure. Ion affinities to different tissues vary—elements like lead bind to bone, whereas mercury and cadmium localise in the kidney and liver.

● While the toxicities of different metals have individual characteristics, metals as a group have a propensity to interact with particular metabolically active groups, which are often associated with amino acids. Thiol (or sulphydryl) groups are of particular importance.

The onset of severe gastrointestinal symptoms (for example, bloody diarrhoea, abdominal pain, nausea, vomiting) and upper gastroinstestinal haemorrhage together with a metallic taste in the mouth is indicative of metal poisoning. Long-term effects of absorption of metal and metallic compounds are varied, and are related to effects in many body systems. The metals reviewed below are those metals which cause adverse effects in occupational situations. Other metals, such as copper, gold, iron, potassium, and so on, also cause adverse effects in other applications (for example, in therapeutic use of paediatric poisoning).

Metal toxicity: specific metals

Not all metals are of toxicological concern, and not all of these are important from the perspective of occupational toxicology. Some metals, such as arsenic, lead and mercury, have a long history, mainly from their use as poisoning agents, but also as they are now recognised as classic causes of particular occupational diseases. Other metals have come to the fore as new technologies and processes require their use (for example, beryllium, chromium and uranium).

The amount of information on the health effects of metals varies from metal to metal, and of course is dependent on a number of factors, including inherent toxicity, availability to workers, the volume of production and the types of processes for which the metal is employed. Some of the more important workplace metals are described briefly below.

Aluminium

Aluminium exposure may occur in a variety of workplace situations from mining, refining and smelting through to use of the metal and its compounds. The study of aluminium toxicity has been related to the study of patients with chronic renal failure on long-term dialysis. These patients develop high aluminium concentrations. Orally, about 12% of aluminium hydroxide is retained, with most body aluminium residing in bone tissue. The main route of excretion appears to be through bile, with renal elimination being more important after high exposures. Elevated aluminium levels have also been found in the autopsy material taken from the brains of individuals with Alzheimer's disease, though its role as a neurotoxic factor is yet to be clarified.

The lungs and the nervous system appear to be main organs of toxicity following occupational exposure. Pulmonary fibrosis has been reported in workers exposed to fine aluminium dust (aluminosis), and aluminium related fumes may exacerbate asthma. Neurological effects have also been reported, including encephalopathy, tremor, incoordination and cognitive defects.

Antimony

Antimony oxide and other compounds can cause a benign pneumonoconiosis, a severe pulmonary oedema and cardiomyopathy following severe exposure. Skin burns, including pruritic papules progressing to pustules known as 'antimony spots' are also observed.

Stibine gas (SbH_3) exposure produces effects similar to that of arsine gas (AsH_3) exposure.

Arsenic

Arsenic has been used in the production of pesticides, although this is declining. Other uses include in glassware, alloy and pigment production, and the use of arsine gas (AsH_3) in the semiconductor industry. Arsenic is a by-product of the extraction of a number of metals, including lead, copper and gold. Intense abdominal pain, bloody diarrhoea and a garlic-like smell on the breath are suggestive of arsenic absorption.

Arsenic compounds present a wide range of toxicities. The most acutely toxic arsenic compound is arsine gas, which is a colourless, non-irritating gas evolving from the mixing of arsenic compounds with acid:

$$A-AsX + H-Y \rightarrow AsH_3 + A-X + A-Y$$

(generic equation)

Where A is an anion of arsenic salt, H is an acid, AsX is a cation of arsenic salt, and Y is a salt of the acid.

The organic arsenic (V) (arsenate, As^{5+}) forms are less toxic than the inorganic arsenic (III) (arsenite, As^{3+}) forms; this is based on their lower solubility.

As^{5+} compounds are well absorbed thought the gut, though As^{3+} are more lipid soluble (dermal absorption). Arsenic replaces phosphorus in bone and binds to sulphydryl groups on proteins. It also disrupts metabolic pathways, including inhibition of oxidative phosphorylation and pyruvate metabolism. Almost all of the absorbed arsenic is excreted by the kidney within 4–10 days.

Arsenic toxicity is well studied, owing to its frequent use as a poisoning agent. Many organs and systems are affected:

- Cardiovascular (vasodilation leading to reflex arteriolar constriction, myocardial depression).

- Gastrointestinal (submucosal vesicle formation, bleeding).

- Kidney (acute tubular necrosis, oliguria, proteinuria and haematuria).

- Skin (erythema, brittle fingernails, local oedema, pigmentation, pyoderma and skin cancer).

- Nervous system (degeneration of myelin, encephalopathy, parasthesias).

- Liver (hepatic fatty degeneration, cirrhosis).

Beryllium

The uses of this light metal include nuclear alloys and in space or defence industries. The lung is the major organ affected, with dyspnoea and cough progressing to chronic granulomatous disease similar to sarcoidosis and military tuberculosis.

Cadmium

Cadmium appears in the workplace during electroplating, in solder, alkaline storage batteries production, pigments, stabilisers in plastics and some alloys. It may also occur in fumes from the smelting or welding of other metals. Approximately 5–10% of the available dose is absorbed from the gastrointestinal tract, while up to 50% is absorbed from the lung. Cadmium is transported in the body bound to red blood cells and high molecular weight plasma proteins like albumin. There may be a small amount transported as metallothionein, a low molecular weight protein, and this could be toxicologically significant. Over half the body burden is stored in the kidneys and the liver. Elimination of cadmium is a slow process, with a half-life of 16–33 years. A syndrome of severe arthralgias and osteomalacia called '*itai-itai byo*' (ouch-ouch disease) was observed in postmenopausal women in Japan, caused by a combination of cadmium contamination of diet and low calcium and vitamin D intake.

Acute toxic effects are similar to those for metal fume fever (see zinc below) for inhalational exposure, and gastroenteritis from oral exposure. The lungs and kidneys are the main target organs for chronic exposure. Effects in the lungs, which are mostly associated with inhalational exposures include chronic bronchitis, emphysema and possibly lung cancer. Proteinuria is the most frequent nephrotoxic finding (glycosuria and aminoaciduria are also common). This is due to proximal tubule damage, which is irreversible.

Chromium

There are two major forms of chromium, the hexavalent chromium (VI) (chromous, Cr^{6+}) and trivalent chromium (III) (chromic, Cr^{3+}). Compounds of the latter form are relatively harmless, owing to their insolubility. Chromium exposures are found in a number of industries, including electroplating, concrete use, tanning, safety match and pigment manufacture. Exposure to chromium is also observed with the use of dichromate compounds. Absorption occurs from gastrointestinal tract and lungs, and systemic effects are possible following skin exposure; about 60% of an absorbed dose is excreted in the urine within 8 h of absorption.

The toxicity of chromium compounds appears to be related to powerful oxidising properties of the hexavalent compound, which is reduced to the trivalent form once absorbed into the body. Chromium compounds are both skin and mucous membrane irritants, and skin and pulmonary sensitisers. Dermatitis, chrome ulcers (a penetrating lesion of skin also called 'chrome holes'), corrosion of the nasal septum, conjunctivitis and lacrimation also occur. Hexavalent chromium compounds are carcinogenic (bronchogenic carcinoma). There is some evidence that short-lived pentavalent chromium (V) intermediates are the specific carcinogenic agents as these have been shown to be directly genotoxic.

Cobalt

Chronic exposure to cobalt produces 'hard metal pneumonoconiosis' in industrial workers using cobalt in the manufacture of heat resistant hard metal alloys. A cardiomyopathy has also been observed in workers using cobalt as a defoaming agent (beer drinkers' cardiomyopathy).

Lead

Exposure to lead is possible in a variety of occupations: smelting, ship breaking, welding, plumbing, battery, alloy and pigment manufacture and printing. Exposure is also possible from non-occupational sources, some quite exotic (hair preparations, tonics, cosmetics). Approximately 5–10% of an ingested dose is absorbed, although lung uptake can reach 50–70% depending on particle size, retention and solubility. Most recently absorbed lead is stored in red blood cells (half-life of about 20–40 days) and most long-term body lead (90%) is stored in bone tissue (half-life of the order of 20–30 years). Elimination of lead occurs mainly through the kidney.

Lead toxicity in workers results primarily from inhalational exposure, although oral exposure may be important in cases of poor hygiene. Lead has been shown to induce effects in a number of body systems.

● Haematopoietic system (disruption in porphyrin synthesis, anaemia).

- Nervous system (neurasthenia, slowed conduction velocity, neurobehavioural disturbances, peripheral neuropathy, encephalopathy).

- Gastrointestinal (colic, constipation).

- Kidney (lesions of proximal tubule, Fanconi syndrome, chronic interstitial disease).

- Reproductive system (stillbirth, spontaneous abortion, decreased sperm counts and increased abnormal sperm).

- Development, particularly of the nervous system and of neurobehavioural function.

- Cardiovascular (hypertension).

For a number of these effects there is sufficient evidence to establish exposure effect relationships, based on blood lead values, at or below $50 \, \mu gdl^{-1}$.

Lithium

Although lithium is used industrially as a nuclear reactor coolant and in the manufacture of alkaline storage batteries and alloys, occupational toxicity is rare. Most lithium poisoning occurs through its therapeutic use as an antidepressant.

Manganese

Acute exposure to manganese fumes produces a metal fume fever (see below), which may develop into pneumonitis. A classic occupational condition known as 'manganism' results from chronic exposure to dust from manganese ores or fumes from manganese steels. The features of this condition are neurological and psychological, including apathy, confusion, bizarre behaviour, increased muscle tone, difficulty with speech and fine motor movement and loss of balance. Onset is progressive and insidious. One feature of chronic manganism is Parkinsonian symptoms, due to manganese induced damage to the CNS extrapyrimidal system (notably the highly dopaminergic red nucleus). This lesion is similar to that in Parkinson's disease.

Mercury

Mercury is used in dentistry, battery, medical and scientific equipment manufacture, and in the production of chlorine and caustic soda. The metal is liquid at room temperature, and exists in elemental, inorganic (Hg^+ or mainly, Hg^{2+}) or organic (Hg^{4+}) forms. Absorption and biological effects vary with these forms, and though the latter is biotransformed and bioconcentrated in food chains and can appear in environmental disasters (for instance, the neurological condition Minamata disease), only the first two are important in occupational situations.

- Elemental mercury is well absorbed by the lung as the vapour (80%), but poorly absorbed by the gut (0.01%). Once absorbed, mercury is oxidised to the Hg^{2+} form. This reaction takes place in a number of tissues, especially the brain.

- Moderate amounts of inorganic mercury (7–15%) are absorbed by the gut. These cause most cases of mercury poisoning. Systemic effects are possible from skin and lung exposure. Excretion occurs in urine and faeces, with a half-life of 40–60 days.

- Organic forms of mercury are extremely well absorbed across the gut, although dermal absorption does not appear to be large. Inhalation of methyl mercury compounds results in a classic condition of ataxia, dysarthria and constricted visual fields. The major route of excretion is through the bile.

The main toxic effects are observed in the kidney and gastrointestinal system (inorganic), central nervous system (elemental and organic) and respiratory system (elemental mercury vapour).

- Kidney (oliguria, proteinuria, nephrotic syndrome);
- Central nervous system (psychological changes, erethism, tremor abolished by sleep, polyneuropathy). Insomnia, loss of appetite, loss of memory, shyness and timidity characterise mercury induced psychosis.
- Gastrointestinal system (gingivitis, salivation, stomatitis, severe mucosal necrosis).
- Respiratory system (inflammation, ventilation/perfusion defects, hypoxaemia, progressive fibrosis, pulmonary granulomas).

Nickel

Occupational exposure to nickel and its compounds occurs in mining, refining and smelting as well as electroplating and battery manufacture. The main occupational toxic effects of nickel compounds are its allergenicity (producing a contact dermatitis called 'nickel itch') and nasal and lung cancers. The latter effect has been associated mainly with nickel subsulphide in both epidemiological and experimental animal studies. It is important to recognise that it may be the relative insolubility of this nickel compound that accounts, at least in part, for its carcinogenic effects. It may be that its insolubility increases its residence time at critical sites in the respiratory system, thereby allowing a continuing exposure at that local site.

Nickel carbonyl results from the combination of nickel with carbon monoxide and is found during some refining operations (Mond process). It is highly acutely toxic being much more lipid soluble than other nickel compounds and there have been many human poisonings reported due to exposure to this compound.

Platinum

The main use of platinum is in catalytic converters in motor vehicle manufacture, although the metal and its alloys are also used in jewellery and dentistry, as a catalyst in the chemical industry and in fibre glass manufacture. Cisplatin (*cis*-dichlorodiamine platinum) is a chemotherapeutic agent. Workplace toxicity results from the sensitising properties of platinum salt complexes, but not from platinum. These compounds induce immediate hypersensitivity reactions, and the term 'platinosis' has been applied to the spectrum of effects (asthma, rhinorrhoea, dermatitis). The incidence of occupational asthma by these compounds can reach 100%.

Selenium

Selenium is widely used in the electronics, glass, ceramics, steel and pigment manufacturing industries. It also has applications in shampoos, dietary supplements, and so on. As selenium is an essential mineral, selenium deficiency can occur. The most toxic compound of selenium is Gun blue (2% selenious acid), with a lethal dose of 30–60 ml. Exposure to selenium dusts can cause respiratory tract irritation, nasal discharge, cough, loss of sense of smell and epistaxis. Chronic selenium toxicity resembles arsenic poisoning.

Thallium

Thallium has specialised uses in the manufacture of low temperature thermometers, semiconductors, scintillation counters and optical lenses. The metal has been used as a rodenticide in the past. The average lethal dose for an adult is in the order of 1 g. Thallium is quickly absorbed and distributed widely in the body. Dermal absorption is possible through thallium containing ointments. Elimination is also relatively rapid, with a half-life of about 2 days.

Thallium has an affinity for sulphydryl groups, and inhibits many enzyme reactions. Thallium also exchanges with potassium and interferes with potassium dependent reactions. The onset of poisoning is insidious, with gastrointestinal symptoms such as nausea, vomiting and diarrhoea progressing to nervous system effects (disorientation, lethargy, psychosis, insomnia, neuropathy, convulsions, cerebral oedema and coma), cardiorespiratory effects (tachycardia, hypertension, dysrythmias, myocardial necrosis) and ophthalmological effects (optical neuritis, ophthalmoplegias). Blue-grey lines may appear on the gums, and dark pigmentation around hair follicles may also be seen. Alopecia, especially on the face, and a dry scaly skin, with white lines across the nails are late signs. Central and peripheral nervous system effects may persist (ataxia, tremor, memory loss).

Tin

Inhalation of dusts or fumes of tin and tin oxide result in a benign pneumoconiosis (stannosis). Inorganic tin compounds have relatively low toxicities. Some tin salts can produce gastrointestinal disturbances at high doses, though systemic toxicity is limited, owing to poor absorption.

Some organic tin compounds are potent neurotoxicants, skin irritants and teratogens. These have wide use as fungicides (now prohibited), antioxidants and plastics stabilisers. Cerebral oedema and hippocampal necrosis has been observed following exposure to dialkyl tin compounds. Severe organic tin exposure has resulted in headache, tinnitus, deafness, memory loss, disorientation, psychosis, respiratory depression and coma. A syndrome of permanent neurological sequelae often occurs, including hyperactivity, inappropriately aggressive behaviour and loss of independence.

Uranium

Adverse effects of uranium are related to exposure to gamma radiation (unlikely to exceed time weighted average exposure standards) and inhalation of dust particles containing short-life radon daughters (isotopes of lead, bismuth and polonium). Toxic effects are related to chronic lung disease and lung cancer.

Vanadium

Vanadium is used as an alloying agent in the steel industry and as a catalyst in the chemical industry. The vanadate ion (VO^{3-}) is the most common form in biological fluids, and it is one of the most potent inhibitors of the Na^+/K^+ ATPase pump.

Absorption is primarily through the lungs, and absorbed vanadium is largely excreted by the kidneys. Most exposures occur when workers inhale vanadium pentoxide fumes. As vanadium is present in fuel oils, workers have developed vanadium toxicity while cleaning out gas fired boilers. A green discolouration of the tongue and a metallic taste suggest vanadium exposure.

Vanadium compounds produce dermal, mucous membrane and pulmonary irritation (including rhinitis, wheezing, nasal haemorrhage, cough, sore throat and chest pain). The systemic effects result from the ability of vanadium to oxidise, including the inhibition of oxidative phosphorylation. Long-term effects include chronic bronchitis, conjunctivitis and pneumonia.

Zinc

Exposure to zinc is possible in a wide variety of occupations, including soldering, battery manufacture, dentistry, pharmaceutical manufacture, electroplaters, pigment and rubber workers. Zinc is an essential element and it is fairly well absorbed from the intestine. Most elimination is through the faeces.

The most toxic salt of zinc is zinc chloride ($ZnCl$), though powerful emetic properties limit expression of other toxic effects. This chemical is used in solder fluxes and can be caustic to the gastrointestinal tract. Inhalation of zinc chloride dust has caused pulmonary toxicity and death. Other organs that may be affected by zinc include the kidney (tubular necrosis and interstitial nephritis) and the pancreas (elevated glucose and amylase and lowered calcium).

The most common zinc related condition is metal fume fever, caused by inhalation of zinc containing fumes by welders. This is a flu-like illness, occurring 4–6 h after exposure. Fatigue, chills, myalgias, cough, dyspnoea, thirst, metallic taste and salivation are characteristic, although they tend to resolve within 36 h. Metal fume fever, as the name implies, is associated with other metals such as aluminium, copper, manganese, nickel and so on.

Treatment of metal poisoning by chelation

The first 'antidote' specifically designed to antagonise metal poisoning was Dimercaprol or BAL (British Anti-Lewisite), which was developed to combat the effects of mustard gas (Lewisite, dichloro-2-chlorovinylarsine) in trench warfare. This was the first chelator (from the Greek *chela* for 'claw'). Chelators are chemicals which bind directly with metal ions to form stable, water soluble complexes which effectively bind the metal and stop it from interacting with biological processes prior to elimination from the body.

Chelators are perceived as having a specific affinity for a particular metal, though this is not the case, and there is a large amount of nonspecific affinity for other metals. For example, ethylene diamine tetra-acetic acid (EDTA) is a chelator used extensivley in metal toxicity (notably lead poisoning), though it will form tight complexes with other metals. When the other metal is calcium (required for physiological control of muscle contraction), hypocalcemic tetany may be produced from chelation of calcium. Nowadays, this problem is removed by administering EDTA as the calcium/sodium salt ($CaNa_2$/EDTA). Common chelators that have been used at one time or another are shown in Table 9.1.

Table 9.1. Chelators used in the treatment of metal poisoning

Chelator	Main use	Metals known to form complexes
CaNa$_2$–EDTA	Pb	Be, Cd, Co, Cu, Fe, Mn, Ag, Ni, Zn
Dimercaprol (BAL)	As	Cd, Pb, Hg
Penicillamine	Oral	Cu, Pb, Hg, Zn
Deferoxamine	Fe	
DMSA*	Pb (paediatric)	

*DMSA, *Meso* 2,3-dimercaptosuccinic acid.

Bibliography

Ellenhorn, M. J. and Barceloux, D. G., 1988, Metals and related compounds, in *Medical Toxicology: Diagnosis and Treatment of Human Poisoning*, Chap. 37, pp. 1007–66. New York: Elsevier.

Friberg, L., Nordberg, G. F. and Vouk, V. B. (Eds), 1979, *Handbook on the Toxicology of Metals*. Amsterdam: Elsevier/North Holland.

Goyer, R. A., 1991, Toxic effects of metals, in Amdur, M. O., Doull, J. and Klaassen, C. D. (Eds) *Casarett and Doull's Toxicology. The Basic Science of Poisons*, 4th Edn, pp. 623–80. New York: Pergamon Press.

WHO, 1986, *Early Detection of Occupational Diseases*, Chaps 7–15, pp. 44–90. Geneva: World Health Organisation.

WHO, *Environmental Health Criteria* (document series). Geneva: World Health Organisation.

Chapter 10

Toxicity of Pesticides

A. Moretto and M. Lotti

Production and Uses

Pesticides are used in agriculture and public health to control insects, weeds, animals and vectors of disease. *The Pesticide Manual* lists about 600 active ingredients currently used as pesticides (Worthing and Hance, 1991); 75% of total amount used is made up of about 50 active ingredients (Salem and Olajos, 1988). Information on global production and uses of pesticides is scarce, while sales data are more readily available. Pesticide sales doubled between 1972 and 1985, and it has been estimated that world production of formulated pesticides increased from about 400 000 in 1955 to over 3 million tonne in 1985 (WHO, 1990). In 1985 herbicides, insecticides, and fungicides represented 46%, 31% and 18% of all pesticides used, respectively. About 75% of the total amount was used in Western Europe, the USA and Japan. However, 50% of insecticides were used in developing countries (IARC, 1991). The fastest growing market is Africa (an increase of 182% between 1980 and 1984) followed by Central and South America (32% increase), Asia (28% increase) and the eastern Mediterranean region (26% increase) (WHO, 1990).

Organophosphorus compounds are likely to continue to be the most used insecticides in developing countries and it has been estimated that demand for these compounds will more than double in the next 10 years (WHO, 1990). Moreover, the use of carbamates and pyrethroids will increase, while that of organochlorine compounds will continue to decline. The use of herbicides (mainly carbamates and triazines) will also increase.

New application techniques are developing and include new mixtures or formulations (e.g. water-wettable powders) and higher concentrations of the active ingredients. This, together with the use of more selective and potent formulations, will allow a reduction in the dosage per unit of area.

Classification

In most countries, pesticides are classified according to their mammalian toxicity, as suggested by WHO (WHO, 1988a) (Table 10.1). The classification refers to the technical compounds, and for each active ingredient it may vary according to the formulation. Different criteria are used when neither the oral nor the dermal is the most relevant route of absorption (e.g. fumigants). This classification is useful for identifying pesticides posing a hazard of acute poisoning, which still represents a major problem in developing countries. However, possible effects of chronic exposure to lower levels as well as the reversibility of acute effects are not taken into account by this classification.

Table 10.1. Classification of pesticides according to hazard* (WHO1988a)

Class	Rat LD_{50} (mg/kg body weight)			
	Oral		Dermal	
	Solids	Liquids	Solids	Liquids
1a Extremely hazardous	⩽5	⩽20	⩽10	⩽40
1b Highly hazardous	5–50	20–200	10–100	40–400
II Moderately hazardous	50–500	200–2000	100–1000	400–4000
III Slightly hazardous	>500	>2000	>1000	>4000

*The terms 'solids' and 'liquids' refer to the physical state of products and formulations.

Pesticides can also be classified according to their chemical structure or according to the target pest, as reported in Table 10.2 (Plestina, 1984). Application of pesticides against individual pests implies the use of various different types of equipment and work practices and, therefore, different kinds of exposure.

Epidemiology of acute poisoning

Acute poisoning can derive from intentional, occupational or accidental exposure to pesticides. The WHO (1990) estimates an annual incidence of unintentional acute poisoning of about 1 million, with an overall mortality rate of about 1% (of which only 1% is in developed countries). The majority of unintentional pesticide poisonings are occupational. Population-based studies in 17 countries gave annual incidence rates of unintentional pesticide poisoning of 0.3–18 per 100 000 (Jeyaratnam, 1990).

The estimated annual incidence of intentional acute poisoning is about 2 million, with a 5.7% mortality rate (WHO, 1990). Such poisoning is more frequent in developing than in developed countries. In Indonesia, Malaysia and Thailand suicide attempts (usually with organophosphorus compounds) represent 60–70% of acute pesticide poisonings (Jeyaratnam, 1990), whereas in California all non-occupational pesticide poisonings represent only about 5% of the total (Mehler *et al.*, 1990).

Table 10.2. Classification of pesticides
according to the target pest (Plestina, 1984)

Acaricides	Larvicides
Attractants	Miticides
Defoliants	Molluscicides
Desiccants	Nematocides
Fungicides	Plant growth regulators
Herbicides	Repellents
Insecticides	Rodenticides

Occupational exposures

Application of pesticides has become progressively safer due to technological improvements, to increasing awareness, and to the fact that pesticides are often applied by professional operators. In developing countries, however, pesticides are often applied by farmers who might use poorly maintained equipment, inefficient hand-sprayers, inadequate protection, and have insufficient training and education. Furthermore, in developing countries about 63% of the active population works in agriculture as compared with 11% elsewhere.

Threshold limits

The American Conference of Governmental Industrial Hygienists (ACGIH) has proposed threshold limit values for about 80 active ingredients (ACGIH, 1991). About half of them have the notation 'skin' since dermal exposure entails significant absorption. With regard to biological exposure indexes (BEIs), only limited indications have been given; in most cases the metabolism of the active ingredient is not well understood and the relationship between urinary levels of a metabolite and the toxic effect of the parent compound is not known. ACGIH has established BEIs only for parathion and pentachlorophenol (see below).

Re-entry times

Pesticide residues on plants, fruit, soil, and buildings may cause significant exposure in farm and pest-control workers, and inhabitants of the buildings. Cases of poisoning after exposure to residues have been reported (Spear *et al.*, 1975; Hodgson *et al.*, 1986; Mehler *et al.*, 1990; Currie *et al.*, 1990). The extent of exposure to residues depends on the formulation and the amount of pesticide applied, the time elapsed from application and the persistence of the active ingredient (Davis *et al.*, 1981). Climatic conditions may influence both degradation of the active ingredient and the exposure to foliar dust particles (Nigg *et al.*, 1984). It is also possible that degradation products are more toxic than the parent compound (e.g. parathion which might degrade to paraoxon) (Spear *et al.*, 1977). General rules cannot therefore be established, and mathematical models to calculate re-entry times are difficult to apply (Popendorf and Leffingwell, 1982).

Mixtures and impurities

Simultaneous exposures to two or more active ingredients is increasingly frequent for agricultural workers and might influence the toxicity of individual chemicals. For instance, concomitant exposure to two or more anticholinesterase agents (i.e. organophosphorus compounds) usually produces an additive effect, but potentiation may ensue. Potentiation might be due to inhibition of carboxylesterase which prevents inactivation of organophosphorus compounds containing a carboxylester function. For instance, DEF (*S,S,S*-tri-*n*-butylphosphorotrithioate), EPN (*O*-4-nitrophenylphenylphosphothioate) and parathion potentiate malathion toxicity because they inhibit its hydrolysis by carboxylesterases (WHO, 1986a). Certain impurities (isomalathion and possibly *O,S,S*-trimethylphosphorodithioate) also increased malathion toxicity by similar mechanisms (Baker *et al.*, 1978; Talcott *et al.*, 1979). Pyrethroids are metabolised by esterases, which are probably the same carboxylesterases (Miyamoto, 1976), and potentiation of their toxicity might occur with combined exposure to certain organophosphorus compounds.

A number of organochlorine compounds are inducers of mixed-function oxidases in mammalian liver and this may explain why, when given in combination, they might change the toxicity of an organophosphorus compound (Keplinger and Deichmann, 1967).

Impurities can be present in commercial pesticides, and their nature and amount are influenced by a number of factors: the process of synthesis and production, coformulants, condition of storage, etc. Impurities might either enhance toxicities (higher toxicity of impurities or potentiation) or induce a different kind of toxicity.

It should also be considered that toxicity of some solvents may approach or exceed the toxicity of the active ingredient e.g. DDT (1,1,1-trichloro-2,2-bis(4-chlorophenyl)ethane dissolved in kerosene or other compounds dissolved in xylene).

Long-term effects

The identification of subjects who have been chronically exposed to pesticides is relatively easy, but biochemical evidence of exposure is seldom available. Moreover, extrapolation from current biomonitoring data to assess past occupational exposures as well as the risk associated with a given pesticide are difficult since most workers use several active ingredients and work practices are different and often changing. Attention has been focused on the carcinogenicity of pesticides, but the long time taken for the disease to develop further hampers these studies. Evaluations of the carcinogenic potential of relatively few pesticides have been performed by the International Agency for Research on Cancer (IARC), even though carcinogenicity studies in animals are available for all pesticides. However, most of them have not been published in the open literature. The results obtained so far by the IARC are summarised in Table 10.3. Several criteria are used by the IARC for choosing the compounds to be evaluated and include:

Table 10.3. The IARC evaluation of pesticides

Compound	Year	Degreee of evidence for carcinogenicity*		Overall evaluation
		Human	Animal	
Insecticides				
Agents and groups of agents				
Aldicarb	1991	ND	I	3
Aldrin	1987	I	L	3
Aramite	1974	ND	S	2B
Arsenic and arsenic compounds	1987	S	L	1‡
Carbaryl	1976	ND	I	3
Chlordane/heptachlor	1991	I	S	2B
Chlordimeform	1983	ND	I	3
Chlorobenzilate	1983	ND	L	3
DDT	1991	I	S	2B
Deltamethrin	1991	ND	I	3
Dichlorvos	1991	I	S	2B
Dicofol	1983	ND	L	3
Dieldrin	1987	I	L	3
Endrin	1974	ND	I	3
Fenvalerate	1991	ND	I	3
Hexachlorocyclohexanes (HCH)	1987	I		2B
Technical-grade HCH			S	
α-HCH			S	
β-HCH			L	
γ-HCH (Lindane)			L	
Malathion	1983	ND	I	3
Methoxychlor	1979	ND	I	3
Methylparathion	1987	ND	ESL	3
Mirex	1979	ND	S	2B
Parathion	1983	ND	I	3
Permethrin	1991	ND	I	3
Piperonyl butoxide	1983	ND	I	3
Tetrachlorvinphos	1983	ND	L	3
Trichlorfon	1983	ND	I	3
Zectran §	1976	ND	I	3
Mixtures				
Terpene polychlorinates (Strobane)	1974	ND	L	3
Fungicides				
Captafol	1991	ND	S	2A
Captan	1983	ND	L	3
Chlorophenols	1987	L		2B
Pentachlorophenol	1991	I	L	3
2,4,5-Trichlorophenol ¶			I	
2,4,6-Trichlorophenol ¶			S	
Chlorothalonil	1983	ND	L	3

Table 10.3. (*Contd.*)

Compound	Year	Degreee of evidence for carcinogenicity*		Overall evaluation
		Human	Animal	
Copper 8-hydroxyquinoline	1977	ND	I	3
Ferbam	1976	ND	I	3
Maneb	1976	ND	I	3
o-Phenylphenol	1983	ND	I	3
Quintozene (pentachloronitrobenzene)	1974	ND	L	3
Sodium o-phenylphenate	1987	ND	S	2B
Thiram	1991	I	I	3
Zineb	1976	ND	I	3
Ziram	1991	ND	L	3
Herbicides				
Amitrole	1987	I	S	2B
Atrazine	1991	I	S	2B
Chlorophenoxy herbicides	1987	L		2B
2,4-D			I	
2,4,5-T			I	
MCPA			ND	
Chloropropham	1976	ND	I	3
Diallate	1983	ND	L	3
Fluometuron	1983	ND	I	3
Monuron	1991	ND	L	3
Nitrofen (technical grade)	1983	ND	S	2B
Picloram	1991	ND	L	3
Propham	1976	ND	I	3
Simazine	1991	ND	I	3
Sulfallate	1983	ND	S	2B
Trifluralin	1991	I	L	3
Other				
1,2-Dibromo-3-chloropropane [|]	1987	I	S	2B
Dimethylcarbamoyl chloride**	1987	I	S	2A
Ethylene dibromide [††]	1987	I	S	2A
Naphthylthiourea (ANTU) [‡‡]	1987	I	I	3

ANTU, α-naphthylthiourea; 2,4-D, 2,4-dichlorophenoxyacetic acid; 2,4,5-T, 2,4,5-trichlorophenoxyacetic acid; DDT, 1,1,1-trichloro-2,2-bis(4-chlorophenyl)ethane; HCH, hexachlorocyclohexane; MCPA, 4-chloro-2-methylphenoxyacetic acid.
*I, inadequate evidence; S, sufficient evidence; L, limited evidence; ND, no data; ESL, evidence suggesting lack of carcinogenicity.
[†] 1, The agent is carcinogenic to humans; 2A, the agent is probably carcinogenic to humans; 2B, the agent is possibly carcinogenic to humans; 3, the agent is not classifiable as to its carcinogenicity to humans; 4, the agent is probably not carcinogenic to humans.
[‡] This evaluation applies to the group of chemicals as a whole and not necessarily to all individual chemicals within the group.
[§] Also a molluscide.
[¶] Primarily used as chemical intermediates.
[\|] Soil fumigant/nematocide.
**Pesticide intermediate.
[††] Soil fumigant.
[‡‡] Rodenticide.

● Evidence of human exposure.

● Some experimental evidence of carcinogenicity and/or some evidence or suspicion of a risk to humans.

Contrary to other national and international committees and agencies, the IARC evaluates data published in the open literature only. In addition to compounds reported in Table 10.3, 'occupational exposure in spraying and application of insecticides' has also been considered by the IARC; the conclusion as based on a few epidemiological studies was that 'spraying and application of insecticides entail exposures that are probably carcinogenic to humans (Group 2A)' (IARC, 1991). It is not clear, however, what the basis is for such a generalisation—several chemicals were applied in different ways and settings, using different mixtures and the assessment of exposure was vague or anecdotal. The statement also seems not to be consistent with the evaluations reported in Table 10.3.

Toxicology

Organophosphates

Most organophosphorus compounds (OPs) are used as insecticides, while a few are used as fungicides, nematocides or plant regulators. The chemical structure of OPs is shown in Figure 10.1. According to the atom (oxygen or sulphur) that is double-bonded to the phosphorus, OPs are called 'phosphates' or 'phosphorothioates', respectively. The latter need to undergo oxidative desulphuration to inhibit esterases. Most commercial OP insecticides are phosphorothioates since the P=S form is more stable and more lipid soluble; their oxidised forms (P=O) are commonly referred to as the 'oxon' (e.g. parathion/paraoxon or chlorpyrifos/chlorpyrifos-oxon). Moreover, dimethyl(thio)phosphates are thought to be less toxic than diethyl(thio)phosphates because of the higher rate of reactivation of dimethylphosphorylated acetylcholinesterase (AChE).

Thousands of cases of acute poisoning by OPs have been reported. The majority of cases were suicidal or accidental, but several, including some fatal ones, were occupational in origin, mainly due to dermal exposure. OP poisoning generally represents a high percentage of total systemic pesticide poisoning, varying from about 30% in California (Mehler *et al.*, 1990) to 77% in China (WHO, 1990).

OPs exert their lethal toxic effect to both insects and mammals through inhibition (phosphorylation) of AChE activity at nerve endings (Lotti, 1991a). AChE inhibition leads to accumulation of acetylcholine, which is responsible for the cholinergic syndrome (see Table 10.4). Symptoms and signs may occur in various combinations and at different times after exposure. An 'intermediate syndrome', apparently non-cholinergic, has been described in some patients acutely intoxicated with OPs (Senanayake and Karalleide, 1987). After the cholinergic phase, the patients developed paralysis of the proximal limb muscles, neck flexors, motor cranial nerves, and respiratory muscles. The syndrome may lead to death if artificial respiration is not provided.

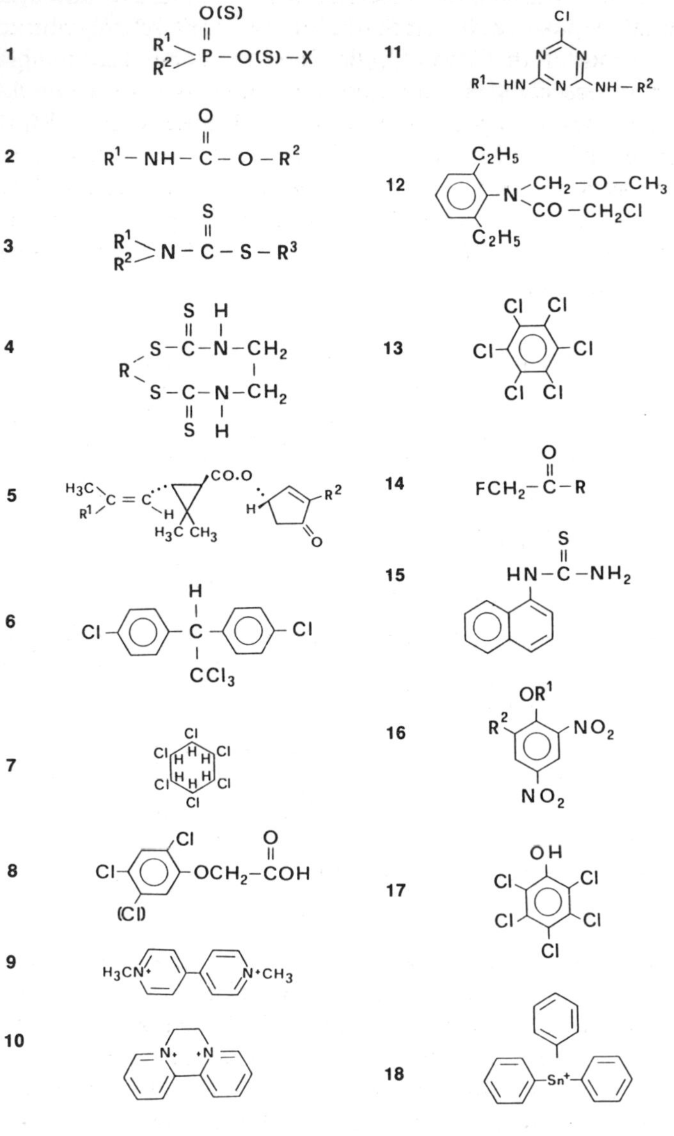

Toxicity of Pesticides

1    $\begin{matrix} R^1 \\ R^2 \end{matrix} \!\! > \!\! P \overset{\underset{\|}{O(S)}}{-} O(S)-X$

2    $R^1-NH-\overset{\underset{\|}{O}}{C}-O-R^2$

3    $\begin{matrix} R^1 \\ R^2 \end{matrix} \!\! > \!\! N-\overset{\underset{\|}{S}}{C}-S-R^3$

4    $R\!\! < \!\! \begin{matrix} S-\overset{\underset{\|}{S}}{C}-\overset{\underset{|}{H}}{N}-CH_2 \\ S-\overset{\underset{\|}{C}}{\underset{S}{}}-\overset{\underset{|}{N}}{\underset{H}{}}-CH_2 \end{matrix}$

5    $\begin{matrix} H_3C \\ R^1 \end{matrix} \!\! > \!\! C=C \cdots \overset{CO.O}{\underset{H_3C\ CH_3}{\triangle}} \cdots H \cdots R^2$

6    $Cl\!\!-\!\!\bigcirc\!\!-\!\!\overset{\underset{|}{H}}{\underset{CCl_3}{C}}\!\!-\!\!\bigcirc\!\!-\!\!Cl$

7   (hexachlorocyclohexane structure)

8    $Cl\!\!-\!\!\bigcirc\!\!-\!\!OCH_2-\overset{\underset{\|}{O}}{C}OH$ (Cl)

9    $H_3CN^+\!\!-\!\!\bigcirc\!\!-\!\!\bigcirc\!\!-\!\!N^+CH_3$

10   (diquat structure)

11   R^1-HN (triazine with Cl)$-NH-R^2$

12    $\begin{matrix} C_2H_5 \\ \\ C_2H_5 \end{matrix}$ ring $-N\!\!<\!\!\begin{matrix} CH_2-O-CH_3 \\ CO-CH_2Cl \end{matrix}$

13   (hexachlorobenzene structure)

14    $FCH_2-\overset{\underset{\|}{O}}{C}-R$

15    $HN-\overset{\underset{\|}{S}}{C}-NH_2$ (naphthalene)

16   R^2 (ring) $\overset{OR^1}{}NO_2$ / NO_2

17   (pentachlorophenol structure)

18   (fentin structure, Sn^+)

Figure 10.1. 1, Organophosphorus compounds; 2, carbamates; 3, dithiocarbamates; 4, EBDC (ethylene-bis(dithiocarbamate)); 5, pyrethroids; 6, DDT (1,1,1-trichloro-2,2-bis(4-chloro-phenyl)ethane); 7, HCH (hexachlorocyclohexane); 8, 2,4,(5)-di(tri)chlorophenoxy acetic acid; 9, paraquat; 10, diquat; 11, triazines; 12, alachlor; 13, HCB (hexachlorobenzene); 14, fluoro-acetic acid derivatives; 15, ANTU (α-naphthylthiourea); 16, 2,4-dinitrophenol derivatives; 17, PCP (pentachlorophenol); 18, fentin.

Some OP insecticides (i.e. chlorpyrifos, dichlorvos, methamidophos, tri-chlorfon and trichlornat) caused a sensory-motor polyneuropathy known as 'organophosphate-induced delayed polyneuropathy' (OPIDP) (Lotti, 1992).

Most cases of OPIDP were suicidal, and only a few involved careless occupational exposures to methamidophos. OPIDP is characterised by flaccid paralysis of the lower limbs, but the upper limbs might also be affected in severe cases. Histopathology shows degeneration of long and large-diameter axons in peripheral nerves and spinal cord. OPIDP development is unrelated to inhibition of AChE and the putative molecular target is a nervous system protein called 'neuropathy target esterase' (NTE) (Lotti, 1991b). Since all commercial OP insecticides display a high potency for anticholinesterase, OPIDP always developed after doses causing severe cholinergic syndrome.

Table 10.4. Signs and symptoms of OP poisoning (from Lotti, 1991a, modified)

Severity of poisoning	Symptoms and signs		
	Muscarinic	Nicotinic	Central nervous system
Mild (RBC AChE > 40%)	Nausea, vomiting, diarrhoea, salivation/lachrymation, bronchoconstriction, increased bronchial secretions, bradycardia		Headache, dizziness
Moderate (20% < RBC AChE < 40%)	Same as above plus meiosis (unreactive to light), urinary/faecal incontinence	Muscle fasciculation (fine muscles)	Same as above plus dysarthia, ataxia
Severe (RBC AChE < 20%)		Same as above plus muscle fasciculation (diaphragm and respiratory muscles)	Same as above plus coma, convulsions

AChE, acetylcholinesterase; RBC, red blood cell.

Repeated exposures to OPs at doses not causing AChE inhibition do not cause either neuropsychiatric disorders or behavioural disturbances (Lotti, 1991b). Persistent electroencephalogram (EEG) changes have been reported in industrial workers who had repeated accidental exposures to sarin (a nerve agent OP). The exposures caused symptoms and significant inhibition of red blood cell (RBC) AChE. The toxicological significance of these EEG changes has, however, been questioned (Lotti, 1991b).

Urinary dimethyl(thio)phosphates and diethyl(thio)phosphates (metabolites of dimethoxy and diethoxy OPs, respectively), which represent the majority of OP insecticides, can be measured. Since OPs with different toxicity may give similar levels of urinary dialkyl(thio)phosphates, hazard can only be determined if such levels are calibrated against AChE inhibition. The time-course and peak of excretion of metabolites vary according to the compound (different rate of absorption, distribution and metabolism) (WHO, 1986a). The leaving group (X) is also excreted and it can be measured in urine. Since it is typical of one or two compounds only, its determination in the urine is specific. The time-course of urinary excretion of the leaving group can be different from that of the alkylphosphates deriving from the same molecule (Morgan *et al.*, 1977). The ACGIH proposes a biological exposure index (BEI) only for parathion by means of measuring *p*-nitrophenol at the end of a shift, the level of which should be less than 0.5 mgl^{-1} (ACGIH, 1991).

RBC AChE is biochemically similar to the synaptyc enzyme. High RBC AChE inhibition is diagnostic of acute OP poisoning. Interindividual variability of RBC AChE is high (coefficient of variation 13–16%) and pre-shift measurements are necessary to assess occupational exposure. The minimal differences for statistical recognition of inhibited RBC AChE vary from about 15% with one to about 12% with five pre-exposure values (Gallo and Lawryk, 1991). A 20–25% RBC AChE reduction of pre-shift values is diagnostic of exposure but is not indicative of hazard; 30–50% indicates overexposure; more than 50% may be accompanied by symptoms of intoxication (see Table 10.4) and the worker(s) must be removed from further exposure until AChE activity returns to within normal values (Plestina, 1984).

Plasma also contains pseudocholinesterases (butyrylcholinesterase), which can be inhibited by OPs. No physiological substrate for this enzyme is known and its inhibition has no known toxicological significance. Measurements of plasma pseudocholinesterase activity, however, can be used to monitor exposure to OPs, and its sensitivity to OP inhibition may be different from that of AChE, depending on the OP involved (Gallo and Lawryk, 1991). Interindividual variation of plasma pseudocholinesterase is similar to that of AChE.

Neuropathy target esterase (NTE) is present in peripheral lymphocytes and its inhibition predicts the development of OPIDP. The interindividual variation of lymphocyte NTE activity requires baseline values to evaluate the effects of exposures and situations are known where false positive and false negative results might arise (Lotti, 1989).

In acute OP poisoning the muscle response to single stimulation is repetitive while the nerve conduction velocity is usually normal or slightly slowed and the amplitude of the compound action potentials are very mildly reduced (Waida *et al.*, 1987). However, no such alterations were seen in exposed workers (Verbeck and Sallé, 1987; Stålberg *et al.*, 1978; Jušić *et al.*, 1980) or in subjects treated with an OP at doses causing about 50% of RBC AChE inhibition (Le Quesne and Maxwell, 1981). Thus, it appears that electromyography (EMG) is not a sensitive measurement of exposure to OPs, given also the low reproducibility of these methods in field conditions.

OPIDP patients may display small compound action potentials, prolonged terminal motor latencies, and electromyographical evidence of denervation with relative preservation of maximum motor conduction velocities (Lotti *et al.*, 1984).

Carbamates

The chemical structures of carbamates and dithiocarbamates are shown in Figure 10.1. Depending on the nature of the R^1 group, carbamates are divided into three groups as follows:

- R^1, methyl: insecticides and nematocides.

- R^1, aromatic group: herbicides and sprout inhibitors.

- R^1, benzimidazole group: fungicides.

Carbamate insecticides inhibit AChE, while herbicides and fungicides do not. Carbamylation of AChE is short lasting and regeneration of enzyme activity is rapid (reversible inhibition) when compared with that of phosphorylated AChE. Human exposure to carbamates is therefore less dangerous than that to OPs. Several cases of carbamate poisoning have been described; symptoms usually recover within a few hours after the end of exposure and parallel the reappearance of RBC AChE activity (WHO, 1986b).

Carbamates with herbicidal activity are not inhibitors of AChE because they have a bulky R^1 group attached to the nitrogen atom (see Figure 10.1). No characteristic toxic effect has been described in mammals for carbamate (phenmedipham, chlorpropham and others), thiocarbamate (molinate, diallate and others) and dithiocarbamate (sulphallate) herbicides. High doses of molinate given to rats have a reversible effect on sperm morphology and reproduction. However, in exposed workers no such alterations were found (WHO, 1987a).

Data on urinary metabolites of carbamates in humans are available for carbaryl and propoxur. Measurement of 1-naphthol in workers exposed to carbaryl should be carried out in urine voided 4–8 h after the end of exposure. Levels of 30 mgl^{-1} of urinary 1-naphthol after a 8 h shift are expected following exposures to 5 mgm^{-3} carbaryl (Maroni, 1988). Following exposure to propoxur, depression of RBC AChE is expected at urinary concentrations of 2-isopropoxyphenol higher than 5 mgl^{-1} (Maroni, 1988).

When exposures to carbamates are monitored by measuring RBC AChE, analytical methods must allow for spontaneous reactivation of AChE. Therefore, a short time of hydrolysis, minimal dilution of the sample and special care in the storage of blood are needed.

Dithiocarbamates

Dithiocarbamates are mainly used as fungicides, but they have other industrial uses (e.g. antioxidants, accelerators and slimicides). Few of them are also used as insecticides or herbicides. The chemical structure of dithiocarbamates is shown in Figure 10.1. Either R^1 or R^2 or both are

alkyl groups: the most used compounds are thiram, ziram and fer-
bam. When diamines are used for the synthesis, two terminal groups
are then linked via an ethylene bridge (ethylene-bis(dithiocarbamates)
(EBDC)) (see Figure 10.1): the most used compounds are maneb (R = Mn),
zineb (R = Zn) and mancozeb (R = Mn; a polymeric complex with zinc
salt). Under certain conditions (presence of oxygen and moisture), dithiocarbamates may decompose to, among other things, ethylenethiourea
(ETU).

The acute toxicity of dithiocarbamates is low and equivocal cases of
human intoxication have been reported. Dithiocarbamates cause alcohol
intolerance by interfering with alcohol metabolism (WHO, 1988b). High
doses of dithiocarbamates cause antithyroid effects in animals, possibly by
interfering with iodination of thyroxine precursors. Workers exposed to
dithiocarbamates have been studied in this respect, but neither alterations
of thyroid function (WHO, 1988b; A. Moretto and M. Lotti, unpublished
results) nor an increased incidence of thyroid tumours (IARC, 1987) were
found.

EBDCs are metabolised to ETU, carbon disulphide (CS_2), hydrogen
sulphide and many other compounds. From studies performed in alcoholic
subjects given disulphiram, it was concluded that measurement of blood
CS_2 levels may be useful for biological monitoring of exposure to dithiocarbamates (Maranelli *et al.*, 1991). Mean urinary excretion of ETU in workers
exposed to mancozeb or maneb was 2–4 mg per 24 h (Kurttio and
Savolainen, 1990). The half-life of urinary ETU was found to be about 100 h.
However, such a long half-life may have been due to occasional exposures
after completion of application (Kurttio *et al.*, 1990).

Pyrethroids

Pyrethroids are synthetic derivatives of the natural pyrethrins from *Chrys-
athemun cinerariaefolium* (see Figure 10.1). Characteristics include high
stability in the field (greater than that of OPs and carbamates), persistence
in soil lower than that of organochlorines, greater insecticidal potency and
low mammalian toxicity (rat LD_{50}/insect LD_{50} ratios are generally higher
than 1000, whereas they are in the range 1–50 for other pesticides) (Elliot,
1976).

Acute intoxication is characterised by dizziness, headache, nausea, muscular fasciculation, convulsive attacks and coma (He *et al.*, 1989; Chen *et
al.*, 1991). Two patterns of symptoms are described in rats after acute
intoxication, depending on the presence or the absence of an (α)cyano-
group substituent: the so-called 'T-syndrome' (aggressive sparring, sensitivity to external stimuli and tremor) and the 'CS-syndrome' (choreathetosis,
salivation and seizures), respectively. Sometimes, however, the two syndromes may combine to give a more complex one (Aldridge, 1990). Cases
of acute pyrethroid poisoning in China have been recently reviewed, but it

was not possible to differentiate the two syndromes in humans (He *et al.*, 1989).

Occupational exposures often result in abnormal skin sensations mainly of the face described as burning and tingling (He *et al.*, 1988; Chen *et al.*, 1991; Moretto, 1991; Zhang *et al.*, 1991). Symptoms appear shortly after beginning work and disappear within 24 h. Most pyrethroids cause these sensations with the following order of decreasing potency: deltamethrin > flucythrinate > cypermethrin = fenvalerate > permethrin (Aldridge, 1990). This neurotoxicity is due to a local effect because only unprotected parts of the skin are affected. Pyrethroids are known to act on sodium channels, thereby causing repetitive firing of sensory nerve endings of the skin (Aldridge, 1990).

Electrophysiological studies performed in the arms and legs of exposed subjects complaining of cutaneous sensations were negative (Le Quesne *et al.*, 1980).

Measurement of urinary levels of the parent compound and/or of metabolites after occupational exposure have been performed, but no correlation with the degree of cutaneous sensations was found (He *et al.*, 1988; Zhang *et al.*, 1991). This is consistent with the local nature of this type of neurotoxicity.

Organochlorines

Organochlorine (OC) insecticides include:

● Ethane derivatives (DDT and its analogues).

● Cyclodienes.

● Hexachlorocyclohexane (HCH) (or benzene hexachloride (BHC)) and lindane.

● Toxaphene (camphechlor) and related chemicals.

● Mirex and chlordecone.
  Chlordecone, mirex and toxaphene are no longer produced in significant amounts.

Different acute toxicities and toxicokinetics are displayed by individual OCs. In general, signs of acute poisoning are related to neuronal hyperexcitability. In the case of DDT and its analogues, for instance, signs of hyperexcitability are due to slowed repolarisation of neuronal membrane and appear in both the peripheral and the central nervous system. They are due to effects on sodium channels, thereby interfering with Na^+/K^+ flow across the membrane (Coats, 1982) with a mechanism similar to that of pyrethroids. The onset of DDT poisoning is characterised by mild effects that progress gradually to convulsions, whereas other OCs may induce convulsions without preceding signs (Smith, 1991).

DDT and its derivatives

DDT (1,1,1-trichloro-2,2-bis(4-chlorophenyl)ethane) (see Figure 10.1) has been extensively used, even by direct application to humans. Because of its accumulation along the food chain DDT was banned in many countries, but it is still used for vector control in many tropical countries. As extrapolated from human exposures, 10 mgkg^{-1} of DDT produces illness in some subjects (Smith, 1991). However, heavy exposure to concentrated DDT dust, as evidenced by workers being covered with DDT dust while working, did not cause adverse effects. Induction of liver microsomal enzymes was demonstrated in some heavily exposed workers (WHO, 1979). 2,2-bis(4-Chlorophenol)acetic acid (DDA) is the main urinary metabolite of DDT. DDA excretion peaks a few hours after intake and continues for several days (Roan *et al.*, 1971). Among workers whose DDT intake was of the order of 35 mg day^{-1}, urinary DDA was found to be 1.7 ppm on average. 1,1-Dichloro-2,2,-bis(4-chlorophenyl)ethylene (DDE) is the metabolite which is preferentially stored in fat. Low DDE as compared with total stored DDT residues indicates high and recent intake of DDT. Occupational exposure can be monitored either by measuring DDT and/or DDE in plasma or by measuring DDA urinary excretion (WHO, 1979).

TDE (tetrachlorodiphenylethane, sometimes called DDD (dichlorodiphenyldichloroethane), when a metabolite of DDT), ethylan, methoxychlor, chlorobenzilate and dicofol are less toxic than DDT, and cases of human poisoning have been reported only for chlorobenzilate (one case) and dicofol (one case) (Smith, 1991).

Cyclodienes

The cyclodienes used as insecticides include chlordane, heptachlor, endosulphan. Aldrin, isodrin, dieldrin, endrin and isobenzan are now banned or severely restricted in most countries. All cyclodienes are easily absorbed through the skin. These compounds differ in their toxicity, endrin being the more potent (rat oral LD$_{50}$: 10–40 mgkg^{-1}). Serious poisoning by these compounds usually causes convulsions which may appear without other preceding signs of illness (Rowley *et al.*, 1987).

Hexachlorocyclohexane and lindane

Both lindane (which is the γ-isomer of hexachlorocyclohexane (HCH) (see Figure 10.1) and HCH are absorbed through the skin. Lindane is rapidly excreted while the β-isomer, which is a CNS depressant, accounts for most of HCH residues in the organism. There are few reports of mild acute intoxication following occupational exposure to HCH or lindane: it is characterised by headache, tremors, vomiting, prostration, and convulsion (Smith, 1991). Studies on workers exposed to lindane for many years did not demonstrate any long-term adverse effect. Abnormal EEG patterns have been reported in workers exposed to HCH (Müller *et al.*, 1981), but not to lindane (Baumann *et al.*, 1981).

Chlorophenoxy compounds

2,4-Dichlorophenoxyacetic acid (2,4-D), 2,4,5-trichlorophenoxyacetic acid (2,4,5-T), 4-chloro-2-methylphenoxyacetic acid (MCPA) and 2-(2,4,5-tri-chlorophenoxy)propionic acid (silvex) are the most used chlorophenoxy herbicides (see Figure 10.1). The use of 2,4,5-T is restricted in several countries because commercial formulations might contain 2,3,7,8-tetrachloro-dibenzo-*p*-dioxin (TCDD) as an impurity. However, TCDD contamination has greatly diminished over the years due to improved industrial technology (IARC, 1986). These herbicides act against growth hormones in plants, but there is no known hormonal effect in mammals. Both 2,4-D and 2,4,5-T have moderate oral toxicity. Signs of toxicity include nausea and vomiting, myalgia, muscular hypertonia, headache, and changes in the electrocardiogram (WHO, 1984a). Chloracne has also been observed in workers exposed to 2,4,5-T, but this effect was thought to be due to 2,3,7,8-TCDD (see Table 10.5). Peripheral neuropathy in workers exposed to 2,3-D or 2,3,5-T has also been reported with slowed nerve conduction velocity in sural and median nerves (WHO, 1984a; Murphy, 1987).

Table 10.5. Pesticides causing allergic contact dermatitis (ACD) or orthoergic dermatitis (OD)*

	Type of dermatitis
Insecticides	
Organophosphorus compounds	
Dichlorvos	ACD
Naled	OD/ACD
Thiometon	ACD
Organochlorine compounds	
Aldrin	OD
DDT	OD †
Dicofol	ACD
Lindane and BHC	OD/ACD ‡
Pyrethrum	ACD
Herbicides	
2,4-D	OD ‡/ACD
2,4,5-T	OD §/ACD
Allidochlor	ACD
Atrazine	ACD
Cynazine	ACD
Dichlobenyl	OD

Table 10.5. (*Contd.*)

	Type of dermatitis
Diquat	OD ¶
MCPA	OD
Metholachlor	ACD
Nitrofen	OD
Paraquat	OD ¶
Phenmedipham	ACD
Propanyl	OD ‖
Propazine	OD ††
Simazine	OD
Fungicides	
1-Chlorodinitrobenzene	ACD
Benomyl	ACD
Captan	ACD
Captafol	OC/ACD
Chlortalonil	ACD
Dinocap	ACD
Imazalil	ACD
Mancozeb	ACD
Maneb	OD/ACD
Pentachlorophenol	OD §
Thiophanate-methyl	OD/ACD
Thiram	ACD
Zineb	OD/ACD
Ziram	OD
Rodenticides	
ANTU	ACD
Solvents and fumigants	
Kerosene	OD
Tetralin	OD
Xylene	OD
Inorganic and organometallic pesticides	
Arsenic and its compounds	OD
Chromium (sodium dichromate)	OD/ACD
Copper (cupric sulphate)	OD
Zinc (zinc chloride)	OD
Miscellaneous pesticides	
Chlorfenson	ACD
Propargite	ACD

DDT, 1,1,1-trichloro-2,2-bis(4-chlorophenyl)ethane; 2,4-D, 2,4-dichlorophenoxyacetic acid; 2,4,5-T, 2,4,5-trichlorophenoxyacetic acid; ANTU, α-napthylthiourea.
*Summarised from Hayes and Laws (1991).
† Due to solvents, mainly xylenes.
‡ Probably due to contaminants.
§ Chloracne was also described but it was likely caused by the contaminant TCDD (2,3,7,8-tetrachlorodibenzo-*p*-dioxin).
¶ Nail lesions also described.
‖ Also chloracne caused by impurities.
‡‡ Probably caused by intermediates in the synthesis.

Case-control studies have shown an association between cancer and occupational exposure to chlorophenoxy herbicides. However, elevated odd ratios for cancer at some sites were not consistent in independent studies as reviewed by IARC (IARC, 1986). Subsequently, more studies have been published showing variations in relative risk estimates for soft-tissue sarcomas, non-Hodgkin's lymphomas and Hodgkin's disease (Pearce and Reif, 1990). Recently, in a mortality study among farmers, a significant dose–response relationship was found between risk of non-Hodgkin's lymphoma and the use of some herbicides (Wigle *et al.*, 1990). The percentage of non-Hodgkin's lymphoma attributable to herbicide exposure was estimated to be 22% in this study. A cancer mortality study on an international cohort of workers exposed to chlorophenoxy herbicides showed a significant excess of mortality for soft-tissue sarcomas, but not for non-Hodgkin's lymphomas occurring in the period 10–19 years after the beginning of exposure (Saracci *et al.*, 1991).

Phenoxy acids can be absorbed through the skin and are mainly excreted unchanged in the urine (Lavy and Mattice, 1989). Concentration of 2,4-D or 2,4,5-T in urine after occupational exposure ranged from 1 to 32 mgl^{-1} in the absence of signs or symptoms of poisoning (IARC, 1986).

Bipyridyl compounds: paraquat and diquat

Paraquat (1,1'-dimethyl-4,4'-bipyridylium salts) and diquat (6,7-dihydro-dipyrido-1,1'-ethylene-2,2'-bipyridylium salts) are non-selective contact herbicides (see Figure 10.1). In cells, they undergo a single electron addition to form a free radical which reacts with molecular oxygen to reform the parent compound and concomitantly produce a superoxide anion. This oxygen radical may then be responsible for cell death.

Several cases of suicidal or accidental acute paraquat poisoning have been reported. The clinical picture is characterised by kidney and liver necrosis which is followed within a few weeks by pulmonary fibrosis. Lung toxicity is related to selective paraquat accumulation in the lung by an energy-dependent process (Smith *et al.*, 1979). Fatal poisoning was also associated with ingestion of the liquid concentrate which caused ulceration of the upper digestive tract. A small number of occupational poisonings have been described and were due to skin absorption (WHO 1984b; Hart, 1987; Smith, 1988). Biological monitoring of exposure may be carried out by measuring urinary paraquat excretion. Paraquat levels up to 0.76 mgl^{-1} have been found in exposed workers (Swan, 1969; Chester and Woolen, 1981). These values are more than one order of magnitude lower than those found in cases of acute poisoning (Hart, 1987). Pulmonary function in those workers was not affected.

Diquat poisoning is much less common than paraquat poisoning and causes kidney and liver necrosis, diarrhoea also being a prominent feature (WHO, 1984b). Lung fibrosis was never reported. Urinary diquat lower than 0.047 mgl^{-1} was found in workers with a dermal exposure up to 1.82 mgh^{-1} (Wojeck *et al.*, 1983).

Triazines

Figure 10.1 shows the chemical structure of the substituted *S*-triazine. The most used triazines are atrazine, cynazine, propazine and simazine. All compounds have low acute toxicity and no case of systemic poisoning has ever been described. In exposed workers atrazine is rapidly excreted both unmodified and as delkylated metabolites, the latter in much greater amounts (Catenacci *et al.*, 1990).

Amides

Alachlor and metholachlor (see Figure 10.1) are the most used herbicides. They have a very low acute toxicity (rat oral LD_{50} values are >1800 $mgkg^{-1}$) and cutaneous absorption is negligible (Stevens and Sumner 1991). Cases of accidental acute, non-lethal metholachlor intoxication have been described; symptoms were nausea, vomiting or diarrhoea, and headache (Stevens and Sumner, 1991).

Arsenical herbicides

Dimethylarsinic acid and methylarsonic acid are the only two arsenical compounds still in use as pesticides (Worthing and Hance, 1991). Their toxicity is low and neither acute nor long-term effects have been described in workers exposed to these compounds (WHO, 1981). These two arsenic derivatives are not carcinogens. However, they may contain inorganic arsenic (a recognised human carcinogen) as an impurity.

Dicarboximides

Captan, captafol and folpet belong to this group of fungicides. The use of captafol has been restricted or banned in many countries. Because of some structural similarities with thalidomide, these compounds were suspected teratogens, but animal studies were negative (Edwards *et al.*, 1991). Dermatitis was reported as a consequence of single exposures (Table 10.5). Although epidemiological studies are not available, captafol is classified in group 2A by IARC (1991) because of its carcinogenic effects in mice and rats.

Hexachlorobenzene

Hexachlorobenzene (HCB) (see Figure 10.1) is still used in some countries as a fungicide for seed treatment. Cases of poisoning following occupational exposure have not been reported. The epidemic of HCB poisoning (porphyria turcica) in Turkey during the 1950s was due to ingestion of wheat seedlings treated with HCB (Morris and Cabral, 1985).

Anticoagulant rodenticides

Anticoagulants used as rodenticides are antimetabolites of vitamin K and inhibit the synthesis of prothrombin (Echobichon, 1991). Warfarin was the first compound to be introduced; other anticoagulants include: coumafuryl, diphacinone, chlophacinone. The risk for workers is associated with accidental ingestion of massive doses.

Fluoroacetic acid and its derivatives

The most common compounds are (see Figure 10.1): sodium fluoroacetate (R = ONa), 2-fluoroacetamide (R = NH$_2$) and MNFA (R = N-methyl-N-1-naphtyl). These are among the most potent rodenticides (rat oral LD$_{50}$ 0.2 mgkg^{-1} for fluoroacetate and 4–15 mgkg^{-1} for fluoroacetamide) which are also highly toxic to man. The active compound is fluoroacetate which inhibits the citric acid cycle, thereby lowering energy production. The heart and central nervous system are the target organs and symptoms of severe poisoning include cyanosis, convulsions and alteration of heart rate. The cause of death is usually ventricular fibrillation or respiratory failure. There are no reports of occupational poisoning, but non-specific symptoms such as nausea, weakness, fatigue and minor electrocardiogram (ECG) alterations (bradycardia, prolonged PQ segment, U waves) in the absence of evident overexposure to MNFA have been reported (Pelfrene, 1991).

ANTU (α-naphtylthiourea)

ANTU (see Figure 10.1) is used as a rodenticide. Poisoning by ANTU is characterised by massive pulmonary oedema and pleural effusion. There is great variability in species' sensitivity to ANTU and humans appear to be relatively resistant. Neither death nor permanent sequelae have been described after accidental or intentional human poisoning with ANTU (IARC, 1983; Pelfrene, 1991). In some countries it has been withdrawn from use because of the presence of carcinogenic impurities such as β-napthylamines (Worthing and Hance, 1991).

1,2-Dibromo-3-chloropropane (DBCP)

DBCP (CH$_2$ Br–CHBr–CH$_2$Cl) is a soil fumigant and nematocide. DBCP is readily absorbed through the skin. Male rats repeatedly exposed for 7 h to 5 ppm of DBCP developed degeneration of seminiferous tubules, increased number of Sertoli cells, reduced sperm counts and abnormal sperm morphology (Torkelson *et al.*, 1961). A group of workers involved in DBCP production became aware that only a few of them had fathered children: 13% were found to be azoospermic, 17% oligospermic and 16% had low normal counts (Whorton *et al.*, 1979). Studies performed in another factory (Egnatz *et al.*, 1980) and in agricultural workers (Takahashi *et al.*, 1981) confirmed the effect of DBCP exposure on testicular function. The levels of DBCP in air of the two factories were reported to be 1 ppm or less. A 7-year follow-up showed that no major improvements in testicular function of the azoospermic/oligospermic workers took place (Eaton *et al.*, 1986).

1,2-Dibromoethane

1,2-Dibromoethane (CH_2Br–CH_2Br), also known as ethylene dibromide (EDB), is used as a crop and soil fumigant. EDB is readily absorbed from the skin, lung and gastrointestinal tract. EDB is metabolised either to bromoacetaldehyde, or to (2*S*)-bromoethylglutathione which is responsible for hepatotoxicity (White *et al.*, 1983).

Workers of the papaya fumigation industry exposed to EDB had statistically significant decreases in sperm count and motility, and increased morphological sperm abnormalities (Ratcliff *et al.*, 1987). This is consistent with experimental data (Short *et al.*, 1979). Workers had an average duration of exposure of 5 years and a geometric mean breathing zone exposure to EDB of 88 ppb (8 hours time weighted average) with peaks up to 262 ppb. In five other epidemiological studies no significant reproductive effect of exposure to EDB was demonstrated, but the potency of these studies was questioned (Dobbins, 1987).

Hydrogen cyanide

Hydrogen cyanide (HCN) is an insecticidal fumigant. Toxicity is due to the block of cellular respiration (Smith, 1991). Occupational exposure occurs through inhalation, while accidental and intentional poisoning usually involves ingestion of a cyanide salt. Lower doses cause at first, stimulation of respiration and heart rate; venous blood remains oxygenated and the patient is not cyanotic. Then respiration becomes slow and gasping until it stops. In the past some applicators died after careless handling of cyanide, but when used by trained applicators its safety record is good. Biomonitoring of cyanide exposure can be carried out by measuring urinary excretion of thiocyanates (Lauwerys, 1983). However, thiocyanates are present in variable amounts in non-exposed subjects, and higher levels are found in smokers (Bertelli *et al.*, 1984). The suggested limit for post-shift urinary thiocyanates is 2.5 mgg^{-1} of creatinine for non-smokers (Lauwerys, 1983).

Dinitrophenols

Derivatives of 2,4-dinitrophenol ($R_1 = R_2 = H$ in Figure 10.1) are used as herbicides, fungicides or insecticides. All share the same mechanism of toxicity in mammals, although they may differ in their ability to be absorbed through the skin (Gasiewicz, 1991). These compounds exert their toxic effect by uncoupling oxidative phosphorylation. The most used compounds are 2,4-dinitrophenol (wood preservative and woodworm insecticide), DNOC ($R_1 - H$, $R_2 = CH_3$, insecticide and fungicide; no longer used in many Western countries), dinocap (R_1 = H, R_2 = 1-methyl-n-heptyl, acaricide and fungicide), and dinoseb (R_1 = COCH=CHCH$_3$, R_2 = sec-butyl, herbicide). The best known of these compounds is DNOC which is easily absorbed by the skin: signs and symptoms of acute DNOC and 2,4-dinitrophenol intoxication include fatigue, restlessness and excessive sweating. Fatal hyperthermia may occur. Biological monitoring of workers exposed to DNOC involves the measurement of the parent compound in the blood. A 10 ppm threshold in blood has been suggested (Lauwerys, 1983). Symptoms appear at or above 30 ppm, while 50 ppm is considered dangerous (Gasiewicz, 1991). Dinocap and dinoseb have a lower acute toxicity.

Pentachlorophenol and related compounds

The structural formula of pentachlorophenol (PCP) is shown in Figure 10.1. The technical product is a mixture of PCP, tetrachlorophenol and traces of chlorinated dibenzo-p-dioxins, polychlorinated dibenzofurans and polychlorobenzenes (WHO, 1987a). In recent years, improved technologies have led to a decreased concentration of impurities (Smith, 1991; Gasiewicz, 1991). PCP and its salts (mainly Na-PCP) have a variety of applications in industry and in agriculture as algicides, bactericides, fungicides, herbicides, insecticides, and molluscicides, but their main use is as wood preservatives. Recently, strict limits on PCP uses other than wood preservative have been established in many countries because of concern for the effects both to humans and to the environment (especially on aquatic organisms) (WHO, 1987b). Several cases of human poisoning have been described, mainly after skin exposure. In workers exposed to a mixture of tetrachlorophenol (20%) and PCP (3%), it was calculated that 30–100% of the dose deposited on the skin was absorbed (Fenske et al., 1987). Acute signs of intoxication resemble those elicited by nitrophenolic compounds, being characterised by a marked increase in metabolic rate due to the uncoupling of oxidative phosphorylation. Fatal cases are always associated with a marked rise in temperature and terminal spasm (Wood et al., 1983; WHO, 1987b). Reversible and non-specific liver and kidney functional changes have been described after exposure to PCP (WHO, 1987b). Monitoring of exposure can be performed by measuring urinary excretion of PCP; post-shift levels of 1 mgg^{-1} of creatinine (Lauwerys, 1983) or 2 mgg^{-1} of creatinine prior to the last shift of the workweek (ACGIH, 1991) have been proposed as permissible values. ACGIH (1991) also proposed an end-of-shift free PCP plasma concentration of 5 mgl^{-1}.

Triphenyltin compounds

Triphenyltin (fentin) acetate and triphenyltin hydroxide (see Figure 10.1) are used as fungicides and molluscicides. Few cases of human poisoning have been described. Symptoms were dizziness, nausea, skin irritation and liver damage. Recently, a case of acute dermal poisoning by fentin acetate has been described (Colosio *et al.*, 1991). The prominent features were urticaria on trunk and arms and genital oedema. The patient suffered from periodic urticaria during the following 5 months. Patch tests with the commercial formulation and the pure component of the formulation were negative. During the acute phase EEG alterations were also observed. Urinary excretion and blood levels of tin showed biphasic kinetics suggesting the possibility of accumulation.

Sources of further information

Books

The most comprehensive book on pesticide toxicology is the *Handbook of Pesticide Toxicology* (Hayes Jr, W. J. and Laws Jr, E. R. (Eds), Academic Press, San Diego, 1991). The edition published in 1991 is the updated combination of two previously published books, namely *Toxicology of Pesticides* (Hayes Jr, W. J. (Ed.), Williams and Wilkins, Baltimore, 1975) and *Pesticides Studied in Man* (Hayes Jr, W. J. (Ed.), Williams and Wilkins, Baltimore, 1982). The book reports most of the animal and human toxicological data available in the open literature.

Other reference books include:

- *The Pesticide Manual* (Worthing, C. R. and Hance, R. J. (Eds), British Crop Protection Council, Thornton Heath, UK, 1991, 9th Edn.), which lists all commercially available compounds and for each of them essential information on nomenclature, development, physicochemical properties, uses, toxicology, formulation and method of analysis (with references) is given. A new edition is published at 3/4-yearly intervals.

- *Farm Chemicals Handbook* (Poplyk, J. (Ed.), Meister, Willoughby, OH); it contains a pesticide dictionary where compounds are listed with their common and commercial names, and essential information on chemistry, uses, toxicology. It also contains an extensive list of company addresses. It is published yearly.

- *Pesticides. Synonyms and Chemical Names* (Commonwealth Department of Health, Australia), lists alphabetically all common names (including rejected and discontinued) and trade names, and reports their chemical name.

- *Casarett and Doull's Toxicology. The Basic Science of Poisons* (Amdur, M. O., Doull, J. and Klaassen, C. D. (Eds), Macmillan, New York,

1991, 4th Edn.). A whole chapter by D. Ecobichon is devoted to the toxicology of pesticides.

Series

The United Nations Environment Programme, the International Labour Organisation, and the WHO sponsor, through the International Programme on Chemical Safety, the publication of reports on chemicals, group of chemicals or general toxicological problems in a series called *Environmental Health Criteria*. Some of the volumes deal with a single pesticide or a group of pesticides and review all available data on properties, analytical methods, environmental distribution, effect of residues, kinetics and metabolism, effects on animals and on man. The books may be obtained from WHO, Geneva.

The same Organisations also publish a series called *Health and Safety Guide* where essential information (20–30 pages) on single chemical substances (including many pesticides) is given. The booklets may be obtained from WHO, Geneva.

Each year a Joint Meeting of the Food and Agriculture Organization Panel of Experts on Pesticides Residues in Food and the Environment and the WHO Expert Group on Pesticide Residues is held and a monograph is published afterwards. These monographs summarise for each pesticide considered the safety data (both published in the open literature and confidentially provided by the manufacturer) on which a decision regarding the acceptable daily intake is made. The monographs were published by the FAO, Rome, Italy. Since 1990 they are published by WHO, Geneva, Switzerland.

The International Agency for Research on Cancer (IARC) publishes the *IARC Monographs on the Evaluation of Carcinogenic Risks to Human*. The results of the evaluation of pesticides have been published in Volumes 4, 5, 12, 15, 30, 53 and Supplement 7. The monographs may be obtained from the IARC, Lyon.

References

ACGIH, 1991, *1991–1992 Threshold Limit Values for Chemical Substances and Physical Agents and Biological Exposure Indices*. Cincinnati, OH: ACGIH.

Aldridge, W. N., 1990, An assessment of the toxicological properties of pyrethroids and their neurotoxicity, *Crit. Rev. Toxicol.*, **21**, 89–104.

Baker Jr, E. L., Zack, M., Miles, J. W., Alderman, L., Warren, M., Dobbin, R. D., Miller, S., and Teeters, W. R., 1978, Epidemic malathion poisoning in Pakistan malaria workers, *Lancet*, **i**, 31–4.

Baumann, K., Behling, K., Brassow, H. L. and Stapel, K., 1981, Occupational exposure to hexachlorocyclohexane. III. Neurophysiological findings and neuromuscular function in chronically exposed workers, *Int. Arch. Occup. Environ. Health*, **48**, 165–72.

Bertelli, G., Berlin, A., Roi, R. and Alessio, L., 1984, Acrylonitrile, in Alessio, L., Berlin, A., Boni, M. and Roi, R. (Eds) *Biological Indicators for the Assessment of Human Exposure to Industrial Chemicals*, pp. 1–16. Brussels/Luxembourg: Commission of the European Communities.

Catenacci, G., Maroni, M., Cottica, D. and Pozzoli, L., 1990, Assessment of human exposure to atrazine through the determination of free atrazine in urine, *Bull. Environ. Contam. Toxicol.*, **44**, 1–7.

Chen, S., Zhang, Z., He, F. Yao, P., Wu, Y., Sun, J., Liu, L., and Li, Q., 1991, An epidemiological study on occupational acute pyrethroid poisoning in cotton farmers, *Br. J. Ind. Med.*, **48**, 77–81.

Chester, G. and Woollen, B. H., 1981, Studies of the occupational exposure of Malaysian plantation workers to paraquat, *Br. J. Ind. Med.*, **38**, 23–33.

Coats, J. R., 1982, Structure–activity relationships in DDT analogs, in Coats, J. R. (Ed.) *Insecticide Mode of Action*, pp. 29–43. New York: Academic Press.

Colosio, C., Tomasini, M., Cairoli, S., Foa, V., Minoia, C., Marinovich, M., and Cralli, C. L., 1991, Occupational triphenyltin acetate poisoning: a case report, *Br. J. Ind. Med.*, **48**, 136–9.

Currie, K. L., McDonald, E. C., Chung, L. T. K. and Higgs, A. R., 1990, Concentrations of diazinon, chlorpyrifos, and bendiocarb after application in offices, *Am. Ind. Hyg. Assoc. J.*, **51**, 23–7.

Davis, J. E., Staiff, D. C., Butler, L. C. and Stevens, E. R., 1981, Potential exposure to dislodgable residues after application of two formulation of methyl parathion to apple trees, *Bull. Environ. Contam. Toxicol.*, **27**, 95–100.

Dobbins, J. G., 1987, Regulation and the use of 'negative' results from human reproductive studies: the case of ethylene dibromide, *Am. J. Ind. Med.*, **12**, 33–45.

Eaton, M., Schenker, M., Whorton, M. D., Samuels, S., Perkins, C. and Overstreet, J., 1986, Seven-year follow-up of workers exposed to 1,2-dibromo-3-chloropropane, *J. Occup. Med.*, **28**, 1145–50.

Echobichon, D. J., 1991, Toxic effects of pesticides, in Amdur, M. O., Doull, J. and Klaassen, C. D. (Eds) *Casarett and Doull's Toxicology. The Basic Science of Poison*, pp. 565–622. New York: McMillan.

Edwards, R. I., Ferry, D. H. and Temple, W. A., 1991, Fungicides and related compounds, in Hayes Jr, W. J. and Laws Jr, E. R. (Eds) *Handbook of Pesticide Toxicology*, pp. 1409–70. San Diego: Academic Press.

Egnatz, D. G., Ott, M. G., Townsend, J. C., Olson, R. D. and Johns, D. B., 1980, DBCP and testicular effects in chemical workers: an epidemiological survey in Midland, Michigan, *J. Occup. Med.*, **22**, 727–32.

Elliot, M., 1976, Properties and applications of pyrethroids, *Environ. Health Perspect.*, **14**, 3–13.

Fenske, R. A., Horstman, S. W. and Bentley, R. K., 1987, Assessment of dermal exposure to chlorophenols in timber mills, *Appl. Ind. Hyg.*, **2**, 143–7.

Gallo, M. A. and Lawryk, N. J., 1991, Organic phosphorus compounds, in Hayes Jr, W. J. and Laws Jr, E. R. (Eds) *Handbook of Pesticide Toxicology*, pp. 917–1123. San Diego: Academic Press.

Gasiewicz, T. A., 1991, Nitro compounds and related phenolic pesticides, in Hayes Jr, W. J. and Laws Jr, E. R. (Eds) *Handbook of Pesticide Toxicology*, pp. 1191–269. San Diego: Academic Press.

Hart, T. B., 1987, Paraquat: a review of safety in agricultural and horticultural use, *Human Toxicol.*, **6**, 13–18.

Hayes Jr, W. J. and Laws Jr, E. R. (Eds), 1991, *Handbook of Pesticide Toxicology*. San Diego: Academic Press.

He, F., Sun, J., Han, K., Wu, Y., Yao, P., Wang, S., and Liu, L., 1988, Effects of pyrethoid insecticides on subjects engaged in packaging pyrethoids, *Br. J. Ind. Med.*, **45**, 548–51.

He, F., Wang, S., Liu, L., Chen, S., Zhang, Z. and Sun, J., 1989, Clinical manifestations and diagnosis of acute pyrethroid poisoning, *Arch. Toxicol.*, **63**, 54–8.

Hodgson, M. J., Block, G. D. and Parkinson, D. K., 1986, Organophosphate poisoning in office workers, *J. Occup. Med.*, **28**, 434–7.

IARC, 1983, *IARC monographs on the Evaluation of Carcinogenic Risks to Humans, Vol. 30, Miscellaneous Pesticides*, Lyon: IARC.

IARC, 1986, *IARC Monographs on the Evaluation of Carcinogenic Risks to Humans, Vol. 41, Some Halogenated Hydrocarbons and Pesticide Exposures*. Lyon: IARC.

IARC. The IARC monographs on the evaluation of carcinogenic risks to humans. Overall evaluations of carcinogenicity: an updating of IARC Monographs Volumes 1 to 42. Lyon, France, IARC, 1987.

IARC, 1991, *IARC Monographs on the Evaluation of Carcinogenic Risks to Humans, Vol. 53, Some Pesticides and Occupational Exposures in Insecticide Application*. Lyon: IARC.

Jeyaratnam, J., 1990, Acute pesticide poisoning: a major health problem, *World Health Stat. Q.*, **43**, 139–44.

Jušić, A., Jurenic, D. and Milic, S., 1980, Electromyographical neuromuscular synapse testing and neurological findings in workers exposed to organophosphorus pesticides, *Arch. Environ. Health*, **35**, 168–75.

Keplinger, M. L. and Deichmann, W. B., 1967, Acute toxicity of combinations of pesticides, *Toxicol. Appl. Pharmacol.*, **10**, 586–95.

Kurttio, P. and Savolainen, K., 1990, Ethylenethiourea in air and in urine as an indicator of exposure to ethylenebidithiocarbamate fungicides, *Scand. J. Work Environ. Health*, **16**, 203–7.

Kurttio, P., Vartiainen, T. and Savolainen, K., 1990, Environmental and biological monitoring of exposure to ethylenebisdithiocarbamate fungicides and ethylenethiourea, *Br. J. Ind. Med.*, **47**, 203–6.

Lauwerys, R., 1983, *Industrial Chemical Exposure: Guidelines for Biological Monitoring*. Davis: Biomedical Publications.

Lavy, T. L. and Mattice, J. D., 1989, Biological monitoring techniques for human exposed to pesticides. Use, development, and recommended refinements, in Wang, R. G. M., Franklin, C. A., Honeycutt, R. C. and Reinert, J. C. (Eds), *Biological Monitoring for Pesticide Exposure. Measurement, Estimation, and Risk Reduction (ACS Symposium Series 382)*, pp. 192–205. Washington, DC: American Chemical Society.

Le Quesne, P. M., Maxwell, I. C. and Butterworth, S. T. G., 1980, Transient facial sensory symptoms following exposure to synthetic pyrethroids: a clinical and electrophysiological assessment, *Neurotoxicology*, **2**, 1–11.

Le Quesne, P. M. and Maxwell, I. C., 1981, Effect of metrifonate on neuromuscolar transmision, *Acta Pharmacol. Toxicol. Scand.*, **49** (Suppl. 5), 99–104.

Lotti, M., 1989, Neuropathy target esterase in blood lymphocytes. Monitoring the interaction of organophosphates with a primary target, in Wang, R. G. M., Franklin, C. A., Honeycutt, R. C. and Reinert, J. C. (Eds), *Biological Monitoring for Pesticides Exposure: Measurement, Estimation and Risk Reduction (ACS Symposium Series No. 382)*, pp. 117–23. Washington, DC: American Chemical Society.

Lotti, M., 1991a, Treatment of acute organophosphate poisoning, *Med. J. Aust.*, **154**, 51–5.

Lotti, M., 1991b, Central neurotoxicity and neurobehavioural toxicity of anticholinesterases, in Ballantyne, B. and Marrs, T. C. (Eds), *Basic and Clinical Toxicology of Organophosphates and Carbamates*, pp. 75–83. London: Butterworths.

Lotti, M., 1992, The pathogenesis of organophosphate induced delayed polyneuropathy, *Crit. Rev. Toxicol.*, **21**, 465–87.

Lotti, M., Becker, C. E. and Aminoff, M. J., 1984, Organophosphate polyneuropathy: pathogenesis and prevention, *Neurology*, **34**, 658–62.

Maranelli, G., Perbellini, L., Romeo, L., Caroldi, S., Bassi, G., Betta, A. and Brognone, F., 1991, Solfuro di carbonio ematico nel monitoraggio biologico dell'esposizione a ditiocarbammati, in Giuliano, G. and Paoletti, A. (Eds), *Proceedings of the LIV National Meeting of the Società Italiana di Medicina del Lavoro e Igiene Industriale*, pp. 1251–6. Bologna: Monduzzi Editore.

Maroni, M., 1988, Carbamate pesticides, in Alessio, L., Berlin, A., Boni, M. and Roi, R. (Eds), *Biological Indicators for the Assessment of Human Exposure to Industrial Chemicals*, pp. 27–54. Luxembourg: Commission of the European Communities.

Mehler, L., Edmiston, S., Richmond, D., O'Malley, M. and Krieger, R. I., 1990, Summary of illnesses and injuries reported by California physicians as potentially related to pesticides—1988, *HS-1541*. Sacramento: California Department of Food and Agriculture.

Miyamoto, J., 1976, Degradation, metabolism, and toxicity of synthetic pyrethroids, *Environ. Health Perspect.*, **14**, 15–28.

Moretto, A., 1991, Indoor spraying with the pyrethroid insecticide λ-cyhalothrin: effects on spraymen and inhabitants of sprayed houses, *Bull. World Health Org.*, **69**, 59–94.

Morgan, D. P., Hetzler, H. L., Slach, E. F. and Lin, L. I., 1977, Urinary excretion of paranitrophenol and alkyl phosphates following ingestion of methyl or ethyl parathion by human subjects, *Arch. Environ. Contam. Toxicol.*, **6**, 159–73.

Morris, C. R. and Cabral, J. R. P., 1985, *Hexachlorobenzene: Proceedings of an International Symposium*. Lyon: IARC.

Müller, D., Klepel, H., Macholz, R. and Knoll, R., 1981, Electroneurographic and electroencephalographic finding in patients exposed to hexachlorocyclohexane, *Psychiatr. Neurol. Med. Psycol.*, **33**, 468–72.

Nigg, H. N., Stamper, J. H. and Queen, R. M., 1984, The development and use of a universal model to predict tree crop harvester pesticide exposure, *Am. Ind. Hyg. Assoc. J.*, **45**, 182–6.

Pearce, N. and Reif, J. S., 1990, Epidemiologic studies of cancer in agricultural workers, *Am. J. Ind. Med.*, **18**, 133–48.

Pelfrene, A. F., 1991, Synthetic organic rodenticides, in Hayes Jr, W. J. and Laws Jr, E. R. (Eds), *Handbook of Pesticide Toxicology*, pp. 1271–316. San Diego: Academic Press.

Plestina, R., 1984, Prevention, diagnosis and treatment of insecticide poisoning. *WHO/VBC/ 84.889*. Geneva: WHO.

Popendorf, W. J. and Leffingwell, J. T., 1982, Regulating OP pesticide residues for farmworker protection, *Res. Rev.*, **82**, 125–201.

Ratcliff, J. M., Schrader, S. M., Steenland, K., Clapp, D. E., Turner, T. and Hornung, R. W., 1987, Semen quality in papaya workers with long term exposure to ethylene dibromide, *Br. J. Ind. Med.*, **44**, 317–26.

Roan, C., Morgan, D. and Paschal, E. H., 1971, Urinary excretion of DDA following ingestion of DDT and DDT metabolites in man, *Arch. Environ. Health*, **22**, 309–15.

Rowley, D. L., Rab, M. A., Hardjotanojo, W., Liddle, J., Burse, V. W., Saleem, M., Sokal, D., Faik, H., and Head, S. L., 1987, Convulsions caused by endrin poisoning in Pakistan, *Pediatrics*, **79**, 928–34.

Salem, H. and Olajos, E. J., 1988, Review of pesticides: chemistry, uses and toxicology, *Toxicol. Ind. Health*, **4**, 291–321.

Saracci, R., Kogevinas, M., Bertazzi, P. A., *et al.*, 1991, Cancer mortality in workers exposed to chlophenoxy herbicides and chlorophenols, *Lancet*, **338**, 1027–32.

Senanayake, N. and Karalleide, L., 1987, Neurotoxic effects of organophosphorus insecticides. An Intermediate syndrome, *N. Engl. J. Med.*, **316**, 761–3.

Short, R. D., Winston, M., Hong, C. B., Minor, J. L., Lee, C. C. and Seifter, J., 1979, Effects of ethylene dibromide on reproduction in male and female rats, *Toxicol. Appl. Pharmacol.*, **49**, 97–105.

Smith, A. G., 1991, Chlorinated hydrocarbon insecticides, in Hayes Jr, W. J. and Laws Jr, E. R. (Eds), *Handbook of Pesticide Toxicology*, pp. 731–95. San Diego: Academic Press.

Smith, J. G., 1988, Paraquat poisoning by skin absorption: a review, *Human Toxicol.*, **7**, 15–19.

Smith, L. L., Rose, M. S. and Wyatt, I., 1979, The pathology and biochemistry of paraquat, in *Oxygen Free Radicals and Tissue Damage (Ciba Foundation Series 65 (new series))*, pp. 321–47. Amsterdam: Excerpta Medica.

Smith, R. P., 1991, Toxic responses of the blood, in Amdur, M. O., Doull, J. and Klaassen, C. D. (Eds), *Casarett and Doull's Toxicology. The Basic Science of Poison*, pp. 257–81. New York: McMillan.

Spear, R. C., Jenkins, D. and Milby, T. H., 1975, Pesticide residues and field workers, *Environ. Sci. Technol.*, **9**, 308–13.

Spear, R. C., Popendorf, W. J., Leffingwell, J. T., Milby, T. H., Davies, J. E. and Spencer, W. F., 1977, Fieldworkers' response to weathered residues of parathion, *J. Occup. Med.*, **19**, 406–10.

Stålberg, E., Hilton-Brown, P., Kolmodin-Hedman, B., Holmstedt, B. and Augustinsson, K. B., 1978, Effect of occupational exposure to organophosphorus insecticides on neuromuscular function. *Scand. J. Work Environ. Health*, **4**, 255–61.

Stevens, H. T. and Sumner, D. D., 1991, Herbicides, in Hayes Jr, W. J. and Laws Jr, E. R. (Eds), *Handbook of Pesticide Toxicology*, pp. 1317–468. San Diego: Academic Press.

Swan, A. A. B., 1969, Exposure of spray operators to paraquat, *Br. J. Ind. Med.*, **26**, 322–9.

Takahashi, W., Wong, L., Rogers, B. J. and Hale, R. W., 1981, Depression of sperm counts among agricultural workers exposed to dibromochloropropane and ethylene dibromide, *Bull. Environm. Contam. Toxicol.*, **27**, 551–8.

Talcott, R. E., Mallipudi, N. M., Umetsu, N. and Fukuto, T. R., 1979, Inactivation of esterases by impurities isolated from technical malathion, *Toxicol. Appl. Pharmacol.*, **49**, 107–12.

Torkelson, T. R., Sadek, S. E., Rowe, V. K., Kodama, J. K., Anderson, H. H., Loquvam, G. S. and Hine, C. H., 1961, Toxicologic investigations of 1,2-dibromo-3-chloropropane, *Toxicol. Appl. Pharmacol.*, **3**, 545–59.

Verberk, M. M. and Sallé, H. J. A., 1987, Effects on nervous function in volunteers ingesting mevinphos for one month, *Toxicol. Appl. Pharmacol.*, **42**, 351–8.

Waida, R. S., Chitra, S., Amin, R. B., Kiwalkar, R. S. and Sardesai, H. V., 1987, Electrophysiological studies in acute organophosphate poisoning, *J. Neurol. Neurosurg. Psych.*, **50**, 1442–8.

White, R. D., Gandolfi, A. J., Bowden, G. T. and Sipes, I. G., 1983, Deuterium isotope effect on the metabolism and toxicity of 1,2-dibromoethane, *Toxicol. Appl. Pharmacol.*, **69**, 170–8.

WHO, 1979, *Environmental Health Criteria 9. DDT and its Derivatives*. Geneva: WHO.

WHO, 1981, *Environmental Health Criteria 18. Arsenic*. Geneva: WHO.

WHO, 1984a, *Environmental Health Criteria 29. 2,4-Dichlorophenoxyacetic Acid (2,4-D)*. Geneva: WHO.

WHO, 1984b, *Environmental Health Criteria 39. Paraquat and Diquat*. Geneva: WHO.

WHO, 1986a, *Environmental Health Criteria 63. Carbamate Pesticides: A General Introduction.* Geneva: WHO.

WHO, 1986b, *Environmental Health Criteria 63. Organophosphorus Insecticides: A General Introduction.* Geneva: WHO.

WHO, 1987a, *Environmental Health Criteria 71. Pentachlorophenol.* Geneva: WHO.

WHO Regional Office for Europe, 1987b, *Environmental Health 27, Drinking-water Quality: Guidelines for Selected Herbicides.* Copenhagen: WHO.

WHO, 1988a, The WHO recommended classification of pesticides by hazard and guidelines to the classification 1988–1989, *WHO/VBC/88.953.* WHO: Geneva.

WHO, 1988b, *Environmental Health Criteria 78. Dithiocarbamate Pesticides, Ethylenethiourea, and Propylenethiourea: A General Introduction.* Geneva: WHO.

WHO, 1990, *Public Health Impact of Pesticides used in Agriculture.* Geneva: World Health Organisation.

Whorton, D., Milby, T. H., Krauss, R. M. and Stubbs, H. A., 1979, Testicular function in DBCP exposed pesticide workers, *J. Occup. Med.*, 21, 161–6.

Wigle, D. T., Semenciw, R. M., Wilkins, K., Riedel, D., Ritter, L., Morrison, H. I., and Mao, Y., 1990, Mortality study of Canadian male farm operators: non-Hodgkin's lymphoma mortality and agricultural practices in Saskatchewan, *J. Natl. Cancer Inst.*, 82, 575–82.

Wojeck, G. A., Price, J. F., Nigg, H. N. and Stamper, J. H., 1983, Worker exposure to paraquat and diquat, *Arch. Environ. Contam. Toxicol.*, 12, 65–70.

Wood, S., Rom, W. M., White, G. L. and Logan, D. C., 1983, Pentachlorophenol poisoning, *J. Occup. Med.*, 25, 527–30.

Worthing, C. R. and Hance, R. J. (Eds), 1991, *The Pesticide Manual. A World Compendium*, 9th Edn. Thornton Heath, UK: The British Crop Protection Council.

Zhang, Z., Sun, J., Chen, S., Wu, Y. and He, F., 1991, Levels of exposure and biological monitoring of pyrethroid of spraymen, *Br. J. Ind. Med.*, 48, 82–6.

Chapter 11

Toxicity of Solvents

N. H. Stacey

Introduction

A solvent can be defined as a substance that has the power of dissolving. It forms the major part of a solution with the other part being the solute. Thus the solute is the substance that has been dissolved in the solvent. Most often when we refer to a solution we are considering a liquid dissolved in a liquid, a solid dissolved in a liquid or a gas dissolved in a liquid. In occupational toxicology discussion of solvents almost invariably relates to organic rather than aqueous solvents. Accordingly, this chapter is confined to organic solvents.

Organic solvents may be classified into two categories:

● Unsubstituted hydrocarbons.

● Hydrocarbons bearing functional group(s).

Table 11.1. Unsubstituted hydrocarbon solvents

Class	Example	Structure
Straight-chain paraffins	*n*-Hexane	$CH_3CH_2CH_2CH_2CH_2CH_3$
Branched-chain paraffins	Isohexane (2-methylpentane)	$CH_3CHCH_2CH_2CH_3$ 　　$\vert$ 　　CH_3
Olefins	1-Hexene	$CH_2{=}CHCH_2CH_2CH_2CH_3$
Naphthenes	Cyclohexane	
Aromatic compounds	Benzene	

Examples of these are given in Tables 11.1 and 11.2. Organic solvents have a wide range of uses which are summarised in Table 11.3, which also shows the proportion of solvent use in the various major use categories.

Table 11.2. Hydrocarbons bearing functional group(s) as solvents

Class	Example	Structure*
Ketones	Acetone	$CH_3-\overset{\displaystyle \|}{\underset{\displaystyle O}{C}}-CH_3$
Alcohols	Ethanol	C_2H_5-OH
Glycols	Ethylene glycol	$HO-CH_2CH_2-OH$
Ethers	Diethyl ether	$C_2H_5-O-C_2H_5$
Esters	Ethyl acetate	$CH_3-\overset{\displaystyle \|}{\underset{\displaystyle O}{C}}-O-C_2H_5$
Chlorinated hydrocarbons	Trichloroethylene	$Cl-CHC-Cl_2$

*Functional groups are in bold type.

Table 11.3. Uses of solvents*

Application	Percentage use
Surface coatings	43.3
Metal cleaning (degreasing)	10
Household products	8.1
Adhesives	6.7
Pharmaceuticals	6.1
Dry cleaning	3.9
Other	20

*Adapted from Collings and Luxon (1982).

As can be partly predicted from the above pattern of solvent use some of the main workplaces/work activities using solvents include automotive with spray painting, woodworking/furnishing, metal trades, printing, plastics/petrochemicals, dry cleaning, laboratories, building and agriculture.

A wide range of solvents is used in the surface coating industry because of the many different types and requirements of products. For example, toluene and xylene figure prominently in spray painting in the automotive industry. Adhesives also call on the varying properties of the different solvents for various product applications. Metal cleaning is a little more specific in its requirements, with chlorinated solvents such as trichloroethylene and 1,1,1-trichloroethane finding considerable application in vapour degreasing. In dry cleaning, tetrachloroethylene (perchloroethylene) is the most widely used solvent.

It should be noted that for many of the applications to which solvents are put it is their ability to vaporise readily that makes them desirable. This very property and use means that they readily get into the air and, unless contained or removed by ventilation, will be found in the workplace air. This is probably why they form a group of chemicals that are of considerable and continuing concern in the workplace. That is, there is substantial scope for the worker to be exposed, which is a prerequisite to the toxicity of a chemical having the opportunity to manifest its actions.

Apart from the ability of a solvent to vaporise, which is related to its vapour pressure, there are other physical properties that need to be considered when using them in the workplace. These relate to safety aspects particularly and include, for example, boiling range, flashpoint, fire point and flammable range.

To provide an indication of the extent of solvent production figures are provided in Table 11.4 for solvent consumption.

Table 11.4. Consumption of solvents*

Solvent class	Tonnes ($\times 10^3$)
Aliphatic hydrocarbons	1200
Aromatic hydrocarbons	900
Chlorinated hydrocarbons	800
Alcohols	600
Ketones	450
Esters	300
Glycol ethers	150

*Adapted from Collings and Luxon (1982).

Toxicity

In general, solvents cause two main types of toxic response to workers. These are to the skin and to the central nervous system. Both probably relate to the lipophilic nature of organic solvents. With the skin, their ability to dissolve lipid or fatty materials enables them to dissolve the fats in the skin on contact and thereby give rise to a dermatitis. Similarly, this property of solvents predisposes them to crossing the blood–brain barrier where, again due to their lipophilicity, they have the capacity to concentrate in the lipids of the cells of the central nervous system (CNS). Concentration in the lipid bilayer of the cell membranes is thought to be likely to interfere with nerve cell function, thereby resulting in a variety of effects on this important system. It is of interest to note that these effects are likely to be due to the physical properties of the solvents because there is a wide range of structures that are able to cause similar responses. The range of effects is listed in Table 11.5.

Table 11.5. Acute effects of solvents on the CNS

Disorientation
Euphoria
Giddiness
Confusion
Progressive loss of consciousness
Paralysis
Convulsion
Death

A dramatic example of the acute effects of solvents on the CNS can be appreciated from the following situation. Two workers entered a tank to paint it. Being a confined space meant that there was a concentration of solvent from the paint in the air as there was poor ventilation. One of the workers climbed out because he felt dizzy. He then noticed that his workmate had collapsed on the floor of the tank. During a subsequent rescue operation 17 more people were overcome by the toluene vapour. On more than one occasion there were three men lying unconscious or semi-conscious on the floor of the tank. Fortunately, in this case rescue was eventually effected by drilling holes in the tank and inserting air hoses to disperse the vapours and no fatalities were recorded. This is a common scenario when the combination of solvent vapours and confined spaces occurs and has been the cause of many deaths. As can be appreciated, this is another example of the mix of toxicity and exposure being required before a toxic response can be realised.

More recently, the effects of chronic exposure to solvents has become an area of attention, contention and concern. A condition termed 'psycho-organic disease' or 'solvent disease' has been described to result from long-term exposure to solvents such as toluene and xylene. Effects including memory impairment, coordination impairment and deterioration of personality have been indicated as important features of this condition. Not all investigators have come to the same conclusion, however, and the reader is referred to the papers by Baker (1988) and Grasso (1988) for further information on this issue.

As well as the general toxic effects of solvents there are also several important specific effects of particular solvents that require attention. Examples of some of these are provided in Table 11.6. As an example, *n*-hexane will be dealt with in more detail. It will also be used to illustrate the importance of understanding various aspects of the toxicity of chemicals so that appropriate decisions can be made about their use and the use of those chemicals that are structurally related to them.

Table 11.6. Specific toxic effects of solvents

Solvent	Specific toxic effects
Benzene	Aplastic anaemia, leukaemia
Methanol	Ocular toxicity
n-Hexane	Peripheral neuropathy

The uses of *n*-hexane have been varied, with it being found in the printing industry, in vegetable oil extraction, in glues, paints, varnishes, plastics and rubber. Large numbers of workers have been exposed in the course of their work and the reports of human peripheral neuropathy are summarised in Table 11.7. There is good correlation between the clinical observations and the observed experimental pathology. The disease process is well-defined with a gradual onset and initial findings in the lower extremities. There is a swelling of the axons, demyelination and degeneration of the nerve fibres of the peripheral nervous system. Once removed from exposure to *n*-hexane there is generally a recovery but it may take months or years. The biotransformation of *n*-hexane is an essential component in the eventual expression of toxicity. This is outlined in Figure 11.1.

Table 11.7. Reports of *n*-hexane peripheral neuropathy in workers

Year	Work activity
1964	Laminating process
1969	Glue in shoemaking
1971	Cabinet making

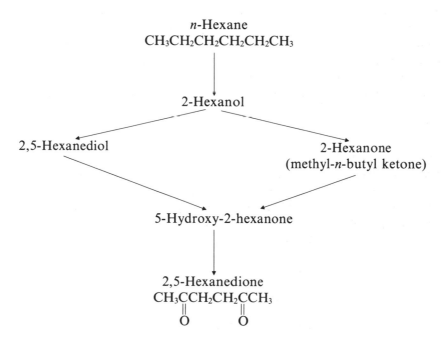

n-Hexane
CH₃CH₂CH₂CH₂CH₂CH₃

2-Hexanol

2,5-Hexanediol

2-Hexanone
(methyl-*n*-butyl ketone)

5-Hydroxy-2-hexanone

2,5-Hexanedione
CH₃CCH₂CH₂CCH₃
‖   ‖
O   O

Figure 11.1. Biotransformation of *n*-hexane.

The key features for the toxicity of this solvent are found in the γ-diketone structure of the metabolite 2,5-hexanedione. Other experimental studies have shown that it is this structural characteristic that is associated with this toxic effect. It can be seen from Table 11.8 that it is only when animals are treated with chemicals bearing this structure that peripheral neuropathy is observed. Thus the five and seven carbon atom chain aliphatic hydrocarbons, pentane and heptane, do not result in peripheral neuropathy because they do not form γ-diketone metabolites. Therefore, a deeper appreciation of the structure involved in this toxic response is required in order that the associated issues are properly understood. Consideration of the biotransformation pathway also indicates that methyl-*n*-butyl ketone, another chemical with considerable occupational use, would be expected to cause peripheral neuropathy, which is indeed the case.

Table 11.8. Peripheral neuropathy

Yes	No
2,5-Hexanedione	2,3-Hexanedione
2,5-Heptanedione	2,4-Heptanedione
3,6-Octanedione	2,6-Heptanedione

From this example of *n*-hexane it can be seen that knowledge of the biotransformation of the chemical is essential to be able to understand what factors are responsible for the peripheral neuropathy and to adequately predict which structurally related chemicals would or would not be expected to cause similar effects.

Apart from the general and specific toxicities listed above there are other toxic effects of particular groups of solvents that need to be considered. These are listed in Table 11.9 for easy reference. It should be noted that, while the effects are generally related to the group, some of them will be found with only some of the solvents within that group. More detail can be found in the publications listed in the Bibliography at the end of this chapter.

Table 11.9. Toxic effects of groups of solvents

Solvent group	Examples	Effects	
		Acute	Chronic
Aliphatic hydrocarbons	Petrol, kerosene, diesel, *n*-hexane	Nausea, pulmonary irritation, ventricular arrhythmia	Weight loss, anaemia, proteinuria, haematuria, bone marrow hypoplasia
Aromatic hydrocarbons	Toluene, xylene, benzene	Nausea, ventricular arrhythmia, respiratory depression	Headache, anorexia, lassitude
Halogenated hydrocarbons	Carbon tetrachloride, dichloromethane, trichloroethane, trichloroethylene, tetrachloroethylene	Irritant, liver, kidney, heart	Fatigue, anorexia, liver, kidney, cancer*
Ketones	Acetone, methylethyl ketone, methyl-*n*-butyl ketone	Irritant, respiratory depression	

Solvent group	Examples	Effects	
		Acute	Chronic
Alcohols	Ethanol, isopropanol, methanol	Irritant, gastrointestinal	Liver, immune function
Esters	Methyl formate, methyl acetate, amyl acetate	Irritant, liver palpitations	
Glycols	Ethylene glycolethens diethylene glycol, propylene glycol	Kidney	Kidney
Ethers	Diethyl ether, isopropyl ether	Irritant, nausea	
Glycol ethers	Ethylene glycolethens monomethyl ether, ethylene glycolethens monoethyl ether, propylene glycolethens monomethyl ether	Irritant, nausea, anaemia, liver, kidney, reproductive system	

*In experimental animals, non-genotoxic.

While the above categories cover the majority of solvents found in workplaces, there are some others that bear mention as they have considerable toxicity. Amongst these are carbon disulphide and dioxane. Carbon disulphide has been clearly associated with neurotoxicity in humans, producing classic symptoms including irritability, violence, sexual difficulties, insomnia and bad dreams. Dioxane is a cyclic ether which produces damage to various organs at high levels of exposure as well as some of the more common symptoms including irritation, headache and nausea. It has been found to be carcinogenic in studies with experimental animals but the applicability of these findings to humans remains contentious.

References

Baker, E. L., 1988, Organic solvent neurotoxicity, *Ann. Rev. Public Health*, **9**, 223–32.
Collings, A. J. and Luxon, S. G. (Eds), 1982, *Safe Use of Solvents*. New York: Academic Press.
Grasso, P., 1988, Neurotoxic and neurobehavioural effects of organic solvents on the nervous system, *State Art Rev. Occup. Med.*, **3**, 525–39.

Bibliography

Amdur, M. O., Doull, J. and Klaassen, C. D. (Eds), 1991, *Casarett and Doull's Toxicology. The Basic Science of Poisons*, 4th Edn. New York: Pergamon Press.

Commission of the European Communities, 1986, *Organo-chlorine Solvents. Health Risks to Workers.* Brussels: Royal Society of Chemistry.

IPCS, *Environmental Health Criteria*, Geneva: WHO. There are several issues in this series on specific solvents that are valuable when requiring detailed and comprehensive information on particular solvents.

MacFarland, H. N., 1986, Toxicology of solvents, *Am. Indust. Hyg. Assoc. J.*, **47**, 704–7.

Patty's Industrial Hygiene and Toxicology, 1981, 3rd Edn. New York: Wiley.

Riihimaki, V. and Ulfvarson, U. (Eds), 1986, *Safety and Health Aspects of Organic Solvents* (*Progress in Clinical and Biological Research*, Vol. 220). New York: A. R. Liss.

Rinsky, R. A., 1987, Benzene and leukemia. An epidemiologic risk assessment, *New. Engl. J. Med.*, **316**, 1044.

Chapter 12

Toxicity of Plastics

R. Drew

Introduction

Plastics have become an integral part of modern life. So diverse are their uses (Table 12.1) it is difficult to imagine being without plastics. The characteristic, specific mechanical and chemical properties of different plastics are a function of the type of polymer(s) from which they are made. The properties are conferred by the arrangement of repeating structural units (monomers) in the polymer chain and the size of the chain. The word polymer is derived from the Greek words poly and meros meaning many parts. Natural polymers include proteins, polypeptides, polysaccharides, DNA, wood, cotton and wool.

Table 12.1. Types of plastic and their uses

Plastic	Uses
Polyethylene	Highly versatile, can be flexible or rigid, transparent or opaque. Used for diverse applications, e.g. shopping bags, power cable insulation, irrigation pipe, milk bottles, waste bins
Polyvinyl chloride	Naturally rigid but can be made flexible. Uses include water pipes, gas reticulation, flooring, gutters, rainwear, footwear, electrical insulation, phonograph records, credit cards, cosmetic bottles
Polystyrene	Used extensively in refrigerator liners. In its expanded (i.e. cellular form) it is used for thermal insulation and freight packaging for fragile products
Polypropylene	Moulded into car battery covers, toilet cisterns, clear film for food packaging, fibre in ropes, carpet
Polyurethane	Flexible foam for cushions, rigid foam as a heat insulator, cast into car bumpers, ski boots
Polyester	Used as resin in combination with glass in 'fibreglass', packaging film, soft drink bottles
ABS	Tough, strong with high gloss finish. Used in telephone handsets, electrical appliance housings, car trim items
Acrylic	Clear, tough; used for outdoor signs, skylights, tail lights, fluoroplastics, non-stick coatings on frying pans

ABS, Acrylamide Butadiene Styrene

213

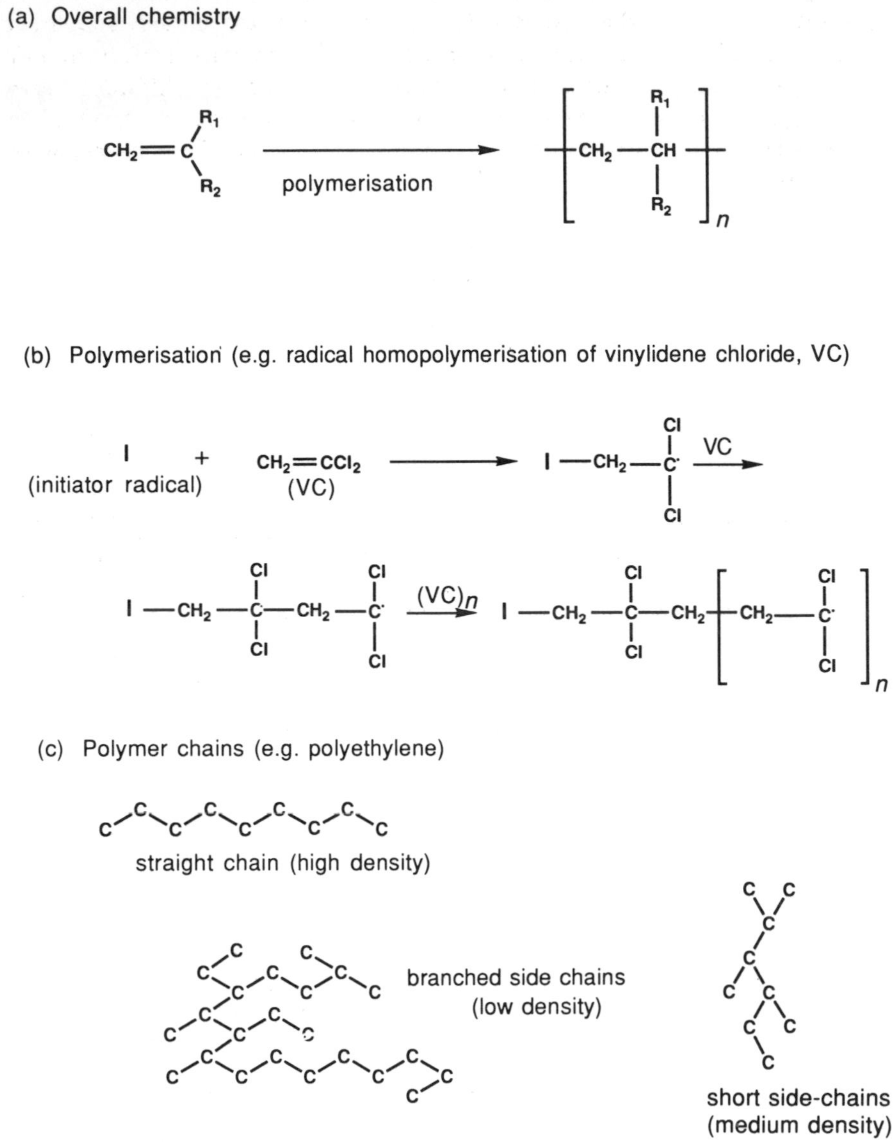
(a) Overall chemistry
polymerisation
(b) Polymerisation (e.g. radical homopolymerisation of vinylidene chloride, VC)
(initiator radical)
(VC)
VC
(c) Polymer chains (e.g. polyethylene)
straight chain (high density)
branched side chains (low density)
short side-chains (medium density)

Figure 12.1. Schematic representation of the chemistry and structure of plastic polymers.

The overall process of synthetic polymer manufacture is shown schematically in Figures 12.1 and 12.2. The basic chemical reaction is essentially addition across the carbon–carbon double bond of a monomer. The polymerisation is achieved in a variety of ways, by using heat, pressure, light or, more frequently, with the aid of a catalyst or initiator. The ensuing chain growth is terminated naturally or by the addition of chain transfer agents which quench the reaction. Conditions are manipulated to achieve straight, medium chain, branch chain or cross-linked polymers. Synthetic polymers characteristically are mixtures of many chains of different molecular weight; the molecular weight of polymers is therefore expressed in ranges. The structural formulae and molecular weights of common plastic monomers and polymers is shown in Table 12.2.

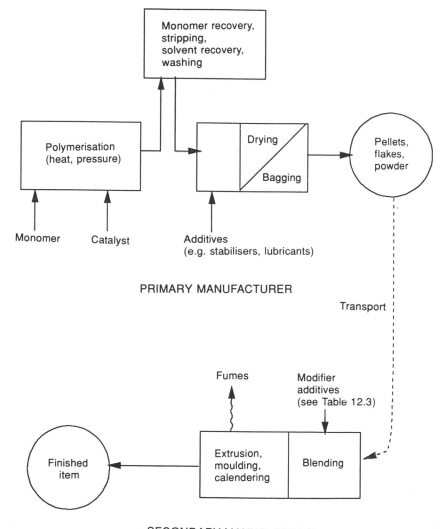

Figure 12.2. Schematic representation of the manufacture of plastic goods. In this scheme the primary manufacturer synthesises the basic polymer and provides it to a secondary manufacturer who turns it into finished goods for sale.

Toxicity of Plastics

Table 12.2. Structural formulae of plastic polymers and their monomers (numbers in brackets indicate molecular weight)

Plastic type	Monomer	Homologous polymer base formula
Polyethylene	$H_2C=CH_2$ Ethylene (28)	$\left[\!\!-CH_2-CH_2-\!\!\right]_n$ (100 000–500 000)
Polyvinyl chloride (PVC)	$H_2C=CCl$ Vinyl chloride (62.5) $H_2C=CCl_2$ vinylidene chloride (96)	$\left[\!\!-CH_2-\underset{Cl}{CH}-\!\!\right]_n$ (60 000–150 000)
Polystyrene	$H_2C=CH-$ ⬡ Styrene (104.1)	$\left[\!\!-CH_2-CH-\!\!\right]_n$ (⬡) (10 000–1 000 000)
Polypropylene	$H_2C=CH-CH_3$ Propylene (42.1)	$\left[\!\!-CH_2-\underset{CH_3}{CH}-\!\!\right]_n$ (>40 000)
Acrylics/acrylates		
Polyacrylic acid	acrylic acid structure $H_2C=CH$ with $\overset{O}{\underset{}{C}}-OH$ Acrylic acid (72.1)	$\left[\!\!-CH_2-\underset{COOH}{CH}-\!\!\right]_n$ (10 000–80 000)
Polyacrylamide	$H_2C=CH$ with $\overset{O}{\underset{}{C}}-NH_2$ Acrylamide (71)	$\left[\!\!-CH_2-\underset{}{CH}-\!\!\right]_n$ with $\overset{O}{C}-NH_2$ (1 000 000–3 000 000)
Polyacrylonitrile	$H_2C=\underset{CN}{CH}$ Acrylonitrile (53.1)	$\left[\!\!-CH_2-\underset{CN}{CH}-\!\!\right]_n$ (100 000–150 000)
Polymethyl methacrylate	$CH_2=\underset{CH_3}{C}$ with $\overset{O}{C}-OCH_3$ Methylmethacrylate (100.1)	$CH_2=\underset{CH_3}{C}-C$ with $\overset{O}{}-OCH_3$ (50 000–1 000 000)
Styrene–acrylonitrile	$\left[\left[-\underset{⬡}{CH}-CH_2-\right]_x\left[CH_2-\underset{CN}{CH}\right]_y\right]_n$	(100 000–400 000)

The manufacture of plastic goods can be conveniently divided into primary and secondary manufacturers. The primary manufacturer creates the polymer plastic and supplies it to the secondary manufacturer in a suitable form to be converted into finished plastic products. Additives (Table 12.3) which enhance the durability, appearance, workability and suitability of a plastic for a particular purpose are combined with the polymer during the primary or secondary manufacturing stages. In the final plastic item, additives are usually present in concentrations typically less than a few percent. The process is shown schematically in Figure 12.2. There are relatively few primary producers of plastics compared with manufacturers making finished items. There is, therefore, a distinction between these two manufacturing sectors in the number of individuals who may be occupationally exposed and the type of chemical to which they may be exposed. Depending upon their job description an individual in the primary sector of the industry may be potentially exposed to monomers, catalysts, initiators, a small range of additives as well as the final polymer. The reactive monomers and catalysts represent the major chemical hazards. By comparison an individual in the secondary sector has far less potential to be exposed to monomers (exposure to these will essentially be as residues in the polymer); there is, however, much greater potential for exposure to a wide range of additives as well as vapours and fumes generated from heating the polymer during moulding or extrusion.

Table 12.3. Additives used to modify plastic polymers

Additive	Uses
Stabilisers	Lead compounds, e.g. oxides, sulphates, phosphates Metal soaps, e.g. Zn, Ca/Zn, Ba/Zn, Ba/Cd carboxylates (stearates, octoates, etc.) Organic tin compounds (dimethyl tin thioglycolate)
Plasticisers	Phthalates and adipates, e.g. diethylhexylphthalate, diethylhexyladipate
Lubricants	Lead stearate, stearic acid, waxes, mineral oil
Catalysts	Hydrogen peroxide, ethyl chloroformate, methylethyl ketone peroxide
Others	Pigments; fillers; bacteriostats; UV radiation absorbers; processing aids and impact modifiers e.g. antistatic agents, surfactants

UV, ultraviolet.

Plastic polymers

General toxicity

Primarily because of their high molecular weight (Table 12.2) and consequential inability to penetrate membranes, polymeric materials *per se* are considered to be biologically inert. The biological effects of plastics are generally attributed to residual monomer, oligomers, additives or ingredient impurities. These compounds are often not chemically bound in the polymer matrix and are able to slowly diffuse from the surface of the plastic. Despite this possibility the overall toxicity of polymers is very low, indeed in long-term animal studies the effects observed are often the result of compromised nutrition due to bulk amounts of polymer physically causing decreased food intake.

Potential adverse effects to the respiratory tract and eye are most likely to be due to physical irritation resulting from exposure to polymer dust. Cases of lung disease have been described after prolonged exposure to high levels of respirable polyvinyl chloride (PVC) dust (Lilis, 1981). The ability of PVC dust to cause respiratory damage is supported by animal experiments (Agarwal *et al.*, 1978; Groth *et al.*, 1981). The pneumoconiosis described indicates a pattern of non-neoplastic effects, a granulomatous reaction with inclusion of PVC particles in macrophages and associated fibrosis which have been found to lead to exertional dyspnoea, diffuse micronodular chest radiographic opacities and restrictive pulmonary dysfunction (Lilis, 1981). This phenomenon is similar to chronic exposure to other particulates as is found in coal miners' disease and farmers' lung. It is probably not unique to PVC, but could also occur with high exposure to other plastic dusts. However, the latter has not been recognised because other plastic dusts have not been as intensely investigated as has PVC manufacture. PVC has been subject to close scrutiny because its monomer, vinyl chloride has been shown to be a human carcinogen.

Good occupational hygiene and maintenance of air dust levels to below the exposure level for nuisance dusts ($10 \, \text{mg m}^{-3}$) is unlikely to present unacceptable risks to workers. Since plastic particles have the ability to generate and hold static electricity, good ventilation and grounding of equipment reduces the risk of electrical discharge and explosion. In addition, exposure to hazardous volatile compounds generated during polymer, processing (see section on 'Fumes During Manufacturing') is reduced by ensuring there is adequate ventilation.

Carcinogenicity

When plastics have been used as food packaging material there has been concern regarding the potential migration of chemicals from the polymer into food, especially since some monomers have carcinogenic potential

Table 12.4. Comparative toxicity and carcinogenicity of some common monomers used to make plastics

	LD$_{50}$* (mgkg^{-1})	Irritancy	Sensitisation	Systemic toxicity	Developmental toxicity	Genotoxicity	Carcinogenicity-IARC Human	Animal	Classification	TWA (ppm)
Ethylene		—	—	L+	—	—	ND	ND	3	
Propylene		—	—	L+	?	—	ND	ND	3	
Styrene	5000	+	?	L+	F+	+++	I	Ld	2B	50
Vinyl chloride	>100 000†	—	—	L+	—	+++	S	S	1	5
Vinylidene chloride	>8000†	+	—	L, K+	—	++	I	Ld	3	5
Acrylic acid	200–2500	+++	±	R, K+	—	±	ND	ND	3	2
Acrylamide	≃ 200	++	?	N+++	—	±	ND	S	2B	0.03 ‡
Acrylonitrile	≃ 100	+++	?	L, R, N+	T+	+	Ld	S	2A	40
Ethyl acrylate	≃ 2000	++	Yes	R+	—	++	ND	S	2B	5
Toluene diisocyanate	≃ 6000	+++	Yes	R+	?	±	ND	S	2B	0.02 ‡
1,3-Butadiene	>2000	—	—	—	F+	++	I	S	2B	10

—, no effect; ± equivocal +, mild; ++, moderate; +++, strong; ?, unknown.
K, kidney; L, liver; N, neurotoxicity; R, respiratory; F, fetotoxic; T, teratogenic.
ND, no adequate data; I, inadequate evidence; Ld, limited evidence; S, sufficient evidence.
1, carcinogenic to humans; 2A, probably carcinogenic to humans; 2B, possibly carcinogenic to humans; 3, not classifiable.
TWA: Time Weighted Average Exposure Standard, Worksafe Australia (1991)
* Rat oral LD$_{50}$.
† LC$_{50}$ in ppm per 4 h.
‡ In mgm^{-3}.

(Table 12.4). Because many implanted prosthetic medical devices contain plastics, the majority of experimental investigations into plastic carcinogenicity have involved implantation of the polymeric material, primarily into subcutaneous tissue. Intraperitoneal, intramuscular and intrauterine implants have also been evaluated. As a general phenomenon any solid material with an uninterrupted, smooth round surface and of a critical size can cause a local tissue sarcoma at the site of implant. The process of such tumour formation is called 'solid state carcinogenesis' (Bischoff and Bryson 1964; Bischoff 1972; IARC, 1979) and is critically dependent on the physical nature of the implant rather than its chemical constituency. Most polymers when they meet the above physical requirements and are implanted cause local sarcomas. While it is highly probable this is the result of solid state carcinogenesis, it cannot be entirely discounted that the carcinogenic effect is not a consequence of the migration of soluble reactive compounds from the implanted plastic into the surrounding tissue. Although there are relatively fewer studies, it is noteworthy that oral or inhalational exposure of animals to plastic polymers (that is, by routes more relevant to the human occupational situation) has not resulted in tumour formation (IARC, 1979; Montgomery, 1982; Maltoni, 1989).

The International Agency for Research on Cancer (IARC, 1979) notes several studies that describe an elevated incidence of digestive system cancers in workers involved in the fabrication of plastics. These studies are considered to be insufficient to evaluate the carcinogenicity of plastics. The problems of such epidemiological studies are illustrated by recent reports (reviewed by Kay (1991)) which investigate an apparent excess of colorectal cancer in workers who handle polypropylene. The studies suffer from the common problems of occupational disease epidemiology, *viz.* adequacy of control groups (colorectal cancer is relatively common in Western society), small exposed groups, multiple exposure to potential causative agents, etc. In particular, continually improving industrial hygiene is removing the risk conditions that existed 20–40 years ago which may have been responsible for the putative association now being investigated. The net result is that on the available evidence the current list of risk factors for colorectal cancer cannot be extended to include the manufacture or use of polypropylene. Indeed, in humans it may never be possible to show a definitive cause and effect relationship between plastic exposure and cancer even in highly exposed populations (i.e. workers); the suggestion of such possibilities therefore resides primarily with experimental animal studies. These show that polymers are not inherently carcinogenic or genotoxic, findings which contrast with some of the monomers (Table 12.4); any potential carcinogenic response is likely to be mediated through 'solid state' mechanisms.

In summary IARC (1979) considers the overall evidence for carcinogenicity of a variety of polymers to be inadequate for determining the carcinogenic potential to humans and has deemed them unclassifiable (IARC group 3).

Monomers

General toxicity

Most monomers used for making plastics are relatively simple mono- or di-substituted alkenes (see Table 12.2). The comparative toxicity and carcinogenicity of some common monomers is summarised in Table 12.4. The chemical reactivity of the monomer carbon double bond and animal species specific metabolism (see the following section) account for differences in toxicological profile among monomers and for differences commonly observed in toxicity between species for a particular monomer. In humans, the systemic toxicity (i.e. organ directed toxicity) of plastic monomers is generally low, it being clinically expressed as reversible liver or kidney damage after very high occupational exposures. Animal studies suggest this is the result of high concentrations distorting the normal metabolism of the monomer (see the following section). Most monomers are not appreciably absorbed through the skin, but can be absorbed very well by the lungs and gastrointestinal tract. Monomers which are relatively unreactive (e.g. ethylene, propylene, vinyl chloride) are of general low acute toxicity, are not irritants and are not sensitisers. These agents are simple asphyxiants and have the ability to cause death by this mechanism. The major biological effect from acute exposure to high concentrations of these monomers is CNS depression —indeed some have been trialled as anaesthetic agents. Thus the major effects experienced by workers exposed to high levels of ethylene and propylene are dizziness, confusion, headache, nausea, light headedness, fatigue, loss of coordination, etc. (Gibson *et al.*, 1987a, b).

In contrast, monomers which are spontaneously highly reactive are moderate to strong skin and eye irritants, and, presumably because of their ability to directly form haptens with tissue macromolecules, tend to be skin and/or lung sensitisers. The injuries to humans resulting from exposure to acrylic acid are due to the strongly corrosive and blistering action of the liquid, vapours and aerosols; severe, painful injuries to the skin, eyes and respiratory tract are described. Pure acrylic acid is not a sensitiser, it appears that the sensitising efficiency of technical acrylic acid depends upon the presence of an impurity, β-diacryloxypropionic acid (Chemie, 1991).

Acrylamide toxicity is different to most monomers. It is efficiently absorbed through the skin and is also a cumulative peripheral neurotoxicant. In common with most monomers, acute exposure to high doses produces signs and symptoms of CNS depression, whereas peripheral neuropathy is a feature of long-term cumulative exposure to smaller doses. The latent period for onset of signs of peripheral neuropathy (paraesthesia, loss of tendon reflexes, impairment of vibration sense and other sensations, peripheral muscular wasting) is dose dependent and decreases with increasing cumulative dose. In animal studies morphological changes are most pronounced in the endings of myelinated sensory neurons and the onset of neuropathy parallels the accumulation of acrylamide bound to protein in the nerves. After stopping exposure to acrylamide most cases recover, however, the recovery period can be prolonged over a number of years depending upon the amount of cumulative damage (IPCS, 1985).

Acrylonitrile also does not fit the general toxicological profile of the monomers. Cyanide is released during acrylonitrile metabolism and thus the acute toxicity of acrylonitrile is similar to cyanide poisoning. Liberation of cyanide, however, cannot entirely account for its CNS toxicity since conventional cyanide antidotes are not completely effective (ASTDR, 1990; Ahmed and Hussein, 1990). It is likely that there are direct CNS depressive effects as with other monomers.

Apart from acrylamide which has some testicular toxicity in mice (IPCS, 1985) it appears that the reproductive effects of monomers in animals are confined to high exposures causing fetotoxic and minor teratogenic effects. These are most likely secondary to maternal toxicity which also occurs at these elevated doses. (IPCS, 1983; HSE, 1985; ASTDR, 1990; Ahmed and Hussein, 1990).

Biotransformation

The primary biotransformation pathways common to most of the substituted alkene monomers are shown in Figure 12.3. The initial metabolism of these compounds occurs in the liver and follows two major competing routes; direct conjugation with glutathione catalysed by glutathione S-transferase, or oxidation by the mixed function oxidase (MFO) enzyme system. Subsequent metabolism by a range of enzymes produces a wide variety of urinary and faecal metabolites. Oxidation by cytochrome P450 isoenzymes in the MFO system may either produce an alcohol or a reactive epoxide. Much experimental evidence indicates that monomer toxicity is the result of adduct formation between the parent molecule, or the epoxide, and critical target tissue macromolecules.

The toxicological profile for a particular monomer in a given species is dependent upon the monomer exposure concentration, the reactivity of the double bond and the balance between the bioactivating and inactivating enzyme pathways.

High concentrations of monomer tend to saturate the major metabolic pathways, and, as a result, many monomers exhibit non-linear toxicokinetics. Metabolic saturation causes increased tissue levels of monomer and increased CNS effects. Manipulation of the metabolic pathways can substantially change the toxicological profile and extent of toxicity. Decreasing available liver glutathione by pre- or co-administration of competitive substrates, inhibiting glutathione S-transferase or inhibiting epoxide hydratase results in greater amounts of epoxide being present and increased hepatotoxicity. Similarly, induction of cytochrome(s) P450 (with phenobarbitone or Aroclor) augments toxicity, whereas inhibition (by SKF 525A) ameliorates toxicity (IPCS, 1983, 1985; Gibson, 1987a, b; ASTDR, 1990, 1992). Co-administration of alcohol with the monomer causes increased CNS effects because the effects of both compounds on the brain are additive. Ethanol also inhibits the metabolism of monomers via the saturable alcohol dehydrogenase pathway; thus ethanol has potentiated the occurrence of vinyl chloride induced liver cancer (Radike *et al.*, 1981) and fetotoxicity (John *et al.*, 1977).

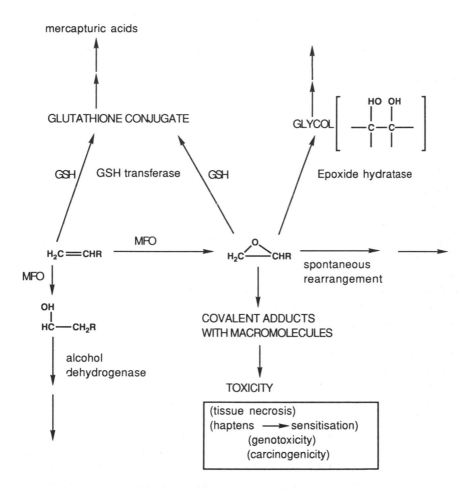

Figure 12.3. Primary biotransformation pathways for substituted alkene monomers. The toxicological profile (see Table 12.4) for a particular monomer in a given species is dependent on the reactivity of the carbon double bond and the balance between bioactivating and inactivating pathways. Monomer structures are given in Table 12.2. For detailed metabolic maps of individual monomers the reader should consult the references cited in the text.

Genotoxicity and carcinogenicity

Vinyl chloride monomer (VCM) illustrates the belated appreciation of potential chronic effects resulting from exposure to monomers of low acute toxicity (Table 12.4). VCM was discovered around 1935, but did not reach appreciable commercial production until after 1945. Prior to acro-osteolysis (dissolution of bone in the distal phalanges of the fingers and toes) being detected and associated with VCM exposure, VCM was considered to be a material of quite low human toxicity and exposures were very high (Wagoner, 1983). Typical exposures to VCM have been retrospectively estimated to be 1000 ppm in 1945–1955, 400–500 ppm in 1955–1960, 300–400 ppm in 1960–1970, 150 ppm in mid-1973, and 5 ppm in 1975 (Barnes, 1976). In 1974, three cases of the rare tumour angiosarcoma (cancer of the blood vessels) of the liver were reported (Creech and Johnson, 1974). Animal studies also show the ability of VCM to cause liver angiosarcoma (Maltoni and Lefemine, 1975, 1981). By 1984, the number of deaths world-wide from liver angiosarcomas in VCM exposed workers was about 120; most of these occurred in individuals whose job it was to remove polymer build-up from the inside of autoclaves; under these circumstances the VCM exposure was likely to be considerably in excess of 1000 ppm (Purchase *et al.*, 1987). The mean time from first exposure to VCM to initial diagnosis of liver angiosarcoma was 22 years. The latency will be much longer at the lower exposures in place since the mid-1970s, indeed the tumours may not be detected at all.

In 1971 a report was published which, in hindsight, points to the tumourigenic potential of VCM (Viola *et al.*, 1971). Although liver tumours were not reported, skin and lung adenocarcinomas developed in rats after 12 months of exposure to 30,000 ppm VCM in air. Depression of the central nervous system begins at VCM concentrations of 8,000–10,000 ppm and it is therefore likely that the very high concentrations of VCM used in this study may have contributed to the apparent lack of concern for carcinogenicity in humans prior to 1974.

The case of VCM has served to focus attention on structurally related chemicals used for similar purposes. While many of the plastic monomers have a structure similar to VCM, this is the only monomer to cause liver angiosarcoma. Some of the other monomers do induce other types of tumour in animals and are genotoxic, but there are no adequate data to indicate they are carcinogenic to humans. Consequently, they are regarded as probably or possibly carcinogenic to humans, i.e. IARC classification group 2A or 2B, respectively (Table 12.4).

The understanding that systemic toxicity, genotoxicity and carcinogenicity of plastic monomers is probably mediated via the formation of a reactive epoxide has provided a rationale for assessing their risk to humans. Those monomers which readily form an epoxide are strongly genotoxic in a variety of test systems, are animal carcinogens and have IARC group 2A or 2B carcinogen classifications. The structural potential, i.e. a carbon double bond, to form an epoxide does not automatically indicate that toxicity will ensue. Ethylene oxide and propylene oxide are genotoxic and are animal carcinogens, but ethylene and propylene monomers are negative in genotoxicity and carcinogenicity tests (Gibson *et al.*, 1987a, b). This suggests that either the epoxides are not formed to any great extent or that they are very rapidly detoxified. Styrene is slightly different; it is strongly genotoxic when metabolically activated to styrene oxide, but only limited evidence exists for its ability to cause tumours in animals. Several studies, however, have indicated an increased frequency of structural chromosomal aberrations in the peripheral blood lymphocytes of animals, or workers exposed to styrene in the reinforced plastics industry (IPCS, 1983). Styrene, therefore, has the potential to affect the genetic material *in vivo* and is classified as being possibly carcinogenic to humans.

The current approach of responsible manufacturers is to handle most monomers which have a reactive carbon double bond as potential cancer causing agents unless there is sufficient evidence to the contrary. As a result many polymerisation reactions are conducted in closed systems, thereby limiting exposure of workers.

Additives

Background

During polymer processing, the polymer, blended with additives, is heated and shaped into the final product. The polymer–additive blending (called 'compounding') may occur to a relatively limited extent during primary production of the polymer. More often, compounding will take place at the secondary manufacturing level before the plastic item is shaped. Table 12.3 shows a list of plasticisers, heat and light stabilisers, impact modifiers, inert fillers, lubricants, fungicides, antioxidants and colourants which may be mixed with the polymer during compounding. This usually involves melting the polymer–additive mix and extruding it as pellets for use in moulding (blow, injection, or compression), calendering or extrusion manufacture of finished items. These latter production techniques require the polymer mix to be heated and melted.

Occupational exposure to plastic additives may occur during the weighing out/mixing phase of the operation, or via off-gassing when heat is applied during manufacture of the final product. It would be expected that unreacted monomer would also tend to volatilise when the compounded polymer is heated. Exposure to off-gas is usually controlled by appropriate mechanical ventilation at the source; regular measurement of air concentrations for selected chemicals that may be present in off-gas provides an indication of the efficiency of ventilation.

Stabilisers

Traditionally, salts or carboxylates of heavy metals (Table 12.3) have been used to stabilise plastics against degradation by heat or ultraviolet (UV) radiation. The use of lead and cadmium containing stabilisers is being phased out of production processes due to potential adverse human and ecotoxicological effects. Where lead compounds are used it is not unusual for workers to be monitored for blood lead levels. In Europe, concern for environmental contamination and subsequent human exposure is such that the use of cadmium compounds in plastics, either as stabilisers or colourants, is severely restricted (EEC, 1991). These compounds are being replaced by stearate and oleate salts of barium/zinc/calcium systems which, although technically less efficient, present a lower risk to workers and the environment.

Organotin compounds have been used for stabilising plastics, especially PVC, since the 1940s. The toxicity of the organotin compounds is mainly determined by the nature of the organic groups linked by covalent bonds to tin; the degree of alkylation confers remarkable differences in toxicity. Recently, organotin mercaptides derived from mercaptoethanol or thiogly-colic acid, e.g. *n*-butyltin- or methyltin-bis(isooctylthioglycolate) have been used. Although the toxicity of these organotin compounds has not been studied in a rigid systematic manner, it is apparent that their toxicity ranking is monoalkyl < dialkyl < trialkyl. The monoalkyl and dialkyl organo-tins have low to moderate mammalian and ecotoxicity. The ability to induce thymus atrophy in rats after chronic oral administration is the most sensitive effect for some of these compounds; the no observed adverse effect level is approximately 1–5 mg/kg body weight per day and the effect is not observed in mice or guinea-pigs (Hyde, 1988; Figge, 1990). Monomethyltin and dimethyltin thioglycolates are approved for use in food contact plastics by the US Food and Drug Administration (FDA) and by authorities in Europe.

There are numerous publications dealing with the mammalian and envir-onmental toxicity of trialkyl organotins, which were widely used as biocides (e.g. trimethyltin chloride). However, they are not relevant to organotin compounds used as plastic stabilisers since this type of organotin is not used as a stabiliser and is present in stabilisers in only extremely small amounts.

Plasticisers

Plasticisers are added to polymers, especially PVC, to confer varying degrees of flexibility to the finished product. Phthalates and adipates are by far the most important and most extensively used plasticisers. These chem-icals have achieved notoriety because they easily off-gas (e.g. from house-hold or car interior plastic products) and can migrate into fatty foods when the food is wrapped in plasticiser containing plastic. Because the acute toxicity of phthalates and adipates is low, relatively large amounts can be administered to animals in medium- to long-term toxicity studies. High doses in excess of $1-2 \text{ g kg}^{-1}$ orally, or greater than 1% in the diet cause testicular atrophy, decreased spermatogenesis and lowered fertility in rats. The hamster, mouse and marmoset are resistant to the testicular effects; this may be due to absorption and metabolism differences (HSE, 1986). Despite the ubiquity of phthalates in the human environment, phthalate induced testicular toxicity has not been observed in humans, probably because the environmental (and occupational) exposure is below the threshold necessary to produce a detectable effect.

Phthalates and adipates also affect the liver of animals, and is manifested by increased liver weight, induction of cytochrome P450 IVA isoenzymes, increased number of peroxisomes and greater specific activity of peroxisomal enzymes (i.e. peroxisome proliferation) (Rao and Reddy, 1987; Sharma et al., 1988). A wide variety of structurally unrelated compounds can also cause peroxisome proliferation; if it is prolonged in rodents, liver tumours can occur. Prior to tumour formation the liver effects are reversible when the inducing agent is removed. Tumours only occur in the liver and it is axiomatic that liver tumour production is absolutely dependent on prolonged peroxisomal proliferation. Observations indicate that rats and mice are the most sensitive animal species to peroxisome proliferation and tumours only occur in these species. Although various hypotheses have been proposed, the precise mechanism by which liver tumours are produced by peroxisome proliferators is unknown. The weight of evidence indicates it is most probably an epigentic mechanism, since peroxisome proliferators are not genotoxic (Reddy and Roa 1986; Moody et al., 1991; Conway et al., 1989; Lock et al., 1989).

The recent discovery of increased DNA transcription mediated by a peroxisome proliferator activated receptor, which is a member of the steroid receptor superfamily, suggests that specific genome activation/suppression may be involved in tumour formation (Green, 1992).

The relevance of hepatic tumour induction in rodents for assessing the risk to humans is questionable, since a growing body of evidence strongly indicates that human and non-human primate livers are non-responsive, or only very weakly responsive to peroxisome proliferators (Bluncke et al., 1983; Hanefeld et al., 1983; Elcombe, 1985; Elcombe and Mitchell, 1986; Makowska et al., 1991). This, and the extremely high plasticiser exposure (12 000–25 000 ppm in diet) required in lifetime studies to produce tumours in mice and rats indicates that humans are at negligible risk of developing cancer as a result of exposure to phthalates or adipates.

Lubricants

Apart from those lubricants which contain heavy metals, most do not present a hazard to humans. Indeed, many are used in the pharmaceutical industry for tablet and capsule manufacture.

Catalysts

Free radical initiators are used to initiate the polymerisation process and are generally consumed during the reaction, they are not therefore; additives in the strict sense. As many of the initiators used are highly reactive peroxides, it is not surprising that they tend to be severely corrosive to the skin and eye. For example, ongoing, chronic and irreversible damage to the eye can result from a single exposure to methylethyl ketone peroxide (Fraunfelder *et al.*, 1990). In many cases, reactivity and acute toxicity of free radical initiators is such that it is not possible to conduct chronic toxicity tests, or to use *in vitro* tests to assess carcinogenicity or genotoxicity potential. Some of the lessor reactive peroxides have been tested. In a two-stage skin bioassay, benzoyl peroxide and lauroyl peroxide were found to promote both papillomas and carcinomas when topically applied to mice after 7,12-dimethylbenz[*a*]anthracene initiation (Slaga *et al.*, 1981). *tert*-Butyl peroxide and cumene hydroperoxide have been found to be mutagenic in bacteria and fungi (Jensen *et al.*, 1951; Chevallier and Luzatti, 1960).

By analogy with less reactive irritants (e.g. formaldehyde, acrolein), it is assumed that tumours of the upper respiratory tract could occur via a mechanism involving prolonged tissue damage and repair should there be chronic exposure of workers to irritant air levels of these agents. Exposure should be kept to a minimum through strict handling techniques, and in many instances the agents are used in closed systems.

Fumes during manufacturing

Typical temperatures used to soften or melt polymers for use in moulding or extrusion range from approximately 150°C to 250°C, occasionally with temperatures as high as 350°C being used. Polymer ingredients, including unreacted monomer and additives, which are volatile have the potential to off-gas during the process. As the temperature is increased the tendency for the plastic to degrade increases. Table 12.5 lists some of the fumes that may be emitted from plastics at operating temperatures above 200°C (Edgerley, 1981). A number of these fumes are moderate to severe irritants and, therefore, have the potential to put the operator at risk. For example, a case of meat-wrappers' asthma has been ascribed to the thermal degradation products of polyethylene coming off at 200–220°C (Skerfving *et al.*, 1980). In general, the gases emitted from polyethylene and polypropylene are less toxic and irritant than those from chlorine and nitrogen containing plastics. Common complaints from workers who have significant exposure include irritation of eyes and nose, headache, nausea and, occasionally, dizziness.

The ability for an additive to off-gas depends on its chemical structure and properties, physical state at the operating temperature, and diffusivity in the plastic matrix.

The major source of exposure to fumes is the hot extrudate leaving the extruder die. Exposure to off-gases depends primarily upon the method used to cool the extrudate; rigid compounds or sheets which are air cooled offer the highest potential for exposure. Since injection moulding, blow moulding and compression moulding are usually done in completely enclosed units the potential for fume exposure is much less. Exposure can occur, however, when the mould is opened or if the hot product is exposed to the environment.

Table 12.5. Fumes potentially emitted* at polymer processing temperatures above 200°C

HCl	Chlorine
CO	Hydrogen cyanide
CO_2	Nitrous fumes
Formaldehyde	Vinyl acetate
Acrolein	Ammonia
Phosgene	Crotonaldehyde

* This is a limited list. The combination of fumes actually emitted will depend upon the polymer being processed. Emission of CO, CO_2, formaldehyde and acrolein occurs with a variety of polymers.

Carefully controlled operating temperatures, and appropriate mechanical ventilation which quickly removes fumes from the operators' breathing zone, are the usual means of reducing occupational exposure to hazardous fumes emitted from hot polymers during manufacture of plastic products. It is prudent that atmospheric monitoring for prominent, potential thermal degradation products be performed regularly to ensure acceptable levels of emissions are not exceeded.

Summary

The plastics industry represents a major segment of the chemical industry in most industrialised countries. The base polymer is manufactured from reactive monomers usually with the aid of free radical initiators. Relatively few chemical companies are involved with this process which is primarily performed in closed systems. The base polymers are used by many smaller manufacturers of finished plastic items after addition of a wide variety of chemical additives. There are thousands of chemicals which can be potentially used as additives for plastics. There is therefore potential for greater numbers of workers to be exposed to a wider range of chemicals in the latter sector of the plastics industry. Major concerns relating to occupational toxicity of chemicals in the plastics industry are those associated with acute exposure to highly reactive chemicals and potential irritancy/corrosivity to tissues. There are also concerns about potential carcinogenic effects, exposure to heavy metals and physical hazards associated with plastic polymers. The systemic toxicity and carcinogenicity of monomers is species specific, and linked to the metabolism of the monomer. Chemicals used in the plastics industry provide examples of a variety of mechanisms by which animal carcinogenicity may occur and a 'classic' example of a human carcinogen. Understanding the metabolism and mechanism of toxicity of chemicals used to make plastics underpins the relevance of animal toxicity studies for human risk assessment. The hazards are primarily controlled by good work practice and occupational hygiene.

References

Agarwal, D. K., Kaw, S. L., Srivastave, S. P. and Seth, P. K., 1978, Some biochemical and histopathological changes induced by polyvinyl chloride dust in rat lung, *Environ. Res.*, **16**, 333–41.

Ahmed, A. E. and Hussein, G. I., 1990, Acrylonitrile, in Buhler, D. R. and Reed, D. J. (Eds) *Ethel Browning's Toxicity and Metabolism of Industrial Solvents. Vol. 2. Nitrogen and Phosphorus Solvents*, 2nd Edn, Elsevier, Amsterdam pp. 306–23.

ASTDR, 1990, *Toxicological Profile for Acrylonitrile*. Agency for Toxic Substances and Disease Registry, US Public Health Service. Cincinnatti.

ASTDR, 1992, *Toxicological Profile for Vinyl Chloride*. Agency for Toxic Substances and Disease Registry, US Public Health Service. Cincinnatti

Barnes, A. W., 1976, Vinyl chloride and the production of PVC. *Proc. R. Soc. Med.*, **69**, 277–81.

Bischoff, F., 1972, Organic polymer biocompatibility and toxicity, *Clin. Chem.*, **18**, 869–94.

Bischoff, F. and Bryson, G., 1964, Carcinogenesis through solid state surfaces, *Prog. Exp. Tumour Res.*, **5**, 85–133.

Bluncke, S., Schwartzkopff, W., Lobeck, H., Edmondson, N. A., Prentice, D. E. and Blane, G. F., 1983, Influence of fenofibrate on cellular and subcellular liver structure in hyperlipidemic patients, *Atherosclerosis*, **46**, 105–16.

Chemie, B. G., 1991, *Toxicological Evaluations 2. Acrylic Acid*, pp. 39–73. Berlin: Springer-Verlag.

Chevallier, M. R. and Luzatti, D., 1960, The specific mutagenic action of 3 organic peroxides on reverse mutations of 2 loci in *E. coli*, *C. R. Acad. Sci.*, **250**, 1572–6.

Conway, J. G., Cattley, P. C., Popp, J. A. and Butterworth, B. E., 1989, Possible mechanisms in hepatocarcinogensis by the peroxidome proliferator di-(2-ethylhexyl)phthalate, *Drug Metab. Rev.*, **21**, 65–102.

Creech, J. L. and Johnson, M. N., 1974, Angiosarcoma of the liver in the manufacture of PVC, *J. Occup. Med.*, **16**, 150–1.

Edgerley, P. G., 1981, A study of fume evolution at polymer processing temperatures, *Plastics Rubber Proc. Appl.*, **1**, 81–6.

EEC, 1991, The Council of European Communities. Council Directive of 18 June 1991, ammendments to Directive 76/769/EEC, *Official Journal of the European Communities*, **L 186/59**.

Elcombe, C. R., 1985, Species differences in carcinogenicity and peroxisome proliferation due to trichloroethylene: a biochemical human hazard assessment, *Arch. Toxicol.*, **8** (Suppl.), 6–7.

Elcombe, C. R. and Mitchell, A. M., 1986, Peroxisome proliferation due to di-(2-ethylhexyl)phthalate (DEHP): species differences and possible mechanisms, *Environ Health Perspect.*, **70**, 211–19.

Figge, K., 1990, Polyvinyl chloride and its organotin stabilisers with special reference to packaging materials and commodities: a review, *Packaging Technol. Sci.*, **3**, 27–39.

Fraunfelder, F. T., Coster, D. J., Drew, R., *et al.*, 1990, Ocular injury induced by methylethyl ketone peroxide, *Am. J. Ophthalmol.*, **110**, 635–40.

Gibson, G. G., Clarke, S. E., Farrar, D., *et al.*, 1987a, Propene, in Snyder, R. (Ed.) *Ethel Browning's Toxicity and Metabolism of Industrial Solvents. Vol. 1. Hydrocarbons*, 2nd Edn, Elsevier, Amsterdam pp. 354–61.

Gibson, G. G., Clarke, S. E., Farrar, D., *et al.*, 1987b, Ethene, in Snyder, R. (Ed.) *Ethel Browning's Toxicity and Metabolism of Industrial Solvents. Vol. 1. Hydrocarbons*, 2nd Edn, Elsevier, Amsterdam. pp. 339–53.

Green, S., 1992, Receptor-mediated mechanisms of peroxisome proliferators, *Biochem. Pharmacol.*, **43**, 393–401.

Groth, D. H., Lynch, D. W., Morrman, W. S., Stettler, L. E., Lewis, T. R., Wanger, D. and Kammineni, C., 1981, Pneumoconiosis in animals exposed to polyvinyl chloride dust, *Environ. Health Persp.*, **41**, 73–81.

Hanefeld, M., Keinmer, C. and Kadner, E., 1983, Relationship between morphological changes and lipid lowering action of *p*-chlorophenoxyisobutyric acid (CPIB) on hepatic mitochondria and peroxisomes in man, *Atherosclerosis*, **46**, 239–46.

HSE, 1985, *Toxicity Review 11. 1,3-Butadiene and Related Compounds.* Health and Safety Executive. H.M.S.O., London.

HSE, 1986, *Toxicity Review 14. Review of the Toxicity of the Esters of o-Phthalic Acid (Phthalate Esters).* Health and Safety Executive. H.M.S.O., London.

Hyde, J. R., 1988, Stabilisers, heat, in *Modern Plastics Encyclopedia.* McGraw-Hill, New York.

IARC, 1979, Some monomers, plastics and synthetic elastomers and acrolein, *Monograph 19.* Lyon: International Agency for Research on Cancer.

IPCS, 1983, *Environmental Health Criteria 26. Styrene.* Geneva: WHO.

IPCS, 1985, *Environmental Health Criteria 49. Acrylamide.* Geneva: WHO.

Jensen, K. A., Kirk, I., Kolmark, G., *et al.*, 1951, Chemically induced mutations in *Neurospara, Cold Spring Harbor Symp. Quant. Biol.*, **16**, 245.

John, J. A., Smith, F. A., Leong, B. K. J. and Schwetz, B. A., 1977, The effects of maternally inhaled vinyl chloride on embryonal and fetal development in mice, rats and rabbits, *Toxicol. Appl. Pharmacol.*, **39**, 497–513.

Kay, S., 1991, Does industrial handling of polypropylene cause colorectal cancer? *Food Chem. Toxicol.*, **29**, 725–6.

Lilis, R., 1981, Review of pulmonary effects of poly (vinyl chloride) and vinyl chloride exposure, *Environ. Health Persp.*, **41**, 167–9.

Lock, E. A., Mitchell, A. M. and Elcombe, C. R., 1989, Biochemical mechanisms of induction of hepatic peroxisome proliferation, *Ann. Rev. Pharmacol. Toxicol.*, **29**, 145–63.

Makowska, J. M., Bonner, F. W. and Gibson, G. G., 1991, Comparative induction of cytochrome P450 IVA1 and peroxisome proliferation by ciprofibrate in the rat and marmoset, *Arch Toxicol.*, **65**, 106–13.

Maltoni, C., 1989, Long term carcinogenicity bioassay of polyvinyl chloride (PVC) administered by ingestion (gavage) on Sprague–Dawley rats, *Acta Oncol.*, **10**, 267–74.

Maltoni, C. and Lefemine, G., 1975, Carcinogenicity bioassays of vinyl chloride: current results, *Ann. NY Acad. Sci.*, **246**, 195–218.

Maltoni, C., Lefemine, G., Ciliberti, A., Cotti, G. and Garretti, D., 1981, Carcinogenicity bioassays of vinyl chloride monomer: a model of risk assessment on an experimental basis, *Environ. Health Perspect.*, **41**, 3–29.

Montgomery, R. R., 1982, Polymers, in *Patty's Industrial Hygiene and Toxicology*, 3rd Edn, pp. 4209–526. New York: Wiley.

Moody, D. E., Reddy, J. K., Lake, B. G., *et al.*, 1991, Peroxisome proliferation and nongenotoxic carcinogenesis: Commentary on a Symposium, *Fund. Appl. Toxicol.*, **16**, 233–48.

Purchase, I. F. H., Stafford, J. and Paddle, G. M., 1987, Vinyl chloride. An assessment of the risk of occupational exposure, *Food Chem. Toxicol.*, **25**, 187–202.

Radike, M. J., Stemmer, K. and Bingham, E., 1981, Effect of ethanol on vinyl chloride carcinogenesis, *Environ. Health Perspect.*, **41**, 59–62.

Rao, M. S. and Reddy, J. K., 1987, Peroxisome proliferation and hepatocarcinogenesis, *Carcinogenesis*, **8**, 631–6.

Reddy, J. K. and Rao, M. S., 1986, Peroxisome proliferators and cancer: Mechanisms and implications, *TIPS*, **7**, 439–43.

Sharma, R., Lake, B. G., Foster, J., and Gibson, G. G., 1988, Microsomal cytochrome p-452 induction and peroxisome proliferation by hypolipidaemic agents in rat liver, *Biochem. Pharmacol.*, **37**, 1193–201.

Skerfving, S., Akesson, B. and Simonsson, B., 1980, 'Meat wrappers' asthma' caused by thermal degradation products of polyethylene, *Lancet*, **i**, 211.

Slaga, T. G., Klein-Szanto, A. J. P., Triplett, L. L., Yotti, L. P. and Trosko, J. E., 1981, Skin promoting activity of benzoyl peroxide, a widely used free radical generating compound, *Science*, **213**, 1023–5.

Viola, P. L., Bigotti, A. and Caputo, A., 1971, Oncogenic response of rat skin, lungs and bones to vinyl chloride, *Cancer Res.* **31**, 516–22.

Wagoner, J. K., 1983, Toxicity of vinyl chloride and poly (vinyl chloride): a critical review, *Environ. Health Perspect.*, **52**, 61–6.

Chapter 13

Toxicity of Gases

C. M. Murdoch

Gases may have both local effects in the respiratory tract and systemic effects after inhalation. Thus the respiratory tract is both a target organ and a point of entry for gases. The local adverse effects relate mainly to irritation. Increased susceptibility to infections, allergic disease, structural disease and cancer also occur in the respiratory tract in response to gases. The systemic effect of gases which is of greatest importance in the workplace is asphyxiation.

The gases treated in the present chapter are:

- The simple asphyxiants—non-toxic gases such as nitrogen, argon and some fuel gases.

- The chemical asphyxiants—carbon monoxide and hydrogen cyanide.

- The common irritant gases—ammonia, chlorine, ozone, nitrogen oxides, sulphur oxides and phosgene.

- Other gases of importance in the workplace, which have both systemic and local effects—hydrogen sulphide, phosphine, formaldehyde and ethylene oxide.

Asphyxiants

Simple asphyxiants

Asphyxiation occurs when the body is deprived of oxygen. Oxygen deprivation may occur because the breathing atmosphere has a lower than normal concentration of oxygen due to dilution with another gas. If this other gas itself has no toxic or other effects on the body, it is referred to as a 'simple asphyxiant'. The simple asphyxiants are colourless, odourless gases, such as nitrogen, hydrogen, helium, argon and methane.

Occupational exposure

Compressed inert gases (nitrogen, argon, helium) are used in welding, for purging storage vessels and pipelines and in the heat treatment of metals.

In liquid form they are used to freeze and preserve foods and other materials, and in situations where very low temperatures are required. The flammable simple asphyxiants (e.g. hydrogen, methane, propane) have a variety of uses, as fuels, and in many industrial processes.

Exposure is most likely to occur by bodily entry into confined spaces containing a gas, or accidental inhalation during activities such as maintenance of pipes or vessels.

Toxicology

Acute asphyxia, from the inhalation of pure asphyxiant gas, results in immediate unconsciousness, followed by death in a few minutes. When oxygen concentration diminishes gradually, symptoms of asphyxiation occur in stages:

- *Stage 1* 16–12% oxygen—increased volume of breathing, accelerated pulse rate, impaired attention and difficulty in thinking clearly, slightly disturbed muscular coordination for fine tasks, increased respiration and hence decreased carbon dioxide in the body.

- *Stage 2* 14–10% oxygen—faulty judgement, altered pain threshold, unusual emotions (e.g. ill temper, pugnacity, hilarity) and mood changes, rapid fatigue from muscular exertion (with possible fainting), intermittent breathing.

- *Stage 3* 10–6% oxygen—nausea and vomiting, loss of muscular control and movement, bewilderment, loss of consciousness, coma.

- *Stage 4* <6% oxygen—breathing reduced to infrequent gasps, convulsive movements, heartbeat stops.

If asphyxia stops after only a short time at stage 4, symptoms are relieved within a few hours. The after-effects may include headache, nausea and general malaise, due to the collection of fluid in brain tissues.

Workers should not be exposed without respiratory protection to atmospheres containing less than 18% oxygen.

Carbon dioxide

Carbon dioxide is a colourless, odourless, unreactive gas. It is heavier than air (relative density 1.53).

Occupational exposure

It is used as a shielding gas in arc welding, for purging tanks and pipes, in fire extinguishers, and for carbonating drinks. In liquid or solid form it is used as a refrigerant for food preservation, and for various chilling operations in laboratories, hospitals and industrial processes. It is produced during combustion, fermentation processes and spontaneous oxidation of organic matter. Thus it may be present in dangerous concentrations in underground mines, drains and sewers, silos, vessels used for brewing, and holds of ships containing foodstuffs or other organic cargo. Exposure in these confined spaces has led to numerous fatalities.

Toxicology

Carbon dioxide acts at low concentrations by stimulating the respiratory centre of the brain. It is normally present in air at a concentration of 0.03% (up to 0.06% in urban areas). If the concentration is increased to about 2%, the breathing becomes deeper and the tidal volume is increased. This effect is marked at 4%, and is distressing to most individuals at 5%, causing breathlessness and headache.

For prolonged exposure, it seems that a level of about 1.5% can be tolerated by normal healthy individuals. However, there are likely to be some metabolic effects, such as acidosis and changes to calcium and phosphorous metabolism.

At concentrations of about 5% and greater, narcotic effects become apparent. Reported effects include headache, somnolence and confusion, and at higher concentrations, tremors, paralysis and unconsciousness. The correlation of concentration with these effects is complicated by the fact that in most incidents of exposure to high levels of carbon dioxide, oxygen levels have been depleted. It has generally been found that if the oxygen concentration remains at 21%, somewhat higher levels of carbon dioxide may be tolerated.

Carbon monoxide

Carbon monoxide is a colourless, odourless, flammable gas, with a relative density of 0.97.

Occupational exposure

Carbon monoxide is produced when organic materials are heated in a limited supply of oxygen; for example, in blast furnaces where coke is used to reduce metal ores (where it is recycled for use as a fuel gas), in the atmosphere present in underground coal mines, particularly after fires and explosions, in coal tar distillation, petroleum refining, vehicle exhausts (and hence in warehouses and other buildings where fork-lift trucks are in use, repair workshops, tunnels and parking stations), in welding gases (especially where carbon dioxide is used as a shielding gas) and in cigarette smoke. It is also produced in a variety of chemical manufacturing processes. Coal gas, supplied for use as a fuel, contains about 7% carbon monoxide. 'Natural gas', which consists mainly of methane and propane, does not.

Toxicology

Carbon monoxide is referred to as a 'chemical asphyxiant'. Its principal effect is on the red blood cell pigment haemoglobin. Haemoglobin is a protein molecule which contains four haem (or heme) units. The haem unit is a ferrous iron complex; the iron atom has a coordination site which reversibly binds molecular oxygen or carbon monoxide. The affinity of the iron for carbon monoxide is 220–250 times that for oxygen. Thus carbon monoxide is bound preferentially and is less readily released than oxygen, with the effect that the haemoglobin molecule has reduced capacity to transport oxygen to tissues. In addition, when a haem unit is bound to carbon monoxide, oxygen bound to the other haem units is held more tightly.

In normal individuals, the carboxyhaemoglobin level is about 1%. About half of this is due to endogenous carbon monoxide produced during the breakdown of haem-containing molecules, and the other half is due to atmospheric pollution.

The initial effects of carbon monoxide exposure are exhibited as slight changes in the function of the central nervous system, such as vigilance, visual and auditory responses, reaction time, hand–eye coordination, mental performance and finger dexterity. There is some controversy about the threshhold levels at which these effects can be detected; they fall in the approximate range 2–5% carboxyhaemoglobin. A 5% carboxyhaemoglobin level could be achieved by exposure at approximately 25 ppm for a full shift (depending on breathing rate and metabolic rate) (Stewart, 1975). The blood of smokers typically contains 5–10% carboxyhaemoglobin.

At levels of 10–20% carboxyhaemoglobin, tightness across the forehead, or a slight headache, may be experienced. At 20–30%, the headache is pronounced, and at higher levels is accompanied by weakness, dizziness, dimness of vision and, eventually, nausea, vomiting and collapse. The fatal level is about 60%.

Workers suffering from ischaemic heart disease are more susceptible to the effects of exposure.

Some chemicals give rise to carbon monoxide during breakdown in the body. The most important of these is dichloromethane, which is used extensively in strippers for varnishes and paints; inhalation of 500–1000 ppm has been observed to give rise to carboxyhaemoglobin levels as high as 10%.

There is some evidence of chronic effects of carbon monoxide exposure. It is generally found to cause increased red cell count. Other effects on the blood and circulation, such as increased reticulocyte count, leakage of albumin from capillaries and changes in clotting time have also been reported.

Some non-specific symptoms suggested to be associated with chronic exposure are headache, dizziness, insomnia, fatigue, loss of memory and mood disturbances.

Exposure to carbon monoxide may be assessed by measuring carboxyhaemoglobin in blood (for example, by spectrophotometric methods) or carbon monoxide in end-exhaled air. Cigarette smoking complicates these measurements, since it is equivalent to intermittent exposure to high concentrations of gas, and the exposure is not simply additive when combined with occupational exposure.

Hydrogen cyanide

Hydrogen cyanide is a colourless, flammable liquid or gas (boiling point 26°C at 1 atmos), with a characteristic odour of almonds. The odour threshhold is about 0.6 ppm; olfactory fatigue occurs quickly.

It is infinitely soluble in water, forming hydrocyanic acid. In aqueous solutions of cyanide salts, there is some free hydrogen cyanide present, and the solutions are alkaline:

$$CN^- + H_2O \leftrightarrow HCN + OH^-$$

This is dependent on pH; raising the pH lowers the hydrogen cyanide concentration in favour of cyanide ion. Aqueous solutions of cyanide salts readily liberate hydrogen cyanide gas if acidified. Solid cyanide salts release small quantities of hydrogen cyanide gas when exposed to moist air.

Occupational exposure

Hydrogen cyanide is used in the synthesis of polymer resin monomers (acrylates, methacrylates, hexamethylene diamine, melamine), nitriles, amino acids, lactic acid and pyrethroid pesticides. It is used as a fumigant for buildings, ships, orchards and foodstuffs, although its use has declined in favour of safer substitutes.

Cyanide salts are used in electroplating baths, in alkaline solution, for the deposition of gold, silver, copper, cadmium, indium, zinc and tin, for the extraction of gold and silver from ores and for refining by froth flotation. Molten sodium cyanide is a component of baths used to case-harden metals. There is some risk of release of the gas, due to accidental acidification or hydrolysis in the presence of water, in most processes utilising cyanide salts. This is probably the most common cause of occupational exposure.

Hydrogen cyanide is a combustion product of many nitrogen containing polymers, such as nylon, polyurethanes, polyacrylonitrile, wool, silk and paper. It is often the cause of fatalities in fires involving these materials. It may also be generated in blast furnaces and coke ovens, from nitrogen containing compounds present in coal or coke.

Toxicology

Hydrogen cyanide is a chemical asphyxiant. The target of the cyanide ion is the enzyme cytochrome c oxidase, the final oxidase in the mitochondrial respiratory chain. It inhibits the enzyme complex by binding to the iron in a haem unit of cytochrome a_3. Thus it inhibits electron transport and oxidative phosphorylation, preventing cellular usage of oxygen, and hence causing cell death. The physiological effects exhibited in cyanide poisoning are disturbances of perception and consciousness and loss of control of the respiratory and cardiovascular systems. Acute poisoning causes giddiness, headache, palpitations, convulsions and coma. Milder poisoning may cause weakness, trembling and headache.

Reported chronic effects of cyanide exposure, typically found in electroplaters, are irritation of the nose and throat, and skin eruptions on the hands, arms and face. The alkalinity of cyanide solutions probably contributes to the skin effects.

Unlike the majority of gases, hydrogen cyanide may penetrate the skin in the gaseous state. In very high concentrations (levels of a few per cent by volume) the absorption of lethal amounts through the skin is possible.

Cyanide is metabolised rapidly to thiocyanate and excreted by the kidney; the elimination half-life is about 3 days.

Antidotes are provided in workplaces where cyanides are in use. Inhalation of amyl nitrite followed by intravenous administration of sodium nitrite then sodium thiosulphate is the most commonly recommended. Nitrites react with haemoglobin to form methaemoglobin, which competes for cyanide and hence restores cytochrome oxidase function; the thiosulphate enhances the conversion of cyanide to thiocyanate. The use of nitrites may be dangerous in patients suffering from heart disease. Other antidotes are dicobalt edetate and hydroxocobalamin.

Irritant gases

The toxicology of these gases is discussed in a single section after the properties and occupational exposures have been treated individually.

Ammonia

Ammonia is a colourless flammable gas, with a characteristic acrid odour (odour threshold approximately 5 ppm). It is very soluble in water (approximately 90 g/100 ml), and gives an alkaline solution:

$$NH_3 + H_2O \leftrightarrow NH_4^+ + OH^-$$

Concentrated solutions containing approximately 28% ammonia are known as 'ammonium hydroxide' (although it is not possible to isolate a salt of that constitution). Aqueous solutions readily release the gas.

Occupational exposure

The gas is manufactured from nitrogen gas and hydrogen (as a gas, or from methane, ethylene or petroleum naphtha) at high temperature and pressure, with a catalyst.

The principal use of ammonia is in the production of ammonium sulphate or nitrate fertilisers; the gas is added to the appropriate concentrated acid. It is also used (compressed to a liquid) as a refrigerant for foodstuffs, and in chemical manufacturing of plastics, explosives, nitric acid, urea, pesticides and detergents.

Exposure typically occurs from accidental leakage or spillage in operations involving bulk quantities of the material, or during repair of pipes. Eye injury from splashes of concentrated solution or liquefied gas is common. Chronic exposure may occur where it is in use in manufacturing or as a refrigerant.

Chlorine

Chlorine is a greenish yellow gas or yellow liquid with a pungent odour. The odour threshhold is about 0.3 ppm; rapid olfactory fatigue occurs. It is slightly soluble in water (approximately 0.5 g/100 ml), forming a solution of hypochlorous and hydrochloric acids:

$$Cl_2 + H_2O \leftrightarrow HOCl + HCl$$

It is a strong oxidant. Salts of hypochlorous acid, hypochlorites, are commonly used as sources of small quantities of free chlorine, for cleaning and disinfection.

Occupational exposure

Chlorine is produced by electrolysis of sodium chloride solution in mercury cells (older process) or diaphragm cells (modern process). It is commonly supplied as a compressed liquid/gas mixture. Its many uses include the synthesis of organic and inorganic chemicals, such as sodium hypochlorite, chlorinated organic solvents, hydrochloric acid, vinyl chloride and polyvinyl chloride (PVC), synthetic rubbers and refrigerant gases, the bleaching of paper and textiles and for water treatment and disinfection.

Exposure most often occurs by accidental loss of containment, through leaking lines, valves or cylinder fittings. Low levels may be present in manufacturing plants. If hypochlorite solutions are used in unventilated spaces, significant concentrations of gas may collect.

Sulphur oxides

Sulphur dioxide is a colourless gas with a pungent odour (odour threshhold approximately 1 ppm). It is heavier than air (relative density 2.21). It is moderately soluble in water (23 g/100 ml), forming an acidic solution which is usually referred to as 'sulphurous acid' (in fact, no free sulphurous acid, H_2SO_3, is present):

$$SO_2 + x\,H_2O \rightarrow SO_2 \cdot x\,H_2O \rightarrow HSO_3^- + H_3O^+ + (x-2)\,H_2O$$

Sulphur trioxide is a solid, with three structural forms, with differing properties. All have relatively high vapour pressures (48–149 mmHg). The vapour is colourless and odourless. Airborne sulphur trioxide reacts vigorously with the water vapour in air to produce sulphuric acid mist. It is present in small quantities in sulphur dioxide produced in combustion processes (see below), and hence contributes to the irritant properties of that gas.

Occupational exposure

Sulphur dioxide is manufactured by the combustion of sulphur or roasting of sulphide ores, for use in the manufacture of sulphuric acid, carbon disulphide, thiophene, sulphones, sulphonates and sulphates, as a bleaching agent for sugar, flour and leather, and a preservative for beers, wines and dried fruit.

Occupational exposures occur most commonly in the refining of metal ores containing sulphides (lead, zinc, nickel, cadmium and copper), and also in the combustion of coal and fuel oils, and in oil refining.

Sulphur trioxide is produced commercially from sulphur dioxide (by reaction with oxygen in the presence of a catalyst), and is used for the manufacture of sulphuric acid, sulphonated oils, detergents, organic acids and dyes.

Ozone

Ozone is a colourless or blue gas with a pungent odour (odour threshhold approximately 0.05 ppm). It is heavier than air (relative density 1.7).

It is a powerful oxidant, and will react with most organic substances at room temperature, often producing radical species. It is an unstable compound, decomposing slowly to oxygen. It is very sparingly soluble in water (< 0.1 g/100 ml).

Occupational exposure

Ozone is produced by the action of ultraviolet (UV) light, electric discharge or ionising radiation on atmospheric oxygen. Hence it is produced during arc welding, particularly metal-inert gas (MIG) welding, by high-voltage electrical equipment, by some photocopying machines, and in nuclear reactors. Natural irradiation of atmospheric oxygen by the sun, and reactions between nitrogen oxides and hydrocarbons in sunlight (producing photochemical smog), give rise to significant background levels.

It is used as an alternative for chlorine as a bleaching agent, for water purification and for sewage treatment.

The most frequent occupational exposures occur during arc welding in unventilated or confined spaces. Heavy usage of some photocopying machines in unventilated rooms may give rise to complaints of irritation.

Nitrogen oxides

The oxides of nitrogen which are of importance in the occupational environment are nitrogen dioxide (NO_2), dinitrogen tetroxide (N_2O_4) and nitric oxide (NO). These occur together as a mixture, which is known as 'NO_x' (pronounced 'nox'), or, incorrectly, as 'nitrous fumes' or 'nitrous gases'.

Nitrogen dioxide and dinitrogen tetroxide exist in temperature-dependent equilibrium. For the pure gases, at 21°C, the proportions are 0.1% NO_2 and 99.9% N_2O_4; at 100°C, 90% NO_2 and 10% N_2O_4. However, dilution with air to parts per million (ppm) levels favours formation of nitrogen dioxide.

Nitrogen dioxide/dinitrogen tetroxide is a brown gas or yellow liquid (NO_2 is brown, N_2O_4 colourless), with a pungent odour (odour threshhold approximately 0.4 ppm). The boiling point is 21°C and the relative density is 1.59.

Nitrogen dioxide is very slightly soluble in water, and in solution, decomposes to form nitric and nitrous acids, the nitrous acid then forming nitric oxide:

$$2 \; NO_2 + H_2O \rightarrow HNO_3 + HNO_2$$

$$3 \; HNO_2 \rightarrow HNO_3 + 2 \; NO + H_2O$$

Nitrogen dioxide/dinitrogen tetroxide are fairly strong oxidising agents in aqueous solution.

Nitric oxide is a colourless gas with a sharp sweet odour. It is not itself an irritant, but reacts in air to form NO_2:

$$2 \; NO + O_2 \rightarrow 2 \; NO_2$$

The rate of this reaction is slow at parts per million levels. For example, 25 ppm NO would form approximately 1 ppm NO_2 in 5 min.

Occupational exposure

The three nitrogen oxides described above are encountered in the workplace mainly as unwanted by-products. Processes giving rise to the gases are the oxidation of organic matter by nitric acid, pickling or etching of metals in nitric acid, gradual decomposition of inorganic nitrates, operations using oxygen/fuel flames such as welding, cutting and brazing, manual metal arc welding, storage of grain and stock feeds in silos, and combustion of petroleum fuels.

Oxyacetylene welding or cutting in unventilated confined spaces has led to many fatalities. Workers entering silos are also at risk of acute exposure. (This may be complicated by the presence of elevated levels of carbon dioxide and depleted oxygen levels.)

Nitric oxide is used in the manufacture of nitric acid. It is manufactured itself by the oxidation of ammonia.

Phosgene

Phosgene is a colourless gas or fuming liquid (boiling point 8°C), with an odour said to be like new-mown hay. The odour threshold is about 0.5 ppm, but the odour may not be recognised; in addition, olfactory fatigue occurs. Its relative density is 3.4.

It decomposes in water, yielding hydrochloric acid and carbonic acid (and hence carbon dioxide):

$$COCl_2 + 2\ H_2O \rightarrow 2\ H^+ + 2\ Cl^- + H_2CO_3$$

Occupational exposure

Phosgene is used for the manufacture of numerous organic chemicals, including barbiturates, carbonates, chloroformates, carbamates, acid chlorides and anhydrides, isocyanates and various types of dyes. It was previously used as a war gas.

It is produced when chlorinated solvents or their vapours are decomposed by contact with flame, very hot metals or ultraviolet (UV) light (as, for example, in arc welding). This hazard is somewhat overrated; it is significant only when relatively large quantities of solvent are involved, and the heating takes place in an unventilated or confined space.

Toxicology of the irritant gases

The irritant gases exert effects on the respiratory tract in a number of ways. Some dissolve to give acidic or alkaline solutions (chlorine, sulphur oxides, ammonia). If the dose is sufficient to exhaust the buffering capacity of the lining of the respiratory tract, immediate sensory effects and increased secretions are produced.

A very water soluble gas, such as ammonia, will interact immediately with the upper regions of the respiratory tract, causing symptoms such as pain, sneezing, nasal catarrh, nosebleeds and sore throat. In the case of ammonia, the irritant effects are usually so severe that dangerous concentrations cannot be tolerated. With increasing dose or continued exposure, the lower parts of the respiratory tract will also be involved. After very high exposure to ammonia, the most likely cause of death is laryngeal oedema. While sulphur dioxide is somewhat less soluble, the immediate effects of exposure are similar to those of ammonia.

A still less soluble gas, such as chlorine, tends to have its first effect in the tracheobronchial region, giving rise to coughing, increased sputum, breathlessness, and possibly laryngospasm and bronchospasm. The oxidising power of chlorine contributes to its effects.

With moderate or severe doses of the acidic and alkaline gases, the pulmonary region of the lungs will be affected, causing pulmonary oedema, dyspnoea, blood-stained frothy sputum, fever and cyanosis.

Chronic exposure to these gases may lead to increased airway hyperreactivity, or increased susceptibility to infection. Ammonia and chlorine have been associated with chronic bronchitis. Chronic exposure to low levels of ammonia leads to acclimation to odour and irritation.

The irritants which are sparingly soluble in water but have appreciable solubility in lipids, namely ozone, nitrogen oxides and phosgene, tend to be deposited in significant amounts in the terminal bronchioles and alveoli, as well as in the upper airways. The oxidising action of ozone and nitrogen dioxide causes degradation of cellular proteins and oxidation of lipids, resulting in pulmonary oedema, usually delayed for up to 30 h. Nitrogen dioxide is particularly hazardous since it is not strongly irritating to the upper respiratory tract, and dangerous levels can be tolerated. Ozone appears to cause systemic effects; drowsinesss and headache can be caused by relatively high exposures.

Phosgene, which yields an acidic solution as it decomposes in water, also gives rise to pulmonary oedema, delayed for 2–24 h after exposure. Chemical reactions causing cellular damage probably contribute to this effect. The sensory effects are relatively mild, and it is not impossible to tolerate dangerous concentrations.

Chronic exposure to the oxidant gases at low levels may lead to emphysema and increased risk of infection.

The approximate concentrations at which effects of the irritant gases occur are summarised in Table 13.1.

Table 13.1. Approximate concentrations at which irritant gases have effects

Gas	Concentration (ppm)				
	Odour threshhold	Minor irritation	Detectible effects on lung function*	Severe effects*	Fatality*
Ammonia	5	30–50	>140	700–1700	2500–7000
Chlorine	0.3	0.2–1	1	10–20	35–50
Sulphur dioxide	1	5	1	20–50	100
Ozone	0.05	0.3–0.8	0.3	10	?
Nitrogen dioxide	0.4	25–50	1–5	50	100–250
Phosgene	0.5	3–5	?	5–20	25–50

*Short exposures (0.5–2 h).

Other gases

Hydrogen sulphide

Hydrogen sulphide is a colourless flammable gas with an unpleasant odour of 'rotten eggs' (odour threshhold approximately 25 ppb). It is slightly soluble in water (approximately 0.3 g/100 ml), and gives a slightly acidic solution. It is heavier than air (relative density 1.19).

Occupational exposure

While hydrogen sulphide is used in chemical manufacturing (of organic sulphur compounds and inorganic sulphides), it is mainly of concern as an air contaminant where sulphur containing materials are present. It is found in pockets, or absorbed in water, in mines where sulphide minerals are present. It is formed during the decay of organic materials, and hence is found in sewers and drains, especially those containing waste water from industries where animal products are processed (tanneries, abattoirs, manure processing). Exposure in these situations has led to fatalities. Chronic exposures occur in the refining of sulphur rich crude oils, in the manufacture of viscose rayon, synthetic rubbers and carbon disulphide, and in the processing of sugar.

Toxicology

Hydrogen sulphide is both a chemical asphyxiant and an irritant. It inhibits cytochrome oxidase in the same way as cyanide, and its toxicity and speed of action are similar to those of cyanide.

Death, caused by asphyxiation, is immediate at levels of about 5000 ppm. High concentrations (500–1000 ppm) cause respiratory paralysis, unconsciousness and, if exposure continues, death. Recovery may be complete, but there is some evidence of neurological damage after exposures sufficient to cause unconsciousness.

At levels of about 250–500 ppm, respiratory irritation is the predominant effect, with pulmonary oedema and bronchial pneumonia resulting from prolonged exposure above 250 ppm.

Moderate concentrations (150 ppm) cause paralysis of the olfactory nerve. Eye irritation is the major effect at low concentrations (about 10–30 ppm), with chronic exposure causing conjunctivitis and keratitis. Other eye symptoms reported are photophobia, blepharospasm, pain, blurred vision and corneal damage. The eye effects are sometimes called 'gas eye'. Occupational exposure limits are based on eye effects.

Other reported symptoms of chronic exposure are headache, nausea, dizziness, digestive disturbances, diarrhoea, nervousness and cough.

Hydrogen sulphide is rapidly metabolised to non-toxic sulphite and sulphate.

Phosphine

Phosphine is a colourless, flammable gas with a relative density of 1.2. The characteristic, unpleasant fishy odour associated with the gas is in fact due to other phosphorus compounds which are always present. The odour threshholds reported for commercial grade gas range from 0.02 to 3 ppm. High concentrations may ignite spontaneously in air at room temperature; this property is also associated with impurities. It is very sparingly soluble in water (0.04 g/100 ml), giving a neutral solution.

Occupational exposure

The major use of phosphine is as a grain fumigant. Solid aluminium or magnesium phosphide is mixed with the grain, and gradually reacts with the moisture present to form phosphine gas. Accidental wetting of the grain/ phosphide mix or of the pure phosphide salt may lead to hazardous concentrations of gas. Workers in grain elevators may be exposed to significant concentrations. Another major use is as a dopant in the electronics industry, where it is used in gaseous form mixed with nitrogen.

It is produced as an unwanted by-product in the manufacture of acetylene from calcium carbide, from the reaction of calcium phosphide impurity with water. It is released by ferrosilicon, probably also from calcium phosphide impurities present. These sources have been the cause of fatalities. The decomposition of phosphate containing rust-proofing on metals during welding is a minor source.

Toxicology

Phosphine is a systemic poison and an irritant. The nature of interactions with the body are not well understood; it probably blocks the respiratory chain by inhibiting cytochrome oxidase in the same way as cyanide. It inhibits other enzymes, and reacts with haem and copper containing proteins.

Acute exposure gives rise to nervous, gastrointestinal and respiratory symptoms, including vertigo, headache, tremor, impaired muscular coordination, drowsiness, nausea, vomiting, liver dysfunction, kidney inflammation, chest pain, shortness of breath and cough. Death is often caused by delayed pulmonary oedema.

There is a scarcity of evidence of symptoms of chronic exposure. Chromosome aberrations in lymphocytes from fumigant applicators exposed to low concentrations have been observed (Garry *et al.*, 1989).

Phosphine is slowly oxidised in the body, and excreted in urine as hypophosphite and phosphite. A significant proportion is eliminated unchanged in expired air.

Formaldehyde

Formaldehyde is a colourless, flammable gas with a pungent odour (odour threshhold approximately 0.1–1 ppm), very soluble in water, with a relative density of 1.0. The pure gas polymerises readily at room temperature. Two mixtures of polymers are commonly used in industry: trioxane, a colourless water-soluble solid; and paraformaldehyde, a polymer mixture of average molecular weight 600, a white crystalline powder or flaky material. When heated to about 100°C, paraformaldehyde decomposes to the monomeric gas. The other form in which formaldehyde is commonly used is in aqueous solution. Solutions containing 37–50% gas by weight are known as 'formalin'. These usually contain 10–15% methanol, added to prevent polymerisation. The gas is readily released from aqueous solutions.

Occupational exposure

Formaldehyde is manufactured by the catalytic oxidation of methanol. It has a large number of uses, in the manufacture of pharmaceuticals, cosmetics, household cleaners, photographic solutions, paper, rubber, dyes, fertilisers, in the treatment of textile fibres, as a disinfectant and fumigant, for the preservation of biological and anatomical specimens, and in the manufacture of polymeric resins (phenol–formaldehyde, resorcinol–formaldehyde, melamine–formaldehyde, urea–formaldehyde), which are used to make glues, laminates, coatings, electrical fittings and domestic tableware.

In addition, it is ubiquitous in the environment. It is produced from the oxidation of methane in the Earth's troposphere, from the burning of wood, refuse, plastics and petroleum fuels, and, in small quantities, from the decomposition of vegetation. Sources in the indoor environment include resins used in furniture and building materials (particularly urea–formaldehyde foam insulation which, for this reason, is now rarely used), cleaning products and cigarette smoke.

Exposures are probably highest in the manufacture of resins, dyes, fertilisers, paper and textiles, in foundries (from resins used as sand binders) and in medical uses.

It is normally present in animal tissues. Both endogenous and exogenous formaldehyde is metabolised by oxidation to formic acid in the liver and red blood cells, then either further oxidation to carbon dioxide, elimination in urine as sodium formate or formic acid, or metabolic transformation into larger molecules.

Toxicology

Formaldehyde is a skin, eye and respiratory irritant. When inhaled, it dissolves and is metabolised rapidly, and hence affects mainly the upper respiratory tract. At concentrations of about 1 ppm, some individuals experience irritation of the eyes, nose and throat. These symptoms are detectable in most subjects at about 3 ppm, and become unpleasant at about 5 ppm; higher concentrations (> 10 ppm) cause severe irritation, difficulty in breathing, coughing and intense lachrymation.

Formaldehyde may give rise to bronchial asthma; this is uncommon, and has resulted only from relatively high exposures. There is some evidence that it can cause respiratory sensitisation, but this is inconclusive.

Sensitisation of the skin, however, is well documented. Formaldehyde is both a primary skin irritant and a powerful sensitiser.

Allergic contact dermatitis results most commonly from repeated contact with aqueous solutions (used for sterilisation and preservation), and also from the handling of paper products and synthetic resins. It most often appears as eczema on the hands, arms, face and eyelids. Once sensitised, individuals may develop a rash even from exposure to small amounts of vapour.

Fabric finishes containing formaldehyde resins (and some free formaldehyde) were once a prominent cause of dermatitis. This is now infrequent, since the newer finishes are less likely to release formaldehyde.

The irritant and sensitising effects of formaldehyde are most probably due to its ability to form chemical links with proteins. Formaldehyde modified proteins have been shown to be antigenic.

Formaldehyde has been classified as an animal (group 2A) carcinogen (IARC, 1987). Rats, but not mice, exposed to high levels of vapour (about 14 ppm for 30 h per week for up to 2 years) developed squamous cell carcinomas of the nose.

In studies of human subjects, there has been limited evidence of excess cancers of several types in workers exposed to formaldehyde. For nasal and nasopharyngeal cancers there is evidence of exposure–response relationships. At the same time, a number of studies demonstrated no excesses of these cancers.

Both positive and negative results have been reported in studies of genetic effects. There is some evidence that formaldehyde gives rise to chromosomal aberrations, sister chromatid exchanges, mutations and DNA damage in human and animal cells.

Ethylene oxide

Ethylene oxide is a colourless, flammable liquid or gas (boiling point 10.4°C), with a slight sweet odour (threshhold about 700 ppm). It is readily soluble in water.

The gas is highly reactive. It decomposes violently when heated, polymerises readily in the presence of a variety of catalysts and undergoes vigorous exothermic reactions with many materials.

Occupational exposure

Ethylene oxide is manufactured from ethylene and oxygen using a catalyst. It is used in large quantities as a chemical intermediate for the production of ethylene glycol (for antifreeze, and synthesis of polyester resins), other glycols and derivatives, non-ionic surfactants and ethanolamines. The other major use is as a sterilising agent in hospitals and in the manufacture of health and medical products. The gas supplied for use in sterilisation is diluted about 10-fold with an inert gas, to reduce the hazards of fire and explosion.

Although the total quantities used in hospitals are typically less than 1% of the total production, the number of exposed workers is probably greater than for all the other uses. The highest exposures usually occur for short periods when steriliser units are opened for unloading.

Toxicology

Cases of acute exposure have been relatively rare. Symptoms reported include nausea, vomiting, headache, dyspnoea, irritation of the eyes, nose and throat, and later, pulmonary oedema, bronchitis and electrocardiograph abnormalities.

Chronic exposure to relatively high levels (at or above the odour threshold) has been observed to cause reversible peripheral neuropathy. Chronic exposure to low levels may cause numbing of the sense of smell, slight eye irritation, and adverse effects on a number of organs, including the liver, kidneys, adrenal glands, testes and central nervous system.

Ethylene oxide has been classified as a class 2A carcinogen (IARC, 1987). It has been found to cause tumours in several organs and systems in rodents. A number of genetic effects, including chromosomal aberrations, sister chromatid exchanges, mutations and DNA damage, have been demonstrated in laboratory animals and cell assays. There is limited evidence of carcinogenicity in humans. Malignancies of the lymphatic and haematopoietic systems have been most common, with a small number of cases of stomach cancer.

In aqueous solution (but not as the pure dry liquid) it is a severe skin irritant, causing reddening, blistering and oedema after a latent period of a few hours. It is absorbed by rubber, plastic and leather; contaminated garments may cause irritation.

References

Garry, V. F., Griffith, J., Danzl, T. J., Nelson, R. L., Whorton, E. B., Krueger, L. A. and Cervenka, J., 1989, Human genotoxicity: pesticide applicators and phosphine, *Science*, **246**, 251–5.
IARC, 1987, *Supplement 7. Overall Evaluation of Carcinogenicity: An Updating of IARC Monographs 1–42*. Lyon: IARC.
Stewart, R. D., 1975, The effect of carbon monoxide on humans, *Ann. Rev. Pharmacol.*, **15**, 409–23.

Bibliography

Haldane, J. S. and Priestley, J. G., 1935, *Respiration*. Oxford: Clarendon Press.
Henderson, Y. and Haggard, H. W., 1943, *Noxious Gases and the Principles of Respiration Influencing their Action*, 2nd Edn. New York: Reinhold.
Shephard, R. J., 1983, *Carbon Monoxide*. Springfield, IL: Charles C. Thomas.

Chemical data, properties

Compressed Gas Association, 1990, *Handbook of Compressed Gases*, 3rd Edn. New York: Van Nostrand Reinhold.
Lide, D. R. (Ed.), 1990, *CRC Handbook of Chemistry and Physics*, 71st Edn. Boca Raton, PL: CRC Press.

Chapter 14

Toxicity of Particulate Matter

A. J. Rogers

The health effects resulting from the inhalation of some toxic dusts were recorded in ancient times in Greek, Roman and Egyptian manuscripts. Agricola, Paracelsus and Ramazzini provided more detailed reviews of the health outcomes of workers in a range of mining, smelting and manufacturing industries in the sixteenth and seventeenth centuries. These accounts include classic descriptions such as

> On the other hand, some mines are so dry that they are entirely devoid of water and this dryness causeth the workmen even greater harm, for the dust, which is stirred and beaten up by digging, penetrates into the windpipe and lungs and produces difficulty in breathing and the disease the Greeks call asthma. If the dust has corrosive qualities, it eats away the lungs and implants consumption in the body. In the Carpathian mines, women are found who have married seven husbands, all of whom this terrible consumption has carried away (Agricola, 1556).

Although dust diseases continued to be widely reported, it was not until the early twentieth century that systematic scientific investigations into the mechanisms, treatment and prevention of these diseases occurred. This was mainly due to dramatic increases in lung diseases associated with the rapid industrialisation and the increased use of coal, precious and base metals, asbestos, uranium and the associated expansion of the agricultural industries with subsequent exposures to grain and animal dusts. Much of our knowledge on the toxic effects of these dusts comes from such early industrial experiences mainly due to the fact that exposure of the workers was excessive and subsequently the extent and severity of disease were easily associated with specific industries and occupations. From these early industrial experiences it was found that the major properties of particulates that affect toxicological outcomes are the size of the particles and the region in which they deposit; the specific composition of the particulates; and the dose which is delivered direct to the lung or indirectly to other target organs.

In contemporary times, due to a series of legislative, political and community attitudes, exposures to toxic dusts have been considerably reduced and hence the dramatic health effects reported in the historical literature are rarely observed. Modern health observations are confounded by the overlap with lifestyle exposures to particulates such as tobacco smoke and recreational contacts with pets and hobbies.

Physical properties of dusts

Dust consists of particulate matter dispersed in air, a so-called 'solid aerosol'. It can originate from natural or synthetic processes, be mineral, animal or vegetable and consist of an organic or inorganic base. The process of dust formation may be via condensation (flocculation) or mechanical means such as breakdown to smaller particles. Dust clouds so generated consist of a wide range of particle sizes which tend towards a log–normal size distribution. The size of particles found in the general and occupational environment range from approximately 0.01 to 1000 μm in diameter; however, only the lower size fraction (less than approximately 200 μm) is relevant in lung disease. Particles have a discrete mass relative to the air in which they are mixed and are subject to physical forces such as gravitation, inertia and diffusion. Subsequently, they are removed rapidly from the air; if inhaled they can be deposited in the respiratory tract and for measurement and control purposes are easily captured by processes such as filtration. For example, a 1 μm particle with a density of 1 deposits out under the influence of gravity at a rate of 2.5 mm min^{-1} or, if inhaled, it has a 50% chance of being deposited in the lung. A 10 μm unit-density particle would fall at 18 cm min^{-1} and, if inhaled, would be likely (because of its size) to be deposited in the upper respiratory tract rather than deeper in the lung.

Deposition of inhaled particles

For a particulate to exert a direct health effect it must first be deposited either on the skin or within the respiratory tract. Inhalation and deposition of dusts can be explained in terms of the physical mechanisms that act on the particles whilst they are in the respiratory tract. The tract can be thought of as a baffled entry chamber leading to a branching system of tubes for transportation of gases which terminate in gas exchange sacks or alveoli. Particles entering into the system must pass through the baffles and approximately 16 bifurcations before entering the dead space of the respiratory bronchioles and alveoli where gas exchange occurs. As such they are subject to the following regional deposition forces:

- Impaction/interception, particularly in the nasopharyngeal region and at bronchial bifurcations, which depends on particle velocity, density and diameter.

- Gravitational settlement in the bronchioles, which is dependent on particle density and the square of the particle diameter.

- Brownian diffusion/impaction, essentially in the alveoli with the rate being dependent on particle size and its area of containment.

These mechanisms have different interactions in each region of the respiratory tract for different sized particles. Uniformity in describing the deposition of non-spherical particles of varying density can be obtained by reference to unit-density spheres (those that exhibit the same terminal velocity in air as do spheres of unit density and hence have equivalent aerodynamic diameters).

Estimates of the size fraction of aerosols that can be inhaled and then deposited at various sites have been obtained from pathological examination of lung deposits, inhalational research and modelling based on depositional forces. One generally accepted respiratory tract depositional curve is shown in Figure 14.1.

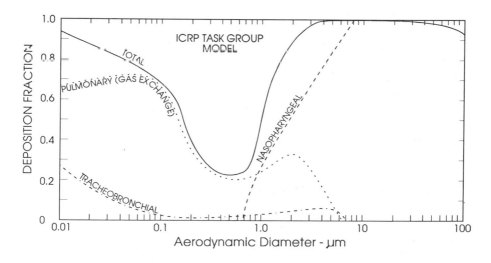

Figure 14.1. Total and regional deposition fractions for various sizes of inhaled airborne particles. (After ACGIH (1985).)

From a toxicological viewpoint there are three important dust deposition regions in the lung:

- The entire respiratory tract where the *inhalable fraction* is deposited.

- The pulmonary or gas exchange region where the so-called *respirable fraction* is deposited.

- The tracheobronchial region where the *thoracic fraction* is deposited.

There are some differences between the European (ISO) and American (ACGIH) definitions of these fractions, as indicated in Figure 14.2. However, given the spacial variability in natural dust clouds and the sampling errors associated with the use of some field measuring instruments, in reality there is little practical difference between the two systems.

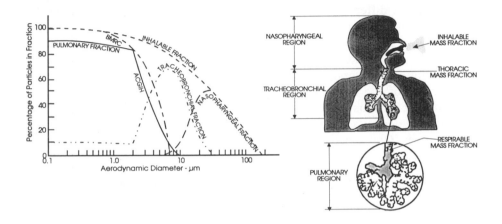

Figure 14.2. Boundaries of the various fractions of dust deposited in the respiratory tract. (After ACGIH (1985) and ISO (1981).)

Clearance and fate of deposited particles

Dust particles deposited in the alveoli are cleared by alveolar macrophages, which engulf and transport the dust to the lower end of the mucociliary elevator in the bronchioles or through the alveolar membrane into the lymphatic system. Those particles deposited higher up on the walls of the conducting airways are simply cleared with the mucus by way of the movement of the ciliated cells. The fate of all these particles is to be expectorated, swallowed into the gastrointestinal tract or to be partly or fully dissolved in the mucus. If swallowed there is the additional chance of dissolution and absorption in the gastrointestinal tract. The ICRP Task Group on Lung Dynamics (1966) have produced a schematic diagram (Figure 14.3) to indicate the complexity of linking lung deposition, clearance, dissolution and transport to other organs all of which affect the short, mid- and long-term toxicological effects of inhaled particles.

Chemical properties of dusts

Having deposited in some region of the respiratory tract, the second most important toxicological factor for particulates is their chemical make-up and the manner in which they present or are released to the body. It is rare to find a dust cloud which is pure in terms of chemical composition—indeed industrial dusts may contain a number of components which have synergistic or differing toxicological effects.

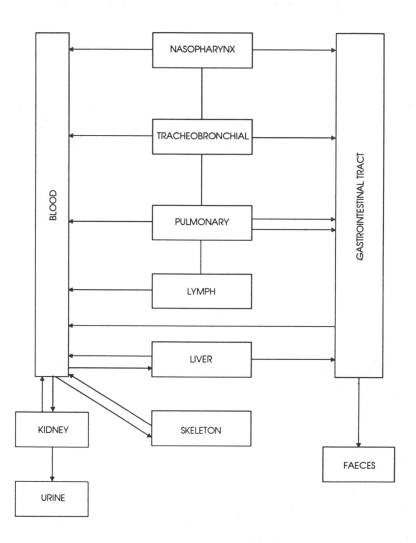

Figure 14.3. Fate of soluble particles. (After ICRP (1966).)

• Each substance under investigation may be a major, minor or a trace component of the dust cloud. For example, in the mining and milling of talc, the presence of minor and trace components such as crystalline silica and asbestos have contributed more to pneumoconiosis cases in the workforce than has the dust created from the talc mineral itself.

- The chemical composition of the dust may also vary with particle size. It is often observed that enrichment or depletion of various toxic components can be found in the various size fractions of the dust, depending on the method of generation of the dust cloud. Crystalline silica is a good example of this process where, because of the relative hardness of silica compared with other minerals, there is a reduced concentration of crystalline silica in the small size fraction of mechanically generated dusts.

- The surface area and surface activity of the dust particles are also important. Consider, for instance, the various forms of silica. Freshly broken crystalline silica dust is well known to be very toxic to alveolar macrophages and results in the build up of collagen in the alveoli eventually resulting in fibrosis (silicosis). As the surface of the silica dust is weathered and aged its biological effects lessen. It is also observed that amorphous silica and non-fibrous silicates do not exhibit such severe toxic effects. A number of authors have suggested that these observed biological differences are due to the amount of surface activity of the dust resulting in free radical formation and the generation of superoxide mechanisms in cells.

- Due to sorting mechanisms such as hardness, density and settling rates it is incorrect to infer chemical composition obtained from bulk material represents the composition of airborne dust or specific fractions such as respirable dust.

Whilst it is relatively simple to follow the toxicological mechanisms by which dusts that are soluble in body fluids exert their effects, the explanation of the effects of seemingly chemically inert dusts is far from complete. Although a considerable amount of toxicological information is available on these types of dust, the overall mechanisms are not fully understood. Theories such as particle size, chemical composition, surface morphology and activity, and bioavailabilty have been presented over the years, but no single factor fully explains the toxicological effects of specific particles such as silica or asbestos. Whilst the above individual factors hold some importance, it is probable that the toxic effects of chemically inert dusts are due to various combinations of these factors which are specific to each dust type.

Part explanation of the different dose–response curves produced in toxicological and epidemiological studies may be that different sources of particulates have different chemical and physical properties that affect the relative biological impact. Asbestos is a well studied example of this phenomenon with the published studies producing a range of dose–response gradients for the different types of asbestos and for the different types of asbestos manufacturing industries.

It should be emphasised that dust is not simply 'dust', silica is simply not 'silica', asbestos is not simply 'asbestos'; each dust type emanating from various processes and industries has specific chemical and physical properties that determine its specific toxicological impact.

For toxicological experimentation and for evaluations, it is important to compare specific dusts against recognised biological dust standards so that any relative differences can be observed and substantiated.

Measurement of dust exposures

In occupational exposure situations it is usual to capture the deposited respirable fraction using miniature cyclones and to measure the deposited inhalable fraction using the modified UK Atomic Energy Authority sampling heads or the Institute of Occupational Medicine inspirable dust sampling head. This inhalable fraction is a combination of respirable, thoracic and nasopharyngeal fractions and is currently used in practical situations to represent either thoracic or nasopharyngeal dust exposures since field sampling instruments for these individual fractions are not commercially available (ACGIH, 1985; SAA, 1987, 1989). Cowled and closed cassette samplers without preselection devices do not collect the correct respirable or inhalable size fractions (Vincent, 1989).

The quantity of specific toxicological agent in the collected fraction is measured via chemical or physical analysis, enzyme activity, etc. Standard methods of analysis have been produced for some industrial dusts (NIOSH, 1984; HSE, 1991). Whilst this approach provides a comparison against recognised occupational or community health based standards it does not necessarily provide adequate information for use in toxicological experimentation where more detailed analysis of dusts may be of value in determining differences in experimental results.

A simple toxicological classification for dusts

Whilst the preceding discussions convey the concept of the toxicological diversity of similar dust types, there are very few guidelines to assist practitioners in determining potential health effects for unknown or uncommon dusts.

The 1991 ACGIH Threshold Limit Value list which is commonly used internationally as a comparison for allowable industrial exposures, lists some 126 specific dusts on which there is available information sufficient to be able to set an industrial exposure limit. This number constitutes only a small fraction of the types of dusts found in industrial situations and partly indicates the difficulties experienced in obtaining specific toxicological data on substances which have a complex chemical composition and variable biological effects on exposed individuals.

It is, however, possible to form a classification of dusts based on a combination of the region in which the dust deposits in the lung and the locality of the resulting biological effect. Many dusts have a number of effects; for example, crystalline silica can cause irritation in high concentrations, may eventually result in clinical silicosis, and also is suspected as being a carcinogen. However even with these multiple effects it is still possible to use the individual effects in this classification as a basis for assessment of exposure standards and the development of a rationale for exposure measurement.

Dusts which have localised toxicological effects on the lung

Respirable dust fraction

Those dusts which exert a toxic effect in the *pulmonary* (gas exchange) area of the lung which can be attributed to the fraction of dust which is deposited directly in this region (*respirable dust fraction*) and result in fibrosis, fever and oedema.

FIBROSIS

This is caused by a wide range of mineral dusts with the type of pneumoconiosis usually named after the associated dust type. As previously mentioned, the most common agent is crystalline silica (silicosis) although other forms of silicates, mixed mineral dusts and coal (coal miners' pneumoconiosis) can produce a milder form of fibrosis given high enough exposures. Asbestos also causes a specific type of fibrosis (asbestosis). These minerals are widespread and are associated with the mining, mineral processing and user industries. Continued exposure to some natural organic dusts may also result in a diffuse interstitial fibrosis. The complete mechanism of fibrosis has not been revealed; however, a number of processes beginning with alveoli macrophage ingestion of the particles, destruction and rupture of the macrophages with migration to alveoli cells followed by tissue reaction and irritation with the eventual formation and build up of reticulin and collagen fibres have all been observed (Morgan and Seaton, 1984). The end result is radiologically observable scarring with reduction of lung elasticity and gas exchange capacity of the alveoli, with subsequent reduced lung function and breathing difficulty, particularly during physical exertion.

FEVER

This specific example of local tissue reaction after deposition of dust in the alveoli is caused by the proliferation of alveolar macrophages and the development of symptoms of fever some 2–8 h after initial exposure. An example commonly encountered in industry is metal-fume fever caused by exposure to a variety of very small freshly formed fumes of metal oxide. Zinc oxide fumes emitted from furnaces or during welding or brazing of galvanised surfaces are particularly noxious from this point of view. Some organic dusts resulting from hypersensitivity also produce a similar reaction which is called 'extrinsic allergic alveolitis'. Repeated episodes may result in low-grade diffuse fibrosis.

OEDEMA

This occurs as a result of parenchymal tissue injury with the subsequent outpouring of cell fluids into the alveoli. Freshly formed cadmium oxide fumes and liquid petroleum droplets are typical examples of particulates that cause this reaction.

Thoracic dust fraction

Those dusts which exert a toxic effect in the *tracheobronchial* region which can be attributed to the fraction of dust deposited directly in this region (*thoracic dust fraction*) and result in allergic reaction and bronchogenic cancer.

ALLERGIC REACTION

Many particulate substances that deposit in the airways can result in sensitisation of the bronchial tissue with the result that subsequent exposures result in a cholinergic bronchospasm or constriction resulting in the common condition called 'asthma'. These particulates include pollens, fungal spores, animal danders, animal proteins, wood and grain dusts which are encountered in a wide range of industries, particularly those involving agriculture and food processing. The composition of these dusts is very complex and the specific chemical agent that causes the reaction is often unknown. Liquid droplets created during the spraying of synthetic paint resins containing unreacted isocyanate groups also cause sensitisation and bronchiospasm. In industries such as coal mining and quarrying, especially where excessive exposure to mineral dusts occurs in workers who are cigarette smokers, increased symptoms of bronchitis with inflammation and excessive secretion of thickened mucus have been reported. It should also be noted that many of the dusts which cause allergic reaction in the bronchi also cause allergic reactions when smaller particles are deposited in the alveoli.

BRONCHOGENIC CANCER

This common cancer of the respiratory tract is known to be caused by a number of aetiological particulates such as tobacco smoke, asbestos, coke-oven emissions, arsenic and radioactive dusts. The site of the development of the cancer is the central bronchi and the bronchial bifurcations, the latter being the main deposition sites for particulates in this region of the lung.

Inhalable dust fraction

Those dusts which exert a toxic effect in the *nasopharangeal* region which can be attributed to the fraction of dust deposited directly in this region (*inhalable dust fraction*) and result in irritation and inflammation.

IRRITATION

Particles deposited in the nose, mouth and throat can cause direct mechanical irritation or chemical irritation of the local tissue. For instance, it has been demonstrated that the degree of a prickling sensation or irritation caused by inhalation of fibreglass is directly related to the diameter of the fibres. Chemical irritants such as acids and alkaline particulates dissolve rapidly in the mucous membrane and have direct chemical contact with the underlying cells causing the sensation of intense impact or irritation as is observed in industries such as cement and soap-powder manufacturing. Individuals usually become acclimatised to this irritant effect but it remains a problem for new workers or those returning after extended periods of absence. Continued contact with high exposures of these irritants may result in nasal bleeding, ulceration and perforation of the septa as has been observed historically in chrome and nickel ore roasting.

INFLAMMATION

This is commonly associated with exposure to organic dusts in natural product industries such as farming and grain handling. The aetiological agent may be from the product debris or from contaminants such as bacterial or fungal fragments or spores. The commonly observed reaction is a localised allergic reaction with inflammation of the nasal membranes and excessive secretion of mucus (rhinitis). This condition may also be observed in those industries such as quarrying where there is excessive exposure to mineral dusts.

Dusts which have a systemic toxicological effect outside the respiratory tract

This category includes those dusts which, having been deposited in either the individual or combined nasopharangeal, tracheobronchial or respiratory tract regions, can be partly or fully dissolved in the mucus membranes or are transported to the gastrointestinal tract followed by translocation to other organs. Heavy metal compounds such as lead oxide are typical of this process. In the lead smelting and remelt industries a combination of lead fume and lead dust can be encountered. These particulates after deposition throughout the entire respiratory tract are partly dissolved in the lung mucus with the rate depending on the size of the particle, site of deposition and the solubility of the lead from the oxide or sulphide. With lead oxide, approximately 35–50% of the amount deposited in the pulmonary region is absorbed by this mechanism. Those particles which are not dissolved, are transported up the mucociliary escalator and eventually ingested into the gastrointestinal tract where they are subject to the acid conditions in the stomach. An additional 10% of the lead oxide is absorbed in this manner and then translocated via the bloodstream to the liver, kidneys, blood and nerve forming tissues where it exerts its toxic influence.

Dusts with minimal or negligible toxicological effect

These have traditionally been labelled as 'nuisance dusts' or more recently as 'particulates not otherwise classified' (ACGIH 1991–1992). All dusts evoke some cellular response in the lung if inhaled in sufficient quantities; however, a considerable number of known dusts have a long history of industrial exposures which result in little adverse effects on the lungs and do not produce significant organic disease or toxic effects when exposures are kept under reasonable control. In terms of the effects on the lung it is known that the architecture of the airspaces remain intact, there is no significant formation of collagen and any tissue reaction caused by the dust is potentially reversible after cessation of exposure. Whilst this lack of long-term effects may be true for almost all the population exposed, some sensitive individuals may be adversely affected by these dusts.

Even though the toxic effects of these dusts may be minor, other considerations such as nuisance factors (i.e. loss of visibility, irritant effects on the eyes, nose, ears and skin, drying or reaction with mucous membranes and mechanical injury caused when cleansing these dusts from the body) may be important. Care should be taken when assigning dusts with limited toxicological data to this 'nuisance' category.

Specific examples of toxic dusts that affect the respiratory tract

Asbestos

'Asbestos' is a general term for a number of fibrous minerals which have found industrial uses such as for fire protection, thermal and acoustical insulation, filtration and providing mechanical support in solid matrices. The asbestos industry was widespread and diversified being in the mining, milling, formulating installation and removal of the various forms of the products and this historically has resulted in considerable disease due to overt dust exposures. The toxic effects of the dust from this mineral assemblage have been studied extensively both in terms of the physics and chemistry of the particles, laboratory cell and animal experimentation and human epidemiological studies. For the three main commercial types (chrysotile, amosite and crocidolite) and the others which are commonly encountered as geological contaminants (tremolite, anthophyllite and actino-lite) it is well documented that, given sufficient exposure, all may cause asbestosis and bronchogenic cancer, whilst for some types of asbestos, mesothelioma is a potential outcome. Asbestosis and lung cancer are diseases caused by deposition of asbestos fibres directly at the site of the resulting tumour, although the exact mechanism of causation is not as yet fully understood (Cotes and Steel, 1987). In addition, as asbestos minerals are relatively inert they do not readily dissolve in the lung mucus and most are too long to be totally engulfed by macrophages; hence a proportion of the deposited load remains in the lung paranchyma. Studies involving examination of historical air monitoring records and examination of lung asbestos burdens indicate that the incidence and severity of each disease can be related to the concentration of asbestos fibres which are inhaled. Airborne exposure can be measured by capturing the total dust cloud using a pump to draw the dust onto a membrane filter which is then prepared as a transparent slide in the laboratory and the respirable size fibres are discriminated by visual comparison, counted and reported as respirable fibres per millilitre of contaminated air.

In all of the studied diseases a dose–response relationship has been found between incidence of the disease and the cumulative exposure expressed as a product of: fibres per millilitre × years. The gradient of the response curve varies depending on the type of disease, asbestos type and industrial situation (McDonald and McDonald, 1987). Legislators have used this information to set occupational exposure standards using available quantitative risk estimates. The first such estimate was made by the British Occupational Hygiene Society in 1968 involving asbestosis risk and chrysotile exposure. Here it was determined that a 1% risk of early signs of asbestosis would occur after a cumulative exposure of 100 fibres per millilitre-years. The standard was then set as 2 fibres per millilitre based on a working lifetime of 50 years. Later examination of this data and additional information indicated that this level of lifetime exposure may also provide a 3% risk of lung cancer. Exposure standards for amphiboles have been set at a much lower value due to their association with mesothelioma. Recently, many countries have adopted lower exposure standards and even prohibitions on some forms such as the amphiboles.

For a variety of technical, social and political reasons, in most countries exposure to asbestos has been reduced or eliminated so that new cases of asbestosis are becoming rare and the risk of lung cancer in the remaining asbestos industry has been reduced to a level where it cannot be distinguished from that of non-asbestos workers. Due to latency effects of around 30–40 years there are still observations of lung cancers and a rising incidence of mesothelioma cases from uncontrolled exposures in the industries that operated in the 1940s to 1960s. It is predicted that due to considerable reduction of exposures in the 1970s to 1990s that this peak will pass by the turn of the century.

Grain dusts

Exposure to grain dusts occurs across the entire grain handling industry including harvesting, transportation and storage. Traditionally it was classified as a 'nuisance dust'; however, a series of surveys on the workforce have indicated widespread symptoms of asthmatic type reactions, flu like illness, rhinitis, dermatitis and conjunctivitis (Dosman and Cotton, 1980). Since these symptoms also exist in sections of the general public due to other agents, it is difficult to attribute specific aetiology for individual cases. There is only limited data on the specific sensitisation agents in the dust. Field surveys have indicated that collected dust consists of a complex heterogeneous mixture of grain debris, pollen, weed debris, arthropods, rodent spore, bird excreta, microbiological growth, fungal spores, soil and silica most of which can cause allergic reactions in individuals. The effects of bronchial restriction occur immediately after exposure and it has been found that disease is related to prior sensitisation which may have occurred over a short time of a few exposures or over many years. The allergic reaction is probably due to a combination of specific agents and occurs primarily in the tracheobronchial region and secondly in the alveoli region of the lung, therefore the method of measurement of exposure is to capture the inhalable dust fraction. Since there is no single chemical agent the results are expressed gravimetrically as the total collected fraction. The current exposure standard for grain dust is a time-weighted average of 4 mg m^{-3}; however, it can be expected that some sensitive or sensitised individuals will react adversely within a very short time to concentrations below this value. Control strategies should be aimed at reducing overall dustiness as it impossible to measure the precise proportion of the dust which is responsible for causing individual reaction and potential sensitisation. Respiratory protection appears to be the most effective means of protection for these workers and experience indicates that powered air purifying types provide the greatest degree of comfort and freedom of movement for this industry.

Crystalline silica

Due to the widespread presence of this mineral, contact with this dust is widespread throughout the mining, manufacturing, construction and demolition industries. For instance in Australia it is estimated that some 140 000 workers have the potential for exposure (NOHSC, 1993). The most common form encountered is quartz but high-temperature polymorphs (cristobalite and tridymite) may occur in hot industries such as glass and metalliferous manufacturing. Long-term exposure to high dust concentrations can result in silicosis which occurs in the pulmonary regions. Lately, evidence has emerged that tracheobronchial effects such as chronic obstructive airways disease and lung cancer may also be caused by crystalline silica. The health effects occur after long-term exposure and it has been found that disease is related to cumulative exposure experienced over a lifetime or at least over many years. Control strategies are based on the prevention of silicosis; hence exposure measurement methods involve the capture of the respirable fraction of the dust using minicyclones. The proportion of crystalline silica in the collected respirable dust is subsequently measured in the laboratory using analysis methods involving techniques such as X-ray diffraction or infra-red spectroscopy. This approach appears to ignore the thoracic fraction of crystalline silica dust, which intuitively is responsible for the airways disease. In practice, however, because of the log–normal distribution of most dust clouds, it is possible to infer that the respirable fraction can be used as an index of the thoracic fraction. There is some limited evidence for a dose–response relationship between exposure to respirable crystalline silica and the development of silicosis and lung cancer. Risk calculations have been applied to the exposed populations; however, the relatively small numbers of additional disease (particularly lung cancers) expected in the population exposed at the current exposure standards is very small compared with the rates of disease found in the general population. Surveillance of the silica industries indicates that in well-controlled situations if exposures are kept below 0.2 mg m^{-3} using such techniques as wet methods and ventilation then debilitating silicosis can be essentially eliminated. In small industries and with contractor services where exposures and medical surveillance are not as well controlled, the situation is different with these groups being responsible for a disproportionate amount of the compensable diseases (NOHSC, 1993).

References

ACGIH (American Conference of Governmental Industrial Hygienists), 1985, *Particle Size-Selective Sampling in the Workplace*. Cincinnati, OH: ACGIH Technical Committee on Air sampling Procedures.

ACGIH (American Conference of Governmental Industrial Hygienists), 1991–1992, *Threshold Limit Values for Chemical Substances and Physical Agents and Biological Exposure Indices, and Documentation of TLV's and Biological Exposure Indices*, 5th Edn with updates. A.C.G.I.H. Cincinnati, OH.

Agricola, G., 1556, De re metallica, in Hoover, H. C. and Hoover, L. H. (Trans.) *The Mining Magazine (London)*, 1912.

Cotes, J. E. and Steel, J., 1987, *Work Related Lung Disorders*. Oxford: Blackwell Scientific.

Dosman, J. A. and Cotton, D. J. (Eds), 1980, *Occupational Pulmonary Disease, Focus on Grain Dust and Health*. New York: Academic Press.

HSE (United Kingdom Health and Safety Executive), 1991, *Guidance Note EH 40/90, Occupational Exposure Limits, and Methods for the Determination of Hazardous Substances MDHS 1–71*. H.M.S.O. London

ICRP Task Group on Lung Dynamics, 1966, International Commission on Radiological Protection, *Health Phys.*, **12**, 173–207.

ISO (International Standards Organisation), 1981, Size definitions for particle sampling—Recommendations of ad hoc working group appointed by Committee TC 146 of the International Standards Organisation, *Am. Ind. Hyg. Assoc. J.*, **May**, A-64–8.

McDonald, J. C. and McDonald, A. D., 1987, Epidemiology of asbestos-related lung cancer in Antman, K. and Aisner, J. (Eds) *Asbestos-related Malignancy*, pp. 57–80. Orlando, FL: Grune and Stratton.

Morgan, W. K. C. and Seaton, A., 1984, *Occupational Lung Diseases*, 2nd Edn. Philadelphia: W. B. Saunders.

NIOSH, 1984, *NIOSH Manual of Analytical Methods*, 3rd Edn. Cincinnati, OH: US Department of Health and Human Services, National Institute of Occupational Safety and Health.

NOHSC (National Occupational Health and Safety Commission), 1993, *Technical Report on Crystalline Silica*. Prepared by the Expert Working Group, NOHSC. Australian Government Publishing Service, Canberra.

SAA (Standards Association of Australia), 1987, *Australian Standard 2985–1987 Workplace Atmospheres—Method for Sampling and Gravimetric Determination of Respirable Dust*. 80 Arthur Street, North Sydney, NSW, Australia: SAA.

SAA (Standards Association of Australia), 1989, *Australian Standard As 3640–1989, Workplace Atmospheres—Method for Sampling and Gravimetric Determination of Inspirable Dust*. 80 Arthur Street, North Sydney, NSW, Australia: SAA.

Vincent, J. H., 1989, *Aerosol Sampling*. Chichester: Wiley.

Fields Interfacing with Toxicology

Chapter 15

Occupational Hygiene—Interface with Toxicology

C. Gray

The scope of occupational hygiene

Assessment and control of toxic substances in the workplace is one of the main roles of the occupational hygiene profession. Although this is by no means the exclusive responsibility of occupational hygienists and is shared with other professionals as well as with workers and management, occupational hygienists have a special combination of skills and knowledge, gained by formal training and/or extensive experience, which equips them for this role. This requires some knowledge of toxicology, occupational diseases, epidemiology, standard setting, occupational health law and management, as well as a thorough understanding of methods of exposure assessment and control. Occupational hygienists are also concerned with physical hazards such as noise and vibration, non-ionising radiation, heat stress and to some extent with biohazards and ergonomics.

They often work in a team along with occupational physicians, occupational health nurses, safety officers, toxicologists and others. Although there is some overlap between the skills of these various professionals their roles are usually quite distinct. The greatest overlap might be found between the occupational hygienist and safety officer. Ideally, an all round safety officer would be able to carry out at least some of the functions of an occupational hygienist. The distinction is usually to be found in the scientific background of the occupational hygienist which enables him/her to understand more deeply the physical, chemical and biological principles that underlie factors which are a threat to health and wellbeing.

Traditionally, occupational safety was concerned primarily with reducing the risk of traumatic injury due to machine accidents, falls, fire, explosion, etc. Occupational hygiene grew out of the recognition of the more insidious effects of repeated exposure to chemicals or other hazards in the workplace. The demarcation which has grown up between these two professions is to some extent artificial, but there is a general and growing recognition of the need for specialists who have sound scientific backgrounds and the appropriate training and experience to equip them to

269

understand and control the increasingly complex hazards in our technically advanced workplaces.

In assessing hazards in the workplace, occupational hygienists are able to draw upon a large store of knowledge built up over many years by the efforts of occupational physicians, toxicologists, epidemiologists and other occupational hygienists. By reference to this knowledge they are able to recognise hazards that may need control or further evaluation.

Measurements can be made of worker exposure to these hazards, for example the airborne concentration of a toxic gas in a worker's breathing zone can be measured and the results can be compared with criteria which allow the risk of disease or injury to be assessed. Appropriate control measures can then be instituted to reduce the risk to the exposed workers. Such controls might involve the substitution of a toxic substance used in a process, or the provision of engineering controls such as ventilation.

This sequence of *recognition, evaluation*, and *control* represents the traditional formula for occupational hygiene practice. A fourth component in the sequence is now recognised and that is *anticipation*. This can involve deliberate consideration of new technology, processes, equipment and materials before they are introduced into the workplace. It can also involve taking account of the consequences of unplanned process changes; the failure of control equipment, the inappropriate use of process chemicals for cleaning purposes and the short cuts in work practice which result in unnecessary exposures.

Occupational hygienists concerned with the assessment and control of chemicals in the workplace would hardly be able to operate without access to toxicological information. They would not know which substances required controlling, nor to what extent. However, this flow of information is not just one way. Occupational hygiene data are an essential part of the toxicological appraisal of industrial substances and are utilised both in epidemiology and in setting of exposure standards. Occupational epidemiology involves examining the relationship between health and workplace exposures and occupational hygienists, or others with relevant experience, are involved in providing assessments of current or historical exposures, depending upon the design of the epidemiological study.

Setting of exposure standards, such as the American Threshold Limit Values (TLVs) and the Australian Worksafe National Exposure Standards, usually draws heavily upon workplace exposure data gathered by occupational hygienists. In fact, the TLVs were developed by technical committees of the American Conference of Governmental Industrial Hygienists (ACGIH). Similarly, various biological limits have been developed based upon biological monitoring techniques such as the measurement of toxic substances or their metabolites in urine. These seek to impose limits on uptake of chemicals by workers rather than on concentrations of substances in the workplace air to which workers are exposed. The ACGIH Biological Exposure Indices (BEIs) are examples of such biological limits. The BEIs are not derived directly from toxicological data as might be expected, but are based on the TLVs and are derived by comparison of occupational exposures and biological monitoring results taking into account the relevant biotransformation and elimination kinetics.

It should be apparent from the foregoing that occupational health involves a complex interplay between toxicology, epidemiology, occupational hygiene and occupational medicine. This is illustrated in a simplified way in Figure 15.1.

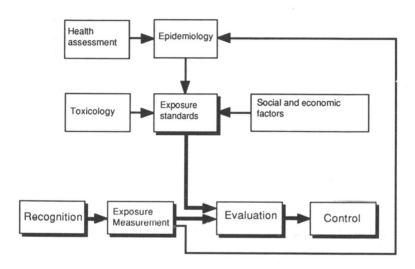

Figure 15.1. Simplified diagram of the relationship between occupational hygiene and occupational epidemiology and toxicology from the occupational hygiene perspective. It should also be borne in mind that clinical or toxicological investigations may be instigated as a result of occupational hygiene or epidemiological observations.

Exposure to chemicals in the workplace

The term 'exposure' implies contact with a substance which can lead to uptake and when we measure exposure in some way we are attempting to measure this potential for uptake.

Airborne gases and vapours and inhalable dusts can enter via the respiratory tract and this is often the most important route of uptake in the occupational setting. Some toxic substances can also be absorbed via the skin and most via the gastrointestinal tract. Lipid-soluble substances including organic solvents and some pesticides readily pass through the intact skin and for some dusty materials hand to mouth contact can result in significant uptake via the gastrointestinal tract. This is thought to be of some importance in the lead industry for example.

Although it is acknowledged that gastrointestinal and skin uptake can be important, exposure limits such as the Australian exposure standards refer only to airborne concentrations of substances which result in uptake via the respiratory tract. The skin notation which is applied to some substances, indicates that there is a potential for systemic toxicity as a result of skin uptake, but there is no exposure limit for this route of entry. Although we have no way of directly quantifying personal exposure by the skin or gastrointestinal routes, biological monitoring can sometimes be used to measure the uptake by all routes including these.

Toxic substances may be present in the air in several physical forms as shown in Table 15.1, the major divisions being: (a) dusts and other particulates; and (b) gases and vapours. Dusts, fumes, fibres, mists and smokes are referred to as 'particulate matter' or 'particulates', whilst a more or less stable suspension of particles in air is referred to as an 'aerosol'.

Table 15.1. Types of air contaminant

Gases	Individual molecules of substances which cannot be liquefied at normal temperatures, e.g. carbon dioxide
Vapours	Individual molecules of substances which are liquid or solid at normal temperatures, e.g. benzene
Total dust	All particles in the air
Inhalable dust	Can be drawn into upper airways
Respirable dust	Can penetrate to alveoli of lungs
Fibres	Elongated particulates (length/breadth > 3:1)
Mist	Airborne liquid droplets
Fume	Solid particles formed by evaporation–condensation processes (e.g. welding fume) or by gas phase reactions (e.g. ammonium chloride)
Smoke	Solid particles or liquid (usually tar like) droplets formed by combustion mechanisms leading to evaporation–condensation, or gas phase reactions leading to condensation

Preliminary assessment

Assessment involves both recognition and evaluation of workplace hazards. Recognition might seem a simple task, after all we could easily observe the use of solvent-based adhesive for example. However, workplaces are usually complex and contain many potential hazards and the problem is to identify all the important ones and to prioritise them for immediate corrective action, further evaluation or for attention at some later date.

In the recognition stage, an initial 'walk-through' or preliminary survey is often carried out to assess the potential hazards associated with the workplace. Generally the walk-through survey is carried out without the use of measuring instruments and involves careful observation of processes, raw materials, intermediates, products, by-products, wastes and significant contaminants. By linking a substance inventory with toxicity data and information on the processes and work procedures, hazards can be systematically identified and prioritised. The preliminary survey can also help to identify physical hazards such as noise, heat stress and poor illumination, and adverse ergonomic factors.

The use and adequacy of control measures such as ventilation, personal protective equipment or special work practices can also be noted. As a result of the preliminary surveys, many hazards which may require a full occupational hygiene evaluation may be identified.

Exposure monitoring

The second phase of the assessment procedure is evaluation and commences with monitoring of personal exposures or workplace air concentrations of chemicals identified in the preliminary assessment phase. There are two main reasons for monitoring chemicals in the workplace.

- To estimate personal exposure to hazardous substances.

- To assist in the design or selection of controls to reduce exposure.

The first of these two reasons for monitoring is usually related to assessing compliance with exposure standards. The second is to provide information for control purposes that will help reduce the exposures in some way. This might involve more detailed investigations of exposure patterns in processes in order to identify which process steps give rise to the greatest exposures so that controls can be designed which are most effective.

For example, personal monitoring might have shown that average exposures to solvent vapour in a manufacturing operation are above the exposure standard. Further investigations might reveal that only one or two process steps, such as loading a solvent tank or equipment cleaning, make a major contribution to the overall exposure. Controls (elimination, substitution, ventilation or personal protection) can then be focused on those process steps rather than on the entire manufacturing operation.

Monitoring might also be required for other reasons including:

- Checking confined spaces prior to entry as they might contain toxic, inflammable or explosive atmospheres or be deficient in oxygen.

- To ensure that processes involving highly dangerous substances are under continuous control; that leaks have not developed and that control equipment is working. These usually require the use of direct reading instruments.

Exposure data might also be used for the purposes of epidemiology, to investigate a possible association between medical outcomes and exposures.

There are many methods of monitoring chemicals in air and these fall into two major divisions.

- Air sampling techniques in which a sample of the contaminant is collected for subsequent analysis in the laboratory.

- Direct reading methods in which an analytical instrument is taken into the workplace to obtain 'real-time' measurements.

Most frequently, air samples are taken to determine the exposure levels of a worker or group of workers. This is most effectively achieved by measuring concentrations of substances in the worker's 'breathing zone' where the air is representative of that which the individual worker is breathing; sometimes this is defined as within 300 mm of the nose or mouth. Often it is satisfactory to collect an air sample at the location of the lapel or breast pocket, but in some situations it is necessary to sample as close to the nose as possible. This is the case where a worker wears a visor (e.g. a welder's helmet) but is also necessary when a worker is very close to the source of the emission and the concentration gradients are very steep. To evaluate engineering controls or determine sources of contamination, samples are normally collected in the vicinity of the operation itself.

The duration of sampling is determined principally by the objective of monitoring and must be selected to take account of the requirements of the analytical method. A full-shift personal sample is preferred when results are to be compared to 8 h time-weighted average exposure standards. Where a substance has a short-term limit it is more difficult to demonstrate compliance. In principle, serial 15-min measurements are necessary, although it is possible to employ less frequent sampling with appropriate statistical analysis. It can be even more difficult to satisfactorily demonstrate compliance with a ceiling limit. This requires continuous monitoring using a direct reading instrument, but sometimes short-term sampling of up to 15 min duration has to be used instead.

It is also important to realise that exposures can be highly variable from worker to worker and from day to day, and it can be misleading to put great reliance in a single, or just a few, exposure measurements. Monitoring should follow a carefully considered strategy aimed at answering clearly stated questions about exposure in a given group of workers and the statistical validity of the results should be assessed.

Dust monitoring

Personal sampling most commonly makes use of small portable battery operated pumps which can be worn by the worker and are used to draw air through a sampling device which will collect the contaminant. Dust can be collected in several ways, the most common of which is to draw a measured volume of air through a suitable filter.

Airborne dusts may have a wide range of particle size and very coarse dust which cannot be inhaled is of little toxicological significance. What is important is the fraction of the dust that can be drawn into the airways. For systematically poisonous substances any dust which enters the nose is important; this is the 'inhalable' fraction. If the lung is the target organ, as in the case of fibrogenic dusts such as quartz, then only that fraction of the dust which can penetrate to the deep regions of the lung is important; this is the 'respirable' fraction.

When assessing the inhalability of dusts, the important property of the dust particles is their 'aerodynamic diameter'. This is the diameter measured by the rate of fall of the particles in air rather than their geometric size or shape.

The inhalable dust fraction is defined by the ACGIH as corresponding with the curve shown in Figure 15.2 and can be sampled using the Institute of Occupational Medicine, Edinburgh (IOM) inhalable dust monitor shown in Figure 15.3 or, more approximately, using the modified UKAEA (seven-hole) sampling head.

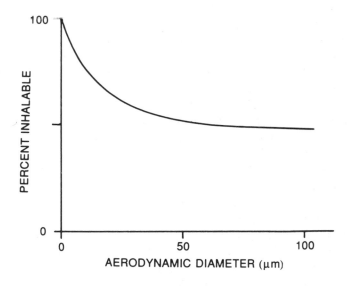

Figure 15.2. The inhalable fraction of airborne dust (ACGIH definition).

The respirable dust fraction is defined by the International Standards Organisation (ISO) as corresponding with the curve shown in Figure 15.4 and is sampled using a suitable cyclone (Figure 15.5) which rejects the

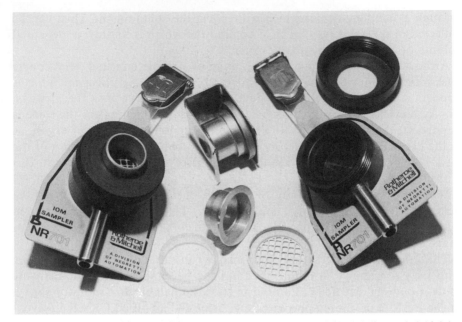

Figure 15.3. The IOM inhalable dust monitor shown assembled (left) and dismantled (right).

non-respirable dust fraction. A different sampling head is used for asbestos monitoring, consisting of a downward facing open face filter holder with a cowl on the inlet to prevent very large particles being collected.

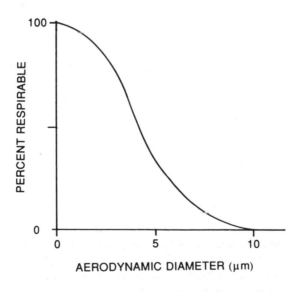

Figure 15.4. The respirable fraction of airborne dust (ISO definition).

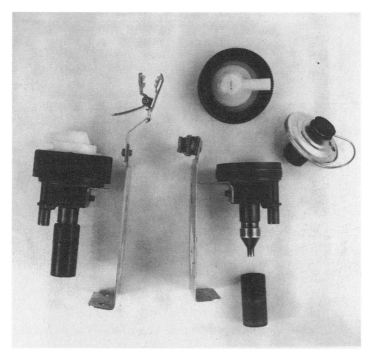

Figure 15.5. A cyclone respirable dust monitor shown assembled (left) and dismantled (right). The filter is mounted in the casette shown held closed by a spring clip.

Once a dust sample has been collected it is then measured or analysed. For example, this might involve accurate weighing, metal analysis by atomic absorption spectrometry (AAS), or asbestos fibre counting by phase contrast optical microscopy (PCOM).

In order to monitor a worker's exposure to dust, a filter is mounted in the sampling head which is then connected to a sampling pump by a length of plastic tubing and the pump is set to the required flow rate ($2 \, \mathrm{l \, min^{-1}}$ in the case of an inhalable dust monitor or $1.9 \, \mathrm{l \, min^{-1}}$ for a cyclone). The sampling head is clipped in the breathing zone of the worker, for example near the lapel, and the pump is hung from a belt or waist band (Figure 15.6). Sampling is then carried out for an accurately timed period which may be a full working day or a shorter interval.

Monitoring gases and vapours

Gases and vapours may be sampled by a variety of different techniques, depending on their physical and chemical properties. It is possible to sample any gas or vapour into a container such as a plastic bag, and special sampling bags made of Teflon (polytetrafluoroethylene) or Tedlar (polyvinylfluoride) are available commercially for this purpose. These have low-permeabilities and adsorptive properties and allow many vapours to be

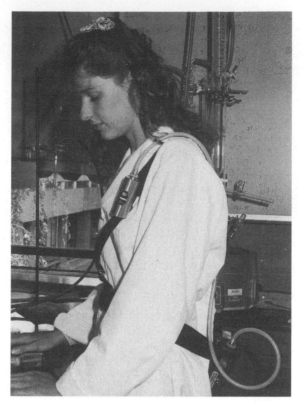

Figure 15.6. A worker wearing a cyclone respirable dust monitor and personal sampling pump.

stored for a day or so with minimal loss. Samples collected in this way are bulky and contain only small amounts of contaminant for chemical analysis, and for these reasons bag sampling is not often used by occupational hygienists. Other techniques of sampling gases and vapours remove the contaminant from the air by trapping it in a sampling device and thereby allow a larger amount to be collected for analysis. Probably the two most important such sampling techniques are *absorption* in a liquid or *adsorption* onto a porous solid such as charcoal.

For many gases and some vapours it is necessary to collect the analyte using liquid absorption. This commonly involves bubbling an air stream through a solution that will dissolve the contaminant or trap it by chemical reaction. For example, alkaline gases such as amines can be trapped in acid solutions and formaldehyde can be trapped as an addition product in aqueous sodium bisulphite solution. The liquid is placed in a glass wash bottle or impinger (Figure 15.7) which can be mounted in the breathing zone of the worker while the pump is attached to the belt or waist band. Contaminants which have been collected in liquids may be analysed by

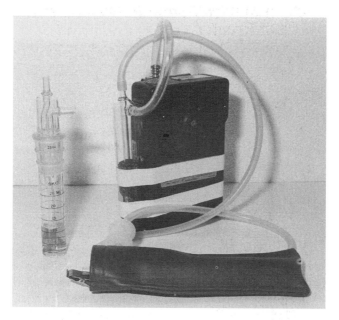

Figure 15.7. Sampling pump and impingers. An impinger is shown strapped to the pump with adhesive tape. The pouch at the forefront is designed to hold and protect an impinger.

a variety of methods depending on the nature of the contaminant and the adsorbing solution. Commonly used techniques are ultraviolet/visible (UV/VIS) spectrometry and liquid chromatography.

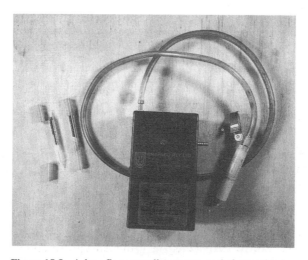

Figure 15.8. A low flow sampling pump and charcoal tubes.

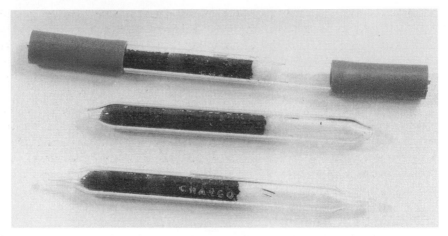

Figure 15.9. Charcoal tubes. Bottom: unused. Middle: tips broken off. Top: capped after use.

For organic vapours, adsorbent sampling onto porous solids such as charcoal is the standard method. A measured volume of air is drawn through a sampling tube made of glass or metal packed with a solid adsorbent and the contaminant vapours are adsorbed from the air stream onto the surface of the adsorbent (Figure 15.8). A typical solid adsorbent tube for organic vapours contains 100 mg of activated charcoal and 50 mg as a back-up section (Figure 15.9). Other solid adsorbent materials include silica gel and a wide range of commercially available porous polymers.

Some examples of solid adsorbents are:

● Activated charcoal—this is by far the most commonly used adsorbent. It has a very large surface area/weight ratio and a high adsorptive capacity. It is non-polar and therefore preferentially absorbs organic vapours rather than polar molecules such as water.

● Silica gel—This is a highly polar adsorbent and efficient collector of polar vapours such as alcohols and amines. It is also hygroscopic and this can cause problems in humid conditions.

● Porous polymers—these, like charcoal are generally non-polar but have lower adsorptive capacity. They are suitable for thermal desorption.

● Molecular sieves—these include zeolites and carbon molecular sieves which retain adsorbed species according to their molecular size.

The adsorbent sampling tube is usually mounted in the wearer's breathing zone, connected to a pump worn on a belt.

After sampling, the tubes are sealed with plastic caps before the tube is sent for analysis. Many variations on geometry and packing are possible. Larger amounts of adsorbent enable sampling to be conducted over longer time periods. Polar adsorbents, such as silica gel, can be used in special applications for polar gases or vapours such as methanol.

A potential pitfall of adsorbent sampling is the phenomenon of 'breakthrough' which occurs after a certain volume of contaminated air has been drawn through the sampling tube. When breakthrough occurs the sample is gradually swept out of the tube with the air stream and is lost. Breakthrough can be avoided if the volume of air that can be sampled before breakthrough occurs (the 'breakthrough volume') is known in advance. Breakthrough volumes for many compounds are published by manufacturers of adsorbent tubes and the back-up section in charcoal tubes is to help indicate when breakthrough has occurred.

Passive sampling

Since the early 1980s, a number of 'passive' sampling devices for gases and vapours have been introduced which do not make use of a pump to collect the sample. These are devices in which the rate at which the gas is absorbed or adsorbed is governed by its rate of diffusion across a well-defined diffusion path. Two general types of passive device are available commercially which are known as 'badges' and 'tubes', respectively. Passive samplers for organic vapours contain an adsorbent material such as charcoal cloth or a porous polymer. For gases a chemically reactive sampling material is used. The adsorbent is located in a small container which is open at one end to allow contaminant molecules in the air to diffuse into the sampler and become trapped on the adsorbent. Tube-type passive samplers such as those marketed by Perkin Elmer have a small frontal area and a relatively small sampling rate. Badge-type samplers have a much larger frontal area and a sampling rate that is considerably higher than for tubes. The effective sampling rate depends on the molecular weight of the contaminant that is being sampled.

Passive samplers are usually calibrated by the manufacturer against standard atmospheres in the laboratory, and users should satisfy themselves that the calibration is suitable for the concentration range and sampling conditions that they are dealing with. Sometimes this requires extensive validation work in the workplace.

Preparation for analysis

Where a vapour has been sampled on to a solid adsorbent, it must be removed from the adsorbent before analysis can take place. The simplest way of removing the vapour is to wash it off with a suitable solvent.

Carbon disulphide is widely used to remove organic vapours from charcoal. The charcoal tube is cut open and the charcoal granules are transferred to a small bottle. A small amount of carbon disulphide is added and the bottle, once capped, is tumbled or otherwise agitated for a short period. A measured amount of the carbon disulphide now containing the contaminant from the charcoal, is then removed using a microsyringe and injected directly into the analytical instrument (usually a gas chromatograph).

A convenient alternative technique for desorption is to heat the adsorbent tube so that the adsorbed vapour is desorbed into a gas stream and passes directly into the analytical instrument. Alternatively the thermally desorbed vapour can be collected in a chamber or by freezing and analysed later. A fully automated thermal desorber is manufactured by Perkin Elmer for desorbing their own design of adsorber tubes.

Some occupational hygienists carry out their own chemical analysis, filter weighing and occasionally asbestos counting, but it is increasingly the case that occupational hygiene samples are analysed by analysts or technicians. When samples must be sent to external laboratories for analysis, the hygienist must satisfy himself or herself that suitable analytical methods are used and that adequate quality control is exercised.

One safeguard that is available for some analyses is to ensure that the laboratory is appropriately registered. The National Association of Testing Authorities (NATA) is the accrediting body for Australian laboratories, and in 1987 set up a technical committee to develop quality standards specifically for laboratories carrying out occupational hygiene measurements.

Direct reading instruments

Direct reading instruments provide an immediate indication (within a fraction of a second up to a few minutes) of the concentration of air contaminants and are available for airborne dusts including fibres, and for many gases and vapours. Direct reading instruments should not be seen simply as an alternative to air sampling techniques. They can provide details of the variation of air concentrations over time and space which can help with the efficient selection of controls and are particularly useful where measurements are required quickly; some can also be used to operate alarms. They also have a number of limitations which can yield misleading results unless these are recognised and taken into account.

The simplest form of direct reading 'instrument' is perhaps the indicator tube (or detector tube). Detector tubes consist of a glass tube initially sealed at both ends and filled with porous granules of an inert material impregnated with a chemical reagent which changes colour in the presence of the contaminant. The actual concentration of the gas is determined either by the length of the stain or by comparing the intensity of the colour with standards. Air is pumped through the tube by means of a small hand-operated pump which may be of a bellows or piston design (Figure 15.10).

Although detector tubes are easy to use with little training, interpretation of the results may require considerable training and experience. Detector tubes may be designed to detect one contaminant or a group of chemically related compounds, but either way the tube may also respond to other contaminants which may be present in the air. This is known as 'cross-sensitivity' and can cause misleading results. For example, benzene detector tubes equally respond to other aromatic hydrocarbons such as toluene and xylene. Before detector tubes are used it is important that the manufacturer's instructions and warnings on cross-sensitivity are studied and account is taken of possible interfering contaminants that may be present.

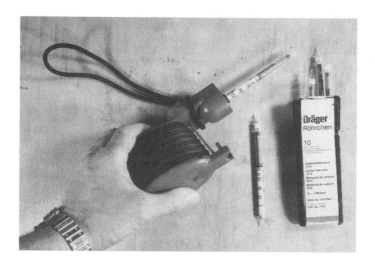

Figure 15.10. Detector tube and bellows-type pump.

Another potential problem with most detector tubes is that they provide a measurement at only one time and place while air concentrations to which workers are exposed may fluctuate widely. It is not possible to have great confidence that a short-term measurement is representative of average conditions or that even a short operation has been adequately assessed. Nevertheless, short-term detector tubes have an important part to play in the assessment of exposures and process emissions. A number of long-term detector tubes are also avaiiable which can be operated over an extended period with a small battery-operated pump. These provide a time-weighted average measurement of contaminant concentration and can be inspected periodically to obtain an up-dated result. Additionally, a number of passive long-term detector tubes are available which operate without a pump and provide a convenient means of personal monitoring for some gases.

Direct reading dust monitors

A variety of direct reading instruments for dusts and other particulates is available. These generally measure the airborne concentration of the particulates but not their composition. They utilise some physical property of airborne particles such as light scattering, although some measure the mass of dust collected on an oscillating quartz crystal.

The main detection principles used in commercially available direct reading dust monitors are:

● Optical—light scattering or obscuration.

● Electrical—e.g. ion interception.

● Piezoelectric—oscillating quartz crystal.

● β Attenuation—attenuation of β radiation by deposited dust.

Examples of direct reading dust monitors commonly used in Australia are the miniature real–time aerosol monitor (MINIRAM) and the fibrous aerosol monitor (FAM).

The MINIRAM is a small forward light scattering dust monitor. Dust laden air diffuses into the sensing zone through which a light beam passes. Dust particles in this zone scatter light which is measured by a photocell and the instantaneous dust concentration is shown on a liquid crystal digital display. Alternatively, the average concentration over a period can be displayed and the data collected during a whole week (40 h) can be stored in internal memory. The MINIRAM is calibrated by the manufacturer against an atmosphere of standard Arizona road dust and this calibration often does not hold for other particulates. In such cases the user must calibrate the instrument for the particulate to be monitored by comparison with a pump and filter technique.

The FAM is also a light scattering dust meter but is designed to detect and count fibrous particles. The air sample is drawn to a sensing zone through which a laser beam passes. A rotating high voltage electrical field causes any fibrous particles present to rotate and they are detected by the varying pattern of scattered light that results. The FAM can be used both to count and measure the size of airborne fibres and is usually calibrated against amphibole asbestos for which it is most reliable.

Direct reading gas and vapour monitors

A large number of types of direct reading instrument for gases and vapours are available. Some of these are highly specific and measure only one contaminant, whilst some are non-specific and will detect any of a wide range of contaminants.

The main principles of detection employed in reading gas and vapour monitors include:

● Colorimetric—detector tubes and paper tape monitors.

● Electrical/electrochemical—conductivity, reactions at an electrode.

● Combustion—oxidation of organic compounds on a catalytic surface.

● Flame ionisation—measurement of the electrical conductivity of a flame in which the air sample is burned.

● Photoionisation—measurement of the conductivity of air due to ions produced from the contaminant by ultraviolet light.

● Infra-red—absorption of infra-red radiation by molecules of the contaminant.

In addition, portable versions of standard laboratory analytical instruments such as gas chromatographs are available.

Two common examples of direct reading gas/vapour monitors are the mobile infra-red analyser (MIRAN) and the total ionisables present (microTIP) photoionisation meter.

The MIRAN is a single beam gas phase infra-red spectrometer with a large sample cell containing a pair of concave mirrors which, by multiple reflections, provides a long optical path length and therefore high sensitivity. The instrument can be set to different wavelengths characteristic of different types of contaminant. This gives some selectivity, for example, ketones could be detected in the presence of hydrocarbons without much cross-sensitivity, however different ketones and other carbonyl compounds would interfere. The MIRAN can be calibrated by the user for a wide range of contaminants.

The microTIP is a small photoionisation monitor employing an ultraviolet light source to produce ionisation in the contaminant which is then measured electrically. Nearly all organic compounds and many inorganic compounds are detected but with different sensitivities and the instrument must be calibrated for each separately. Methane is not detected and can actually suppress the response due to other compounds present.

Caution must be employed in the use of direct reading instruments and in the interpretation of their results. Many of the instruments are nonspecific and the occupational hygienist may often have to verify findings by supplementary sampling and laboratory analyses. Nevertheless, direct reading instruments can provide valuable information supplementary to that which can be obtained by air sampling.

Biological monitoring

Analysis of tissue or body fluids is employed to measure toxic chemicals in the body or to assess biochemical changes which might provide the early signs of toxic damage. These two different objectives may be termed 'biological *exposure* monitoring' and 'biological *effect* monitoring' (Table 15.2).

Table 15.2. Examples of biological monitoring techniques for exposure and effects of various substances

Substance	Biological exposure	Biological effect
Lead	Lead in blood. Lead in urine	Zinc protoporphyrin in red blood cells
Cadmium	Cadmium in urine	Low molecular weight proteins in urine
Carbon monoxide	Carbon monoxide in exhaled breath	Carboxyhaemaglobin in blood
Nitrobenzene	p-Nitrophenol in urine	Methaemaglobin in blood
Toluene	Toluene in blood or exhaled breath. Hippuric acid in urine	
Organophosphate insecticides		Cholinesterase in red cells or plasma

Biological exposure monitoring assesses the uptake of chemicals by measuring the chemical or its metabolites in the body or excreted fluids. These may include blood, fat, bone or organs, urine, faeces, breath, sweat, nails, hair, sputum and breast milk. As discussed earlier, the American Conference of Governmental Industrial Hygienists (ACGIH) has set a number of biological exposure indices (BEIs) which are concentrations of substances or principle metabolites in specified body fluids which would indicate exposures around the corresponding threshold limit value (TLV) concentration.

Biological effect monitoring must be clearly distinguished from biological monitoring of exposure. Whereas the latter technique attempts to quantify the body burden of a substance, biological effect monitoring aims to identify individuals with early signs of adverse health effects, e.g. increased levels of cytoplasmic enzymes in the case of exposure to hepatotoxic chemicals, or increased levels of protein in the urine in cases of exposure to nephrotoxic chemicals. However, not all biological effects can necessarily be described as adverse.

In principle, biological monitoring provides a more accurate assessment of health risk than measurement of air concentrations in the workplace. A biological parameter reflecting the internal dose is necessarily more closely related to systemic adverse effects than is any environmental measurement. Unfortunately, biological monitoring can present practical difficulties and the results are sometimes difficult to interpret. Nevertheless, it has a number of major advantages over exposure monitoring.

In particular, it can provide a measure of uptake by all routes including via the skin and gastrointestinal tract, whereas exposure monitoring can assess only uptake via the respiratory tract. Additionally where workers are using personal protective equipment such as respirators, and monitoring cannot provide a true measure of respiratory exposure, biological monitoring may still give a useful indication of uptake.

When a biological monitoring method is based on the determination of the chemical or its metabolite in biological media, it is necessary to know how the substance is distributed to the different compartments of the body, biotransformed and finally eliminated if we are to correctly interpret the results. For most substances the toxicokinetics are best described by a compartment model consisting of various tissue types with different capacities, perfusion rates and partition coefficients.

Following exposure, the chemical is eliminated from the various compartments with different half-lives. For example, for volatile organic compounds elimination from blood and alveolar air is generally rapid, whereas that from adipose tissue is relatively slow. Consequently, elimination curves from body fluids are composites of several curves with increasing half-life, reflecting the disappearance from the main body compartments (e.g. vascular, extravascular, and fat in the case of a lipid-soluble solvent). When a toxicant is substantially metabolised before elimination the toxicokinetics are also dependent upon the rate of biotransformation. If the toxicokinetics are known, then it is relatively simple to select an appropriate time after exposure when the biological sample should be taken such as end of shift, end of the working week or 16 h post-exposure.

The majority of methods for biological monitoring of exposure rely on the determination of the chemical or its metabolite in blood, urine, or alveolar air.

Blood

The amount of chemical absorbed can sometimes be assessed by measuring its concentration in blood. This technique is suitable for a variety of metals and many organic compounds. In the case of organic compounds, it may be appropriate to measure the unchanged chemical in the blood or a metabolite.

The concentration of a solvent in blood frequently reflects either the most recent exposure, if blood is collected during exposure, or the integrated exposure during the preceding day, if blood collection is performed after the end of exposure (i.e. before the next shift). However, the concentration in blood of some cumulative organic chemicals, such as polychlorinated biphenyls or hexachlorobenzene, mainly reflects stored body burden; the blood level of these chemicals being related to the duration of exposure or to the concentration in the storage compartment (e.g. adipose tissue).

Blood samples may be collected by syringe or a skin prick. Normally venous blood is collected with an addition of an anticoagulating agent and analysed whole or after separating the cells from the plasma. Whole blood may be analysed if the toxic substances are to be found in solution in the plasma. Cell fractions may be analysed if the toxicant is protein bound and is found predominantly in the red blood cells (e.g. lead). If the cellular portion is required then the blood is centrifuged so that the plasma and cells are separated.

Substances commonly assessed in blood samples include cadmium, lead, mercury, styrene, and toluene.

Urine

The most commonly used test in occupational health to assess the internal dose of a chemical is the measurement of a metabolite or the chemical itself in urine. For many organic chemicals, the urinary excretion of the metabolites increases progressively during the workshift to reach a maximum at, or sometimes after, the end of the exposure period; it then declines in an exponential fashion. Depending on the exposure conditions, the biological half-life of the metabolite, and the sensitivity of the analytical method, the metabolite concentration can be determined in the urine collected during the shift, at the end of the shift, or before the next shift.

Urine analysis presents two advantages. First, it is relatively non-invasive and not unduly inconvenient for the worker to provide a sample. Second, when a metabolite is monitored, its level in urine is much less influenced by peak exposures than the concentration of the unchanged chemical in blood or alveolar air. Urine analysis is suitable for many metals and pesticides as well as a range of other substances.

Because urine volume is subject to considerable variation concentrations of excreted substances may be subject to random errors. Two techniques are commonly used to correct for such variations in urine volume.

- *Specific gravity correction*—the specific gravity of the urine is measured and the concentration of the chemical/metabolite is adjusted to a standard specific gravity of 1.02.

- *Creatinine correction*—the creatinine concentration in urine is measured as well as the chemical/metabolite and the results are expressed as grams of substance/gram of creatinine or moles of substance/mole of creatinine.

Chemicals commonly assessed in urine include cadmium, chromium, fluorides, lead, MEK, phenol and trichloroacetic acid for trichloroethylene exposure.

Exhaled breath

For volatile compounds, such as organic solvents, the concentration in alveolar air can be used to estimate current or recent exposure. Several factors influence the concentration of a solvent in alveolar air, the most important being the blood–air partition coefficient. The less blood-soluble the solvent is, the higher will be its concentration in alveolar air compared with that in the blood. Exhaled breath analysis is an attractive method as it is easy to perform and is non-invasive.

Exhaled breath analysis can be performed using direct reading instruments. However it is more common to collect a breath sample in an inert plastic bag and analyse this later. A one-way exhalation valve is often used to collect the sample and a charcoal filter on the inlet prevents contamination. Air contaminants may be transferred onto charcoal tubes for storage.

Chemicals assessed in exhaled breath include benzene, carbon monoxide, *n*-hexane, methylchloroform, styrene and toluene.

Biological monitoring results can often be interpreted on an individual basis and used to identify overexposed workers. In the lead industry high individual blood lead values indicate persons who should be removed from the source of exposure until their blood lead concentration returns to a low value.

It must be kept in mind that in biological monitoring, personal human data are obtained and the ethical aspects must receive attention. In particular, the monitoring procedure itself must be without health risk, sufficient information must be given to the subjects before and after monitoring, and individual results must remain confidential.

Exposure assessment for epidemiology

In epidemiological investigations actual exposure measurements made by occupational hygienists for individuals in the cohort are rarely available. Historical exposure measurements are usually difficult to reconstruct due to insufficient data, incomplete work histories, and changes in manufacturing processes, control technology, and industrial hygiene measurement techniques. Instead, estimates of exposure have to be made in a variety of ways which have considerably less precision than exposure measurements.

If no quantitative exposure data are available, epidemiological investigations are still possible by using exposure surrogates such as:

● Ever/never employed in the industry or in a specific job category.

● Length of service in the industry or in a specific job category.

● Years since first exposure.

These measures are not quantitative and usually do not permit exposure–response analysis.

Some occupational exposure data may be available for the study population, although this is rarely comprehensive. In other circumstances exposures must be estimated in some way.

Historical exposure data

Occupational hygiene exposure data may be available for groups of workers, linked for example to job categories. As an approximation an individual's exposure might be assumed to be equal to the average for his job group. There are several potential sources of error in this approach, including:

- *Intentional bias*—occupational hygienists usually investigate situations they believe give high exposures in order to direct control measures efficiently. Historical exposure data might, therefore, not be representative of average exposures.

- *Changes in technology*—exposure data obtained prior to or following changes to processes or control equipment might be invalid in the study period.

- *Personal protection*—measurements made where the workforce uses respiratory protection are not measures of exposure but only of environmental concentration.

- *Other routes of uptake*—occupational hygiene measurements take no account of skin or gastrointestinal uptake.

These last two problems might be overcome if biological monitoring data are available, but this is not very common.

Exposure estimation

Where no reliable measured exposure data are available for the study population, exposure intensities are often estimated on the basis of job descriptions or simply job title. Such exposure estimates can be obtained in many ways, including:

- Interviews with subjects with the disease being studied, their relatives, and/or their employers.

- Measurements of current exposure (suitable where process and control technology, and work practice have not changed greatly).

- Simulation (repeating historical work practice so that exposure measurements can be performed).

- Exposure panels (teams of experienced hygienists and physicians familiar with the industries being studied) to estimate exposure intensities for industries or job categories.

- Job exposure matrices (a table listing typical exposures against job titles).

Exposures estimated in these ways are usually very imprecise and can often only be used for ranking (e.g. low, medium, high).

Control

It must be remembered at all times that the primary responsibility of the occupational hygienist is to do what is necessary and reasonable to control hazardous exposures, not just to assess them. Control might be achieved in many different ways, ideally at the source of the emission by eliminating or substituting processes or materials, or by process modification. A second option is to try to contain or capture the emission after it has been produced. This might be achieved by ventilation of some sort, or by segregation of the process from the workforce. Generally the least satisfactory option is to try to protect the workers by the use of protective clothing and respirators after their working environment has become contaminated.

All possible routes of exposure (respiratory, skin and gastrointestinal tract) must be identified if adequate control is to be achieved. For example, during the application of some pesticides the major uptake is via skin contact, and efforts to control the airborne substance will not be rewarded by greatly reduced overall exposures. In such cases the control strategy might involve reduced handling, avoidance of spills, suitable clean-up procedures, waste disposal arrangements, protective clothing, washing facilities, provision of work clothes and changing rooms, and a range of operational rules covering food, drink and tobacco use at work.

Several hierarchical schemes are possible, for the control of substances in the workplace, of which the following is an example. The relative order of importance of the various control options can be different in different processes.

- Control at source:
  (a) eliminate or substitute the process or the hazardous substance;
  (b) modify the process to reduce the emissions.

- Transmission control:
  (a) segregation of the process from the workers;
  (b) good housekeeping to prevent re-release from, or contact with, surface contamination;
  (c) local exhaust ventilation;
  (d) dilution ventilation.

- Personal protection:
  (a) personal hygiene;
  (b) respirators;
  (c) gloves;
  (d) impervious clothing, etc.

Summary

This chapter provides an overview of the contribution of occupational hygiene to industrial toxicology in terms of recognition, evaluation and control, and in epidemiology and standard setting. Readers who desire more detailed information on any of the topics are referred to the many excellent texts that are available, some of which are listed in the Bibliography to this chapter, and to the various short training and postgraduate courses which are available.

Bibliography

General occupational hygiene

Occupational Health and Hygiene Guidebook for the WHSO, 1992. Brisbane: David Grantham.

Plog, B. A. (Ed.) 1988, *Fundamentals of Industrial Hygiene*, 3rd Edn. National Safety Council, Chicago USA.

Monitoring

Australian Standards AS 2986–1987 Workplace Atmospheres—Organic Vapours—Sampling by Solid Adsorption Techniques. Canberra.

Gill, F. S. and Ashton, I., 1992, *Monitoring for Health Hazards at Work*. Oxford: Royal Society for the Prevention of Accidents/Blackwell Scientific.

Gray, C. N. and Thomson, J. M., 1984, Passive and active atmospheric monitoring, in Harrington, J. M. (Ed.) *Recent Advances in Occupational Health*, Vol. 2. Edinburgh: Churchill Livingstone.

Hering, S. V. (Ed.), 1979, *Air Sampling Instruments*, 7th Edn. ACGIH. (For evaluation of atmospheric contaminants.) Cincinnati.

Ness, 1991, *Air Monitoring for Toxic Exposures*. New York: Van Nostrand.

Quality control in analysis

NIOSH, 1973, *The Industrial Environment, its Evaluation and Control*, Chap. 22. Washington, DC: US Government Printing Office.

NIOSH, 1984 (3rd edition) Introduction, Section C, in *Manual of Analytical Methods*. Cincinnati, OH: NIOSH.

Whitehead, T. P., 1977, *Quality Control in Clinical Chemistry*. New York: Wiley.

Biological monitoring

Baselt, R. C., 1980, *Biological Monitoring Methods for Industrial Chemicals*. Davis: Biomedical Publications.

Documentation of the threshold limit values and biological exposure indices, in *American Conference of Governmental Industrial Hygienists*, 6th Edn. American Conference of Governmental Industrial Hygienists, Cincinnati, 1991.

Hinch, A. L., 1974, *Biological Monitoring for Industrial Chemical Exposure Control*. Boca Raton, FL: CRC Press.

Ho, M. H. and Dillan, H. K., 1987, *Biological Monitoring of Exposure to Chemicals—Organic Chemicals*. New York: Wiley.

Exposure assessment for epidemiology

ACGIH, 1991, *Exposure Assessment for Epidemiology and Hazard Control*. Michigan: Lewis.

Gerin, M., Siemiatycki, J., Kemper, H. and Begin, D., 1985, Obtaining occupational exposure histories in epidemiological studies, *J. Occup. Med.*, **27**(6), 420–6.

Kauppinen, T. and Partinen, T., 1988, Use of plant- and period-specific job-exposure matrices in studies on occupational cancer, *Scand. J. Work Environ. Health*, **14**, 161–7.

Rosenstock, L., Logfero, J., Heyer, N. J. and Carter, 1984, Development and validation of a self-administered occupational health history questionnaire, *J. Occup. Med.*, **26**(1), 50–4.

Chapter 16

Occupational Medicine—Interface with Toxicology

W. O. Phoon

Although Bernardino Ramazzini (the father of occupational health) lived and died a few centuries ago, the subject with which his name is associated is still relatively new. It is rapidly evolving and has developed more sub-disciplinary areas than perhaps most other health disciplines.

Most of the original pioneers of occupational health, like Ramazzini, were physicians, e.g. Paracelsus, Percival Potts, Charles Thackrah, Alice Hamilton, and Thomas Morrison Legge. Ramazzini himself was Professor of Medicine (Internal Medicine) at different times in the Universities of Padua and Modena, Italy. Cases of poisoning from mercury, lead and other substances and other occupational diseases led him to go out from his consulting room in the hospital to the worksites from which his patients came. This led to his trail-blazing studies on occupational diseases encapsulated in his famous textbook on the subject.

The early years of the development of occupational health focused on the diagnosis and treatment of overt occupational diseases, including those from chemicals. This stage of development was not very different from similar periods in the development of internal medicine. A rich repository of new knowledge about the symptoms and signs of occupational diseases then rapidly accumulated. The nineteenth century and early years of the present century could be termed the 'classical age of clinical occupational medicine' in the sense that the symptom complexes of conditions such as lead poisoning, mercury poisoning and silicosis were all fully documented during those periods.

The input of other sciences, such as nursing, psychology, physiology, biochemistry, pharmacology, chemistry, physics and engineering greatly enhanced the development of occupational health as a scientific discipline. Epidemiology and statistics gave added strength to the systematic detection and quantification of occupational conditions. More recently, the appearance of the newer (and largely applied) professions such as in physiotherapy, vocational therapy and ergonomics have added to the repertoire of skills needed to control and prevent occupational hazards and to rehabilitate victims from them.

Nowadays, occupational health practitioners come from a wide and expanding spectrum of different basic disciplines. Each category of such practitioners has both a unique part to play, drawing upon his or her special skills, as well as a collective part to play, as a member of a multi- or inter-disciplinary team in the prevention, management or rehabilitation of occupational illnesses.

Definition of occupational medicine

As with most other subjects, there are many definitions of occupational medicine. A simple definition is that occupational medicine encompasses the role played by medical practitioners in occupational health. As such, occupational medicine focuses on the prevention, diagnosis and management of occupational injuries and diseases, including health surveillance.

Training for occupational medicine

Occupational medicine should be regarded as an extension of the work of a basic practitioner. The usual period of training of a doctor at medical school is 6 years or longer. After that there is normally a compulsory period of supervised work experience ('housemanship' or 'internship') of at least 1 year. Most occupational physicians undergo a few more years of supervised training work in hospital, community or general practice before embarking upon formal training in occupational health. Professional training for the latter subject is generally relatively brief. In many universities, doctors and others can obtain their Master of Occupational Health and Safety degree or equivalent qualification after approximately only 10 months of full-time work, followed by the part-time preparation of a treatise. Treatise preparation may last 1–2 years or more. In general, however, occupational physicians all over the world require additional (usually 2) years of supervised training in practical situations to qualify for registration as a specialist occupational physician, and that only after an 'exit' examination. Even then, the whole duration of formal training in occupational health (as distinct from experience) is generally appreciably shorter than the whole duration of formal training for medicine as a whole. This is little different from training in other medical specialisations, e.g. surgery or psychiatry.

The training for a medical doctor is fairly homogeneous throughout the world, though the standards may vary. Occupational health, however, as a subject in the curriculum for medical students, varies immensely. Medical schools often provide as few as 10 hours of training throughout the entire course.

The postgraduate training for medical practitioners in occupational health is much more diverse. In certain countries, e.g. the UK, occupational medicine is generally regarded as a 'clinical discipline'. Consequently, there is strong emphasis on clinical teaching. In some other countries there is next to no clinical teaching, and there occupational health, including the role of medical practitioners, is probably best described as a subsegment of public health.

Occupational medicine as applied to toxicology

The medical doctor needs to have at least a reasonable level of competence in general medicine to diagnose and manage toxicological problems. A skill in taking a good medical history, both general and occupational, is essential. Sometimes an exhaustive history is taken, but at all times proper judgement is necessary to sort out 'the wheat from the chaff'. Just as it has been said with some truth that the most important part of a stethoscope is that between the earpieces, good history-taking is an art requiring a high level of deductive reasoning sharpened by knowledge and experience.

Taking a history, however competently done, is nonetheless insufficient in itself. The doctor needs to be able to perform a clinical examination to confirm or refute the provisional diagnosis in his mind after the taking of the history. This is especially important where organ system medical specialists who are particularly knowledgable in occupational health are not easy to find. This situation is often aggravated by overspecialisation (especially in developed countries).

Often toxicological problems may fall between different internal medicine 'stools' because such problems may affect several organ systems in the same case and 'general' internal medicine has lost prestige and become rather unfashionable in many developed countries. The danger of missing the 'wood' because of an overemphasis on looking at individual 'trees' is not very conducive to the detection and management of toxicological problems.

The diagnosis of an intoxication from a poisonous substance should be mainly based on clinical judgement. The history may be typical or suggestive. The clinical examination may reveal positive signs, but sometimes the diagnosis of intoxication can still be justifiably made despite an absence of signs. Sometimes laboratory tests or other investigations, e.g. psychomotor tests, are indicated. Sometimes estimations of the substance or substances in the work environment may be required, although the causal relationship between the present concentration and the onset of the disease can be a very complex one, especially for cases of chronic poisoning or occupational carcinogenesis.

To illustrate the principles in the diagnosis and management of toxicological problems in occupational situations, two examples are discussed here. They relate to inorganic lead and organic solvents, respectively.

Inorganic lead

Lead is, of course, a metal well known to humankind for a very long time. Even in modern times, inorganic lead is still fairly extensively used, for the manufacture of accumulator storage batteries, as alloys (usually mixed with tin), etc. Organic lead is used, though to a diminishing extent, as an anti-knock agent in petroleum.

The diagnosis of inorganic lead poisoning is based on the parameters described below.

History of exposure

Whenever possible, a history of exposure to significant amounts of inorganic lead should be established. It is pointless to talk merely of 'lead exposure', because in almost any environment, especially in urban areas, the exposure to small amounts of the metal is inevitable.

For practical purposes, not only the amount of exposure but also the duration of exposure should be significant in occupational circumstances. It is very rare in those circumstances for a worker to suffer from lead poisoning after an exposure of less than several weeks. A duration of at least several months is more usual.

Possibility of absorption

A worker can be working in an atmosphere heavily laden with lead but may not absorb any because he or she is using completely effective personal protective equipment throughout exposure. However, the use of personal protective equipment is not comfortable, fraught with possibilities of human error (e.g. a respirator not fitting the facial contours well because of wearing a beard), the filter may not be changed regularly, or the person may simply not wear the device except very intermittently. Therefore, personal protective equipment should not be relied on as the main means of preventing lead poisoning. The use of other methods, e.g. exhaust ventilation, to control the concentration in the work environment is more dependable.

High exposure occupations, e.g. lead smelting (primary and secondary), burning off of lead paints, the assembly of lead accumulator batteries, and lead discing, are usually attended by some degree of lead absorption, despite good standards of occupational hygiene. Other exposure situations, e.g. mixing of lead in paints and lead soldering, are associated with lower but not absent risks of lead absorption.

A consistent or suggestive history

The 'classical' syndrome of lead intoxication, with symptoms of weight loss, anorexia, epileptiform fits, constipation, abdominal colic, wrist drop, wasting, anaemia and Barton's line on the gums, is extremely rare. Much more common nowadays would be a history of general ill-health with rather ill-defined symptoms, although the more severe and dramatic symptoms and signs mentioned above can still be seen in some less developed countries. Of particular significance is a temporal history of usually several months after taking employment in a job situation with apparently appreciable exposure to the metal. Poisoning can occur as a result of changes in either the work environment or work conditions. For example, a person might be absorbing more lead than usual when the exhaust ventilation system was not working properly; or he might be working overtime (which means his exposure is proportionately increased with the same ambient concentration of the substance).

Deterioration in health can often be elicited by asking a worker whether he is as well as, say, 1 year or 6 months ago, or what his weight was then compared with now. Vague symptoms such as lassitude, inability to sleep or disturbed sleep, a metallic taste in the mouth, undue tiredness and muscle aches could provide useful clues. Obviously, the physician or nurse taking the history has to be careful not to ask too many leading questions! It is advisable to let the patient describe his or her medical complaints first without any or much prompting and then follow up with questions if necessary.

Physical examination

Signs such as mild anaemia, slight degree of muscle wasting, and evidence of peripheral neuropathy may be present. Depending on the symptoms, the exclusion of other disease should also be borne in mind by the examiner.

Laboratory investigations

A wide spectrum of laboratory investigations can be performed in cases of suspected lead poisoning. They usually fall into the following categories.

1. Concentration of lead in body fluid, e.g. lead in blood or urine.

2. Depression of concentrations of enzymes in the blood relating to haem synthesis, e.g. δ-aminolaevulinic acid dehydrase (ALAD).

3. Excess of excretion in the urine of substances normally used for haem synthesis in the urine because of interference with haem synthesis, e.g. excess of aminolaevulinic acid in the urine.

4. Effects of lead on body systems, e.g. anaemia and reduced packed cell volume due to interference with haem synthesis; reduction in nerve velocity, etc.

In children there is sometimes the presence of a 'lead line' in the shafts of long bones near the epiphyses, but this is not seen in adults. What laboratory investigations are made depends on what the symptoms and signs indicate. The laboratory investigation generally agreed to be most useful (subject to quality control) is the lead concentration in blood (PbB).

The use of the laboratory investigations described in (1) to (3) above is commonly referred to as 'biological monitoring', which can be defined as a regular measuring activity in which selected, validated indicators of the uptake of toxic substances are determined in order to prevent health impairment. The regular use of biological monitoring in combination with medical examination as well as investigative methods for the detection of early effects of toxic substances upon body systems (such as those investigations mentioned under (4) above) is usually collectively referred to as 'health surveillance' (of workers who are exposed to such substances).

Environmental monitoring

For single cases seen at the usual clinic, it is not always practicable either to inspect the worksite or to measure the lead concentration there. For epidemiological studies or the establishment of surveillance for groups of workers, however, measurements of lead levels in the work environment are essential. There is a 'lag period' in the correlation of environmental lead to blood lead levels, as the latter reflects absorption 1–2 weeks previously rather than at the present time.

Organic solvents

Most of the substances used as solvents are organic chemicals used for a large variety of purposes such as degreasing, thinning, extraction or cleaning. As is well known, solvents can cause a wide spectrum of health effects. Solvents are one of the leading causes of occupational dermatitis. The majority of organic solvents are depressants of the central nervous system. Acute exposure may cause narcosis, excitation, headache, dizziness, nausea and confusion. Severe exposure may cause convulsions, coma and failure of the vital brain centres, sometimes with fatal results. Chronic exposure may lead to undue fatigue, headache, disturbed sleep, intellectual impairment, poor memory, impaired vision, reduced manual dexterity and motor weakness. Certain solvents, such as carbon disulphide, methyl bromide, tri-*o*-cresyl phosphate, *n*-hexane and methyl-*n*-butyl ketone, may cause peripheral neuropathy.

Effects on the respiratory system are mainly irritation to mucous membranes of the throat and respiratory passages. Effects on the cardiovascular system can be caused by several solvents, such as carbon disulphide, halogenated carbon compounds and benzene. The risk of angina pectoris increases with carbon disulphide exposure. Benzene, toluene and halogenated carbon compounds can cause cardiac arrhythmia, especially ventricular fibrillation.

Hepatotoxicity is a possibility with sufficient exposure to any organic solvent. Carbon tetrachloride and tetrachlorethane are the most toxic solvents in this regard. Other hepatotoxic solvents include chloroform, tetrachlorethylene, trichlorethylene, diethylene dioxide and diethylene glycol.

Damage to the kidneys, in the form of acute renal failure, can be caused by aromatic hydrocarbons, halogenated carbon substances, and glycols. Aromatic hydrocarbons can cause glomerulonephritis. Acute renal failure due to toluene has been described in glue sniffers.

Bone marrow depression and leukaemia have been associated with benzene.

Carbon disulphide and carbon tetrachloride have been implicated in the reduction of fertility in both sexes in humans. Chromosomal aberrations have been detected following exposure to benzene.

The diagnosis of solvent poisoning can be extremely complex, especially since in many occupational situations, several solvents can be used together. In patients who are seen long after exposure to solvents has ceased, it is not always possible to identify what solvents were actually used by the patients concerned.

The diagnosis of organic solvent poisoning is based on the parameters described below.

History of exposure

The 'index of suspicion' of the medical examiner should be raised if the patient comes from one of the many trades or handles one of the many processes known to be associated with solvent exposure.

Possibility of exposure

Organic solvents are used for many purposes in modern life. Workers can be exposed while using these chemicals as cleaners, degreasers and thinners. The industries using solvents include those related to engineering, printing, painting, construction and repairs. Solvents are also used extensively in the manufacture of different chemicals. Solvents also occur in a wide range of domestic chemicals. Often a distinction must be made as to whether solvent exposure has occurred from occupational or domestic circumstances.

A consistent or suggestive history

Unfortunately, there are no really pathonogmonic symptoms for solvent intoxication. Patients presenting with mild symptoms referrable to the nervous system are often misdiagnosed as cases of psychoneurosis or even malingering. In acute cases, there may be a fairly well-defined correlation between work exposure and the onset and duration of the symptoms. The patient may be quite well when he arrives at his workplace. He may feel more tired and have headache as the working day proceeds. When he returns home at the end of the day, he may feel so tired that he does little else except eat his dinner and go to bed early. If the exposure is intermittent, e.g. the worker may not do spray-painting every day, he may be able to volunteer the information that only on spray-painting days does he suffer from those symptoms. In instances where different substances are used for different forms of spray-painting, the patient may sometimes be able to identify those substances which are more prone to cause his symptoms. Another useful clue is whether or not the patient had similar symptoms before he started his present job. However, enquiry then has to be made whether or not his previous jobs carried similar risks of solvent exposure.

Tiredness, or rather undue tiredness, can be very subjective. Two individuals' degrees of tiredness after the same amount of mental or physical exertion can be very different. In such circumstances, it is often useful to ask the patient whether the volume of work has changed recently. If not, does he feel the same extent of tiredness as, say, 6 months or 1 year ago? Does he feel the same extent of tiredness on weekends or long vacations? It must be remembered, in this connection, that workers sometimes engage in more frenetic activities during their own time than at work. Moreover, the use of organic solvents in domestic or recreational activities must also be considered, e.g. handyman type activities or hobbies involving the use of glues, thinners, etc.

Sometimes, solvent intoxication may be precipitated by an increased volume of work, the introduction of a new substance containing another solvent, or the breakdown or cessation of usage of a normally effective exhaust ventilation system or other preventive measures, such as respirators. Therefore questions directed at eliciting these kinds of information are often necessary. The chronic effects of solvents on the neurological system do not necessarily have time relationships to exposure and its cessation. Effects such as memory loss and intellectual deficit can persist long after cessation of exposure.

If the presentation relates to the liver, a provisional diagnosis of solvent poisoning is generally made on the basis of a history consistent with exposure to a hepatotoxic solvent and the exclusion of other known toxic substances affecting the liver. It must be borne in mind, however, that other agents injurious to the liver, e.g. alcohol and hepatitis virus, could operate synergistically to either provoke or aggravate the liver disease.

A similar process of excluding other causes applies to the diagnosis of cases presenting with skin, respiratory, renal or cardiovascular complaints.

Physical examination

A comprehensive and thorough examination has to be done, since solvent exposure can attack so many organ systems and assume so many forms. In general, special concentration should be on the neurological system and liver, although other systems may be affected at the same time.

Laboratory investigations

There are very few specific tests. The usual laboratory investigations fall into the following categories.

- *Tests for increased levels of metabolites excreted*—for example, in the urine, phenol levels after benzene exposure, trichloroacetic acid and similar compounds after trichlorethylene exposure, hippuric acid after toluene exposure, and methylhippuric acid after xylene exposure.

- *Tests for functions of target organs*—central nervous system: electro-encephalography, psychomotor tests (e.g. memory tests, reaction time, etc.). Peripheral nervous system: nerve conduction velocity, electro-mygraphy, use of evoked potential (visual and somatosensory).

Environmental monitoring

This could be useful but is not always practicable. Moreover, results only refer to the present situation and not necessarily to the past when the concentrations of the solvent (or solvents) could have been quite different.

Medical management of cases of occupational poisoning

The management of occupational poisoning varies not only with the cause of the poisoning but also with other factors such as severity, whether it is acute or chronic, the availability of poisons advisory and treatment centres, the level and nature of nearby health services, and the skill and expertise of the occupational health personnel concerned.

In some cases of occupational poisoning there are fairly specific remedies such as chelating agents. In others, general measures such as supporting treatment, exchange transfusion, dialysis, etc., may be used. Management should include proper attention to electrolyte balance, nutrition and oxygenation. Particularly for severe cases, careful watch should be kept for complications such as chest infections and pulmonary oedema, and liver and kidney failure, and the appropriate treatment promptly instituted.

In the present context, it is not appropriate to discuss in detail the medical management of cases of occupational poisoning. In many countries of the world, poisons advisory centres exist, which can often provide invaluable information concerning antidotes to specific poisons. Just as important perhaps as specific antidotes is supportive treatment, such as the maintenance of vital functions in the victim by resuscitation and assisted respiration, proper nutrition, electrolyte balance, and prevention of secondary infection.

For all serious cases, it is best to admit the patient to hospital for observation or treatment. Pulmonary oedema from chemicals may not manifest itself until several hours after exposure. Therefore it may be wise to err on the side of caution and admit all cases of acute exposure to respiratory poisons for at least 24 h for observation and whatever treatment may be necessary. In cases of chronic poisoning, e.g. lead poisoning, it is prudent, moreover, to treat patients with chelating agents as in-patients. Chelating agents can give rise to severe electrolyte imbalance and may precipitate attacks of acute poisoning from mobilisation of metal stores from the bones into the bloodstream.

Bibliography

He, F. S., 1987, Occupational neurotoxicology: current problems and trends, in *Keynote Addresses of XXII International Congress on Occupational Health*, pp. 48–77. Sydney: XXII ICOH Organising Committee.

Lauwerys, R., 1989, *Detection of the Nephrotoxic Effects of Industrial Chemicals: Assessment of the Current Screening Tests* (*Lucas Lecture*). London: Faculty of Occupational Medicine, Royal College of Physicians.

Phoon, W. O., 1992, Incidence, presentation and therapeutic attitudes to antichollinesterase poisoning in Asia, in Ballantyne, B. and Marrs, T. C. (Eds), *Clinical and Experimental Toxicology of Organophosphates and Carbamates*, pp. 482–9. Oxford: Butterworth-Heinemann.

Phoon, W. O., 1992, Occupational medicine: principles and practice (special article), *CME Rev.*, **2** (1), 16–18.

Phoon, W. O. and Ong, C. N., 1982, Lead exposure patterns and parameters for monitoring lead absorption among workers in Singapore. *Ann. Acad. Med. Singapore*, **11**(4), 593–600.

World Health Organisation, 1986, *Environmental Health Criteria No. 63. Organophosphorus Insecticides. Report of a WHO Task Group on Organophosphorus Insecticides*. Geneva: WHO.

Chapter 17

Occupational Epidemiology— Interface with Toxicology

M. S. Frommer and S. J. Corbett

Introduction

Epidemiology is the study of health-related phenomena in groups of people. The domain of epidemiology is the health of communities or populations. Epidemiology contributes to human well-being by determining the patterns of health and ill-health in populations, identifying factors which influence health, and evaluating the application of this information to the control of health problems.

Epidemiological methods are used to describe health-related phenomena in populations (descriptive epidemiology), and to estimate the strength of associations between putative determinants and health outcomes (analytical epidemiology). Through these approaches, epidemiological practice is concerned with:

- Characterising the occurrence and distribution of hazards, diseases and injuries in populations.

- Describing the natural history of disease states in groups of affected individuals.

- Testing hypotheses of disease and injury causation.

- Investigating clusters or outbreaks of disease.

- Evaluating interventions designed to prevent or modify adverse health outcomes.

Occupational epidemiology is the application of epidemiological methods to work-related health problems. It is largely concerned with investigating the relationship between elements of the work environment (in the broadest sense) and the occurrence of disease or injury. The elements of the work environment which attract particular attention are workers' exposures to substances and forms of energy. Occupational epidemiological practice therefore requires a detailed understanding of workplace exposures and the characteristics of the working populations that encounter them.

Measuring the occurrence of health-related phenomena

Epidemiological thinking starts with a systematic approach to counting relevant health events, such as the number of people having a certain disease within a population. Counts of health events are called *measures of occurrence*. For convenience, the following discussion refers to the 'occurrence' of disease; the same principles apply to the occurrence of other types of health-related phenomena.

At the simplest level, disease occurrence is determined by counting the number of people who have the disease in a population (the *frequency* of the disease). However, in order to understand more about the pattern of the disease occurrence, and to make comparisons with other populations or comparisons within the same population at different times, it is helpful to express the occurrence as a *rate*. This consists of a numerator (the number of cases of disease), a denominator (the number of people at risk of getting the disease), and a time period to which the numerator and denominator refer. Two fundamental types of rate are used:

● Rates that express the current existence of disease in a population. These are called *prevalence* rates. The number of cases of a disease in a population at a specified time point is the *point prevalence*, while the number of cases in existence in a population during a specified time period is the *period prevalence*.

● Rates that express the occurrence of new cases arising in a population during a specified time period. These are called *incidence* rates.

Incidence and prevalence are related insofar as the incidence contributes to the pool of prevalent cases, and prevalence is a function of both incidence and the duration of the disease. Prevalence rates are used to describe the burden of disease in a community, while incidence rates are used when considering disease causation, prevention and related issues.

Most populations are dynamic, i.e. their size and composition are continually changing. In the general community the main forces of change are birth, death and migration, while the main force of change in a dynamic working population is labour turnover. Denominators for incidence and period prevalence rates, i.e. the numbers of people at risk of getting a disease, must make allowance for this. Conventionally the denominator for a period prevalence rate is taken as the magnitude of the population in the middle of the time period. The construction of denominators for incidence rates is often more complex, and two different concepts of incidence are often invoked: the cumulative incidence rate and the incidence density.

Cumulative incidence rate

The cumulative incidence rate is given by the number of new disease cases during a specified time period, divided by the size of the population at the beginning of the time period.

EXAMPLE
An epidemic of hepatitis A occurred in a community over a 12-month period. At the beginning of the period, there were 12 626 people in the community, and 436 new cases were recorded in the 12 months. The cumulative incidence of hepatitis A over the year was 34.5 per 1000.

Incidence density

In incidence density the numerator is the same as that for cumulative incidence. The denominator is calculated by assessing the length of time during which each individual in the population is under observation, and summing the person-time units. If an individual develops the disease of interest, he or she contributes person-time to the denominator only from the beginning of the observation period until the onset of illness.

EXAMPLE
Three of the seven employees in a small printing shop developed contact dermatitis within 1 year of the introduction of a new coloured ink. The three affected individuals had had 1, 3 and 5 months of exposure to the ink prior to developing the condition, and avoided exposure subsequently. Of the four unaffected employees, one changed jobs after 5 months (without further exposure), and the other three worked in the shop throughout the year. Thus there were three cases and $1 + 3 + 5 + 5 + (3 \times 12)$ person-months of exposure. The incidence density was 3 per 50 person-months, or 60 per 1000 person-months.

Epidemiological strategies

Epidemiological objectives can be fulfilled by:

1. Analysing data collected routinely for the explicit purpose of monitoring particular aspects of the health of a population, e.g. government health department data collections on pregnancy outcomes, hospital in-patient diagnoses, and infectious disease notification systems.

2. Using data collected on a routine basis primarily for non-health reasons, e.g. mortality data compiled from death registrations which have primarily a legal and demographic purpose, and work-related injury data compiled from workers' compensation case records.

3. Conducting studies designed to answer specific questions.

Epidemiological surveillance

The use of routinely collected data (as in (1) and (2) above) is the basis of epidemiological surveillance systems. The purpose of disease surveillance is to monitor disease occurrence and detect trends. In general, surveillance data are relatively superficial, and the investigation of any changes in disease occurrence that are detected usually necessitates a more detailed additional data collection. Many epidemiological surveillance systems rely on a requirement, often written in legislation or regulations, to notify a central agency of the occurrence of certain types of events, such as infectious diseases which warrant public health action, cancer, and birth defects. The notification system may be supplemented by various methods of case-finding intended to ensure complete ascertainment of the nominated diseases in the population.

The term *register* is sometimes used to describe a complete repository of case data from a defined population. For example, most Australian states and territories have a cancer register and a birth defects register. Registers of this type have the same purposes as other epidemiological surveillance systems and, in addition, the case data recorded in a register can be used as the basis for analytical studies.

A detailed account of epidemiological surveillance systems is beyond the scope of this chapter. Readers seeking further detail are referred to other texts (e.g. Eylenbosch and Noah, 1988).

Health surveillance and other routinely collected data are often used in *ecological studies*, in which the health experiences of entire groups are compared, and population (rather than individuals') markers of health outcomes and/or putative health determinants are used. For example, it has been suggested that a relative deficiency of dietary selenium may be associated with sudden infant death syndrome (SIDS). Some evidence for this hypothesis comes from the observation of an elevated incidence of SIDS in areas where soil selenium levels are low. In such ecological studies, dietary or tissue selenium levels of individual infants are not assessed.

Descriptive epidemiology

Much of our knowledge of health and disease has been obtained from descriptive studies, which rely on astute observation and careful recording of disease and injury and associated factors. Descriptive studies may be prospective, with data collection on new (incident) events; retrospective, with data collection on events that occurred in the past; or cross-sectional, focussing on current (prevalent) events.

For example, in a retrospective descriptive study, Wagner *et al.* (1960) investigated 33 cases of diffuse pleural mesothelioma in the North Western Cape Province of South Africa. The study was done because one of the authors had become concerned at the number of these unusual tumours among his patients. Detailed information was collected on the past occupation and place of residence of the 33 cases, of whom 32 had probable exposure to crocidolite asbestos.

While descriptive studies often have analytical components, the essence of a descriptive study is that it does not seek to test an hypothesis (such as a causal hypothesis) by comparing the health experience of different subgroups. Rather, it describes the nature of a disease, or the health status of a community or population. Descriptive studies may generate (rather than test) hypotheses.

Analytical epidemiology

By contrast, the purpose of analytical studies is to test hypotheses. Analytical studies examine associations between potential determinants (such as workplace exposures) and health outcomes (such as diseases or injuries) by comparing different subgroups.

There are three fundamental types of analytical design, each being defined by the conceptual basis on which the subgroups for comparison are identified.

Cohort study

In a cohort study, subjects are selected for study on the basis of whether or not they are exposed to the potential determinant of disease. For example, in a study of the relationship between exposure to a chemical in the workplace and the occurrence of a disease, subjects exposed to the chemical and an unexposed comparison group are selected. Both groups are then followed up over time, and the occurrence of the disease in the exposed group is compared with that in the unexposed group. The simplest cohort studies classify exposure dichotomously (exposed versus unexposed). In more complex studies, exposure is classified on several levels or is measured on a continuous scale.

Cohort studies may be prospective or retrospective. In a *prospective cohort study*, the investigator classifies subjects according to their exposure status at the time of the start of the study, and then observes them prospectively into the future to determine their disease experience. In a *retrospective (or historical) cohort study*, the investigator classifies the exposure status of the subjects at some time in the past, and then observes them forward from that time to determine their subsequent disease experience. Many historical cohort studies examine only an exposed group or several exposed groups, and compare their experience of the health outcome with that of the general population or a specified subsection of it.

EXAMPLE
In a prospective cohort study of carbon disulphide exposure and cardiovascular mortality, 343 Finnish men exposed for at least 5 years to carbon

disulphide in a viscose rayon plant were identified in 1967. A comparison group of 343 men (matched for age, district of birth and type of job) were selected from a nearby paper mill. The men in the comparison group had no or insignificant (<6 months) exposure to carbon disulphide or other industrial toxicants. The two groups were followed for 15 years, and their mortality from cardiovascular disease was compared (Nurminen and Hernberg, 1985).

EXAMPLE

In a retrospective cohort study of leukaemia in benzene workers, all white males occupationally exposed to benzene in the production of a natural rubber cast film at two plants in Ohio during 1940–1949 were identified retrospectively. The exposed group comprised 748 men. Their mortality from leukaemia was compared with that of: (1) the American white male general population, taking account of age and the time period over which the benzene-exposed workers lived; and (2) 1447 white men who had been employed in an Ohio fibrous-glass construction products factory during 1940–1949 and who had achieved 5 or more years of employment by mid-1972 (Infante *et al.*, 1977).

Case-control study

In a case-control study (also known as a *case-reference study*), a group of subjects who have experienced the health outcome or disease of interest is identified (*cases*), and a suitable comparison group (*controls* or *referents*) is assembled. The frequency of exposure to one or more hypothesised causal factors in the case group is then compared with that in the control group.

The major design question in a case-control study is how to select a suitable control group. This is usually determined by the method used to select the cases. In a *population-based case-control study*, a search is made for all the cases of the disease of interest which have occurred in a defined population during a specified time period. The case group in a population-based case-control study may comprise either all the cases, or a random sample of them. The controls are then taken as random samples of the population from which the cases came. In case-control studies which are not population-based, cases are usually identified from a convenient source, e.g. the cases presenting to a particular hospital with the disease of interest. A control group of people without the disease is then assembled by one of numerous methods, e.g. patients with other disease in the same hospital as that from which cases were selected are often used as controls.

EXAMPLE

In a population-based case-control study of the hypothesised association between exposure to leather dust and nasal cancer, all incident cases of malignant tumour of the nasal cavity and paranasal sinuses occurring among the residents of Vigevano (in the Lombardy region, northern Italy) during 1968–1982 were identified. Sources of the cases were: (1) records from the local hospitals; (2) the cancer registry of the National Cancer Institute; (3) the Vigevano mortality records; and (4) practising otolaryngologists in Vigevano. The completeness of case ascertainment was checked by examining discharge lists for all hospitals in the Lombardy region. Two controls were matched to each case. Live controls were randomly selected from the Vigevano electoral roll. Dead controls were selected from mortality records, choosing the two nearest subjects with the appropriate matching characteristics who died from non-cancer causes. Exposure to leather dust and other potential nasal cancer risk factors was assessed on the basis of recorded interviews (Merler *et al.*, 1986).

EXAMPLE

In a hospital-based case-control study of the association between exposure to wood dust and nasal cancer, the cases comprised all male patients with malignant tumours of the nose and paranasal sinuses referred to the Ear, Nose and Throat Clinic and Radiotherapy Unit of Siena, Italy, during 1963–1981. Five controls were matched to each case, the controls being randomly selected from men of the same age admitted to the Siena Medical Clinic within 3 months of the respective cases. Subjects were asked to complete a questionnaire which included questions about having ever worked in the wood, furniture, and shoe and leather industry (next-of-kin of deceased subjects were interviewed). Subjects who had been employed as woodworkers or cabinet makers were defined as exposed to wood dust (Battista *et al.*, 1983).

Cross-sectional analytical study

In a cross-sectional study, the association between a potential determinant and the health outcome is examined at the same time. A group of people are identified for study, and their exposure and disease status are assessed simultaneously.

EXAMPLE

Two men working in a factory where epoxy resins, acrylics, phenol formaldehyde, chromates, and polyvinyl chloride were used to coat rolled steel sheets with coloured plastic developed symptoms suggestive of occupational asthma. To establish whether other workers were affected and to identify the cause, a cross-sectional study was done in which the 241 employees were asked to complete a questionnaire and undergo lung function and skin prick tests. Occupational asthma, defined in terms of respiratory symptoms, was reported by 21 of the 221 subjects who responded to the questionnaire. Further investigation suggested that the asthmatic rections were related to toluene diisocyanate released in the coating process (Venables *et al.*, 1985).

Hybrid designs

In some circumstances it can be efficient to use mixtures of different analytical designs, e.g. the *case-control study within a cohort*, or *nested case-control study*. Subjects in a cohort study or individuals in an epidemiological surveillance programme who manifest a health outcome of concern are identified, and together they constitute the case group. A random sample of the other subjects in the study is taken as the control group, and data analysis is done as for a case-control study. The advantages are at least two-fold. First, the need for an external comparison group is eliminated; and second, comprehensive exposure data that may have been collected prospectively in the cohort study eliminate the need for a retrospective reconstruction of exposure information.

EXAMPLE

A cohort of 3916 Swedish copper smelter workers employed for at least 3 months between 1928 and 1967 were followed until 1981. Exposure to arsenic was assessed in detail for each worker. A total of 107 lung-cancer cases were identified in the cohort, and 214 controls were also selected from the cohort. Smoking histories were obtained on all of the cases and controls. A case-control analysis was done of the relationship between arsenic and lung cancer. The interactive effect of arsenic exposure and smoking was also examined (Jarup and Pershagen, 1991).

Intervention studies

The cohort, case-control, cross-sectional analytic and hybrid designs described above are examples of *observational* epidemiological studies. They are observational in the sense that the investigator observes the occurrence of various potential determinants of disease, but does not influence whether or not an individual is exposed to these determinants. By contrast, in *intervention* studies the investigator *assigns* the exposure status of individuals, i.e. individuals are assigned to receive one form of intervention or another, or no intervention. The different intervention groups are then followed up and outcomes are assessed. Thus in concept, intervention studies are the same as cohort studies.

A key feature of intervention studies is the manner of allocation of subjects to intervention groups. The allocation may be done in some systematic fashion, possibly depending on the characteristics of individuals. Alternatively, the allocation may be random. The study is then called a *randomised controlled trial*. Randomised controlled trials are widely used in the evaluation of health interventions and medical therapy, e.g. the efficacy and effectiveness of drugs

Basic concepts in the analysis of epidemiological data

Risk and incidence

Central to the analysis of epidemiological data is the concept of risk. *Risk* refers to the probability of an untoward event, such as the occurrence of disease or injury. While it is impossible to predict whether or not an individual will develop a disease, epidemiological methods can be used to estimate an individual's risk of disease. The extent to which this risk is modified by characteristics of the individual (called risk factors), or exposure experience, can also be estimated.

Incidence (as defined above) is a direct estimate of risk. The incidence of a particular condition in a group of people with known risk factors can be taken as equivalent to the risk faced by an individual in that group. Incidence is therefore sometimes referred to as *absolute risk*.

Measures of association in cohort studies

In a cohort study, the incidence of disease can be measured directly in the exposed and unexposed groups. Where there is just one exposed group and an unexposed group, the incidence in the two groups can be compared. The incidence in the exposed group divided by the incidence in the unexposed group is called the *relative risk*, or *risk ratio*.

$$\text{Relative risk} = \frac{\text{Incidence in exposed}}{\text{Incidence in unexposed}}$$

The relative risk indicates how many times more likely (or less likely) a person with the exposure factor is to develop the disease, compared with unexposed people. The relative risk thus gives an index of the strength of the association between the exposure and the disease. If there is no association between the exposure and the disease, then the risk of disease will be the same in the exposed and unexposed groups, and the relative risk will be 1.0. If the exposure confers an increased risk of disease, the relative risk will be >1.0. If the exposure confers protection, the relative risk will be between zero and 1.0.

It is often convenient to summarise incidence data from a simple cohort study in a 2×2 table in which the determinant (exposure) and the outcome (disease) are cross-tabulated.

EXAMPLE
A group of 50 metal-working apprentices undertook a 3-month training attachment in an aircraft factory in which they were exposed to surface-cleaning agents, while their 120 colleagues had a term of classroom training with no exposure to these agents. During the term, 20 of the group in the aircraft factory and six of the classroom group developed contact dermatitis.

These data are summarised in the 2 × 2 table shown in Table 17.1, with the row and column totals given outside the table, and the grand total at the lower right-hand corner. Here, relative risk = (20/50)/(6/120) = 8.0. Thus, apprentices in the aircraft factory were eight times more likely to develop the dermatitis than those who remained in the classroom.

Table 17.1. The 2 × 2 table summarising the data used for the example given in the text.

	Dermatitis	No dermatitis	
Exposed	20	30	50
Unexposed	6	114	120
	26	144	170

It is evident from this example that unexposed apprentices have a risk of developing dermatitis unrelated to the exposure, i.e. a background risk. The exposed apprentices have a much greater risk, which can be considered as having two components: a background component unrelated to exposure, and an incremental component due to exposure. This incremental component is called *attributable risk (exposed)* or *risk difference*, calculated by subtracting the incidence of the disease in the unexposed group from the incidence in the exposed group.

Attributable risk (exposed) = Incidence in exposed − Incidence in unexposed

Sometimes it is useful to express the incremental component due to exposure as a proportion of the risk experienced by exposed persons. This is called the *attributable fraction (exposed)* or *aetiological fraction (exposed)*.

$$\text{Attributable fraction (exposed)} = \frac{\text{Incidence in exposed} - \text{Incidence in unexposed}}{\text{Incidence in exposed}}$$

If written as a percentage, the attributable fraction (exposed) is called the *attributable risk percent (exposed)*.

Relative risk, attributable risk (exposed) and attributable fraction (exposed) are *measures of individual risk*, in that they estimate the risk to an individual, given exposure to a risk factor. Measures of individual risk do not take account of the prevalence of the exposure or risk factor in the population, and are unaffected by changes in the prevalence of the exposure. The risk to an exposed individual is unaffected by the frequency of exposure in the population (for example, an individual smoker's risk of lung cancer is unaffected by the number of smokers in the population).

A risk factor may be strongly associated with an adverse health outcome (high relative risk), and yet be so rare that it does not have an appreciable impact on the health of the community. Conversely, a risk factor may have a weaker association with an adverse health outcome (lower relative risk);

but if the risk factor has a high prevalence in the population, it may have a big impact on the health of the community.

Measures of population risk assess risk in populations. They take into account the frequency of occurrence of the risk factor as well as the strength of its association with the health outcome of interest. The *attributable risk (population)* is calculated by subtracting the incidence of the disease in the unexposed group from the incidence in the exposed and unexposed groups combined.

Attributable risk (population) = Overall incidence – Incidence in unexposed

Often it is preferable to express this as a proportion (percentage) of the overall incidence. This is the *attributable risk percent (population)*.

Attributable risk percent (population) =

$$\frac{\text{Overall incidence of disease} - \text{Incidence in unexposed}}{\text{Overall incidence of disease}} \times 100$$

This gives the proportion of the community incidence of a disease that can be attributed to exposure to a certain risk factor.

Measures of association in case-control studies

Unlike cohort studies, case-control studies begin with the selection of a group of cases (who have the disease) and a group of controls (who do not). As the numbers of cases and controls are set the investigator, the incidence of disease cannot be directly determined within the study. Therefore a relative risk cannot be calculated directly.

Instead, the relative risk is estimated by examining the relative frequencies of exposure among the cases and controls. This estimate is called the *odds ratio*.

Consider a case-control study in which a cases and b controls are exposed to some risk factor, while c cases and d controls are unexposed. In this study there are $(a + c)$ cases and $(b + d)$ controls, while $(a + b)$ individuals have the exposure factor and $(c + d)$ do not, as illustrated in the 2×2 table given in Table 17.2. Here the *odds that a case is exposed* is given by a/c, and the *odds that a control is exposed* is given by b/d. The *odds ratio* is calculated by dividing these odds:

$$\text{Odds ratio} = \frac{\text{Odds that a case is exposed}}{\text{Odds that a control is exposed}}$$

$$= (a/c)/(b/d)$$

$$= ad/bc$$

The odds ratio indicates how many times more likely (or less likely) a diseased person was to have been exposed to the risk factor, compared with a person without the disease.

Table 17.2. The 2 × 2 table used in the example given in the text

	Cases	Controls
Exposed	*a*	*b*
Unexposed	*c*	*d*

The odds ratio is analogous to relative risk, and conveys the same information, giving an equivalent index of the strength of the association between the exposure and the disease. If there is no association between the exposure and the disease, then the odds of having been exposed will be the same in both the diseased and the non-diseased groups, and the odds ratio will be 1.0. If the exposure confers an increased risk of disease, the odds ratio will be >1.0. If the exposure confers protection, the odds ratio will be between zero and 1.0.

Measures of association in cross-sectional analytical studies

In a cross-sectional study the *prevalence* of disease among the groups under comparison is usually determined, and a *prevalence ratio* can be calculated analogous to the relative risk in a cohort study. However, care must be taken in interpreting a prevalence ratio if the duration of disease differs between the exposed and the unexposed groups. The odds ratio can also be used in cross-sectional analytical studies.

Sources of distortion in epidemiological studies

Because epidemiology is concerned with human communities, methodological compromises are inevitable in the design and execution of studies. The epidemiologist's task is to come up with a design that minimises these compromises, and to conduct and analyse the investigation as tightly as possible. However, numerous potential sources of distortion inevitably persist. An evaluation of the impact of these potential sources of distortion is essential for the interpretation of epidemiological data.

The effect of chance

One of the most important issues in epidemiological investigations is the effect of chance. Implicitly or explicitly, the people selected for study constitute a sample. Because of the influence of chance, an identical study of another sample assembled under apparently similar circumstances is likely to yield results that are at least slightly different. Chance can affect all stages of a study. For example, in a randomised controlled trial, the play of chance (or *random variation*) can affect the selection of subjects for the trial, their allocation to one or other intervention group, and the observations made on them.

A review of the statistical techniques for dealing with chance effects is beyond the scope of this chapter, and the reader is referred to the numerous texts on statistical aspects of epidemiology, such as that by Armitage and Berry (1987). The overriding concern is the chance that a study will falsely conclude that a health hazard exists when in fact it does not (*type I error*) or falsely conclude that a health hazard does not exist when in fact it does (*type II error*). Two related issues warrant mention here. The first is the size of a study. Given type I and type II error levels and making few assumptions, it is quite simple to estimate in advance the number of subjects required to ensure that a firm conclusion can be drawn from the results of the study. Alternatively, if the number of subjects available for study is fixed by circumstances, it is possible to calculate in advance whether or not firm conclusions of the required degree of detail can be drawn. Second, when the results of a study are given, they should be accompanied by estimates of their statistical significance or precision. Preferably confidence limits should be stated.

Bias in epidemiological studies

Just as chance can affect all stages of a study, so can non-random influences. Non-random or systematic influences lead to *bias*. 'Bias' has a specific meaning in epidemiological usage, referring to systematic distortion at any stage of a study. In epidemiology, 'bias' does not carry implication of prejudice or lack of scientific objectivity on the part of the investigator or observers.

Bias can operate in many ways. These can be grouped under three headings: selection bias, information bias and confounding.

Selection bias

This refers to distortions arising from the selection or assembly of subjects for study. Different manifestations of selection bias have been catalogued by Sackett (1979). Selection bias may occur in a cohort study where loss to follow-up occurs unequally in the exposed and unexposed groups. If an exposure truly causes disease and if subjects who develop the disease are more likely to be lost to follow-up than subjects who do not, then the exposure/disease association will be underestimated.

Selection bias does not pose a major problem in population-based case-control studies if there is comprehensive case ascertainment from a population and controls are sampled from the same population. However, if controls are selected on the basis of having other diseases (as in a hospital-based case-control study), selection bias will occur if the other diseases are themselves associated with the exposure.

A frequently encountered selection bias in occupational cross-sectional analytical studies is called *survivor bias*. Because exposure and health outcome status are ascertained simultaneously, subjects who develop the outcome condition as a consequence of the exposure may be unavailable for study because they have sought other employment. For example, workers who develop dermatitis as a result of contact with a workplace solvent may transfer to another plant or resign because of their skin problem. This results in an underestimate of the exposure/outcome association.

Information bias

This arises when observations or measurements of exposures or health outcomes are made incorrectly or inaccurately, and when the quality of observations differ between groups under comparison. Incorrect measurements or differential quality of measurements may be due to observer error, problems with instruments, or disturbances within the person or thing being measured, including disturbance that results from being measured. According to the context, information bias is sometimes called *measurement bias* or *observation bias*.

EXAMPLE
A cross-sectional analytical study of the effect of workplace noise on blood pressure uses two sphygmomanometers, one of which (unbeknown to the investigator) shows lower readings than the other. The blood pressures of a large proportion of subjects exposed to high noise levels happen to be made with the low-reading instrument. Although the subjects exposed to high noise levels really do have higher blood pressures, the results of the study indicate that there is no association between noise exposure and blood pressure, as a consequence of the instrument error.

EXAMPLE
In a population-based case-control study of a possible link between soft-tissue sarcoma and the exposure of agricultural workers to pesticides, information on exposure is obtained by means of a structured interview. Because most of the subjects with sarcoma are manifestly unwell, it is impossible to 'blind' the interviewer (i.e. prevent him from knowing whether he is interviewing a case or a control). Subconsciously or otherwise, the interviewer is slightly more assiduous in seeking exposure information from cases. Furthermore, the cases have an understandable tendency to search for causes of their illness, and are inclined to think about their history of pesticide exposure in more detail than the controls, most of whom are in good health.

Error in the measurement or classification of exposures or outcomes can affect the groups under comparison to differing extents (*differential error*). In other circumstances, measurement error may be *non-differential*, i.e. affect the groups under comparison to the same extent. A source of measurement error which exerts an apparently random influence is likely to be non-differential. It has been shown that non-differential error always biases the estimate of association towards the null, i.e. the relative risk or odds ratio is driven towards 1.0. This is important to consider in the interpretation of negative studies, i.e. studies which show no effect.

Confounding

Confounding is a distortion of the relative risk or odds ratio due to an extraneous factor which has an independent effect on the health outcome and occurs in association with the main exposure.

EXAMPLE

In a case-control study of alcohol consumption and lung cancer, a strong association was found between heavy alcohol consumption and lung cancer. However, the investigators also collected data on smoking, and they observed a much larger proportion of smokers among the heavy alcohol consumers than among more moderate drinkers and non-drinkers. They demonstrated statistically that the apparent association between heavy alcohol consumption and lung cancer was largely due to smoking, and that heavy alcohol consumption did not have an independent association with lung cancer.

For confounding to occur, the extraneous factor (smoking in this example) must: (1) influence the occurrence of the disease (lung cancer), independent of the main exposure (heavy alcohol consumption); (2) be unequally distributed between the exposure groups (e.g. different proportions of smokers among the heavy, moderate and non-drinkers); and (3) not be a consequence of the main exposure (e.g. alcohol consumption does not cause smoking).

Confounding can distort the association between an exposure and a health outcome *positively* (taking the relative risk or odds ratio further from unity) or *negatively* (bringing the relative risk closer to unity).

An extraneous factor that causes confounding is called a *confounder*. Whether or not an extraneous variable is a confounder is specific to the dataset under consideration, and is not a necessary characteristic of that extraneous variable. Extraneous factors which have the potential to cause confounding by virtue of their influence on the occurrence of the health outcome or disease are called *potential confounders*. They exert a confounding effect only if they are unequally distributed among the exposure groups. In the example of alcohol consumption and lung cancer given above, it could have so happened that the proportions of smokers among heavy, moderate and non-drinkers were very similar. Under these circumstances, smoking would not have exerted a confounding effect.

Confounding is a *statistical* phenomenon. It occurs simply because an extraneous factor which influences the occurrence of the health outcome is unequally distributed among the exposure groups, and is not due to any biological interaction between the main exposure and the extraneous factor.

A *biological interaction* between an extraneous factor and the main exposure may also alter the relationship between the main exposure and the outcome. If this occurs it is called *effect modification*. The distinction between confounding and effect modification is important in the analysis and interpretation of epidemiological data.

Minimising bias

The minimisation of bias is one of the most important topics in epidemiological practice.

Selection bias

Selection bias can be minimised only in the study design. For example, in cohort studies and randomised controlled trials, every effort should be made to ensure that follow-up or outcome data are collected on all (or almost all) the subjects originally selected for study. In case-control studies, population-based designs are least susceptible to selection bias; the implications of control selection in other case-control designs must be examined rigorously before a study is carried out. Survivor bias is a typical problem in cross-sectional analytical studies, although other forms of selection bias can also occur. The appropriateness of using a workplace-based cross-sectional design in a workplace with high labour turnover should be questioned.

Information bias

Standard approaches to the minimisation of information bias include careful design of measurement and data-collection techniques, using reliable instruments that can be recalibrated or do not vary in their accuracy. Frequent checking of instruments is mandatory. Observers should be carefully selected and thoroughly instructed in the observation techniques, and their adherence to protocols should be checked on a regular basis. Wherever possible, observers should be unaware of the status of subjects with regard to exposure or disease ('blinded'). Where more than one instrument is used or more than one observer is employed, subjects from all comparison groups should be randomly allocated to the different observers and instruments.

Confounding

The minimisation of confounding depends mainly on investigators' awareness of potential confounders. Known potential confounders can be dealt with either in the study design or in the analysis.

In the study design, the possibility of confounding by an extraneous variable can be eliminated by:

- Matching of the comparison groups with respect to the potential confounder. This ensures that the potential confounder is present in the same proportions of subjects throughout all the groups under comparison. For matching to prevent confounding in a case-control study, a special type of analytical procedure (*matched analysis*) is used.

- Confining the study to individuals with particular characteristics. For example, if sex is known to be a potential confounder, the study could be confined to males or females. If smoking is known to be a confounder, the study could be confined to smokers or non-smokers.

In the analysis, confounding can be controlled for in several different ways, provided that the investigator has collected data on potential confounders. These include:

- Carrying out a separate analysis for each level of the confounder (*stratified analysis*), e.g. if gender is a confounder, the association between the exposure and the disease can be assessed separately for men and women.

- Using an appropriate arithmetic or algebraic method which can take account of (or *adjust* for) the influence of one or more confounders on an exposure/disease relationship. A relatively simple method which is often used to adjust for age is called *standardisation*. If, for example, mortality rates are being compared between two groups which have different age structures, the age-specific mortality rates in each population can be weighted by the age distribution of an arbitrarily chosen reference population. The weighted average mortality rates of the two groups can then be compared. This is an example of *direct standardisation*. In *indirect standardisation*, the age distribution of the groups is weighted by the age-specific mortality rates of the reference population to determine the expected number of deaths in each group. The ratio of the observed number of deaths to the expected number is called the *standardised mortality ratio* (*SMR*). The SMR is often used as an outcome measure in historical cohort studies where the mortality experience of a single exposed group is compared with that of the general population. Standardised morbidity ratios and standardised incidence ratios can be calculated by analogous methods. A full treatment of standardisation, including worked examples, is given by Armitage and Berry (1987).

More complex methods of adjustment make use of a variety of regression models which have become popular with the advent of powerful microcomputer-based statistical analysis packages. These enable an investigator to evaluate the association between a main determinant and a health outcome, and also quantify the contribution of several covariates to the outcome. Some of these covariates may be regarded as confounders, and the main association can be re-examined when they are held constant.

Critical appraisal of epidemiological evidence

As noted above, methodological compromises inevitably arise in the design and execution of epidemiological studies. Users of the information generated in epidemiological investigations must decide whether the information is valid or not. The following questions provide a structure for this appraisal.

● What study design was used? Was it appropriate to resolve the objectives of the investigation? Could a stronger design have been used?

  The strongest evidence about an exposure/disease relationship (or about the efficacy or effectiveness of an intervention) is provided by a randomised controlled trial, because the random allocation favours an even distribution of unknown confounders among the groups under comparison. Cohort studies and population-based case-control studies can also provide strong evidence. The interpretation of other case-control designs and cross-sectional designs must be more circumspect, but these designs can be very efficient if used appropriately.

● Were the exposure and outcome factors relevant to the problem under investigation? How were they measured? Were appropriate steps taken to minimise information bias? If measurement error could have occurred, was it differential or non-differential, and how would it have affected the conclusions of the study?

● Were reasonable steps taken to avoid selection bias in the design and execution of the investigation? What was the likely impact of any residual selection bias?

● Were all relevant potential confounders considered? Were confounders adequately controlled for?

● Were the data presented clearly? Was the analysis adequately described? Were the analytic methods appropriate to the problem under investigation and the nature of the data? Were there sufficient subjects to obtain a conclusive result (especially important in studies which find no association between a putative determinant and a health outcome)? Was there any evidence of errors in the interpretation of the data or the analysis?

Causality

While epidemiological methods can be used to estimate the strength of associations between putative determinants and health outcomes, they do not establish causal relationships. Causality is determined by weighing the evidence, usually from more than one study, and often from different types of scientific investigation (e.g. epidemiological and toxicological). Factors to be considered in weighing the evidence include the following:

- The validity of the epidemiological studies.

- The strength of the epidemiological associations (while weak associations may arise because of biases, stronger associations are less likely to be attributable to biases).

- The existence of a demonstrable exposure–effect relationship, the strength of the epidemiological association increasing in parallel with the level of exposure (this is analogous to a dose–effect relationship).

- Consistency among epidemiological studies (especially among studies conducted in different populations, and/or using different designs); consistency with the results of intervention studies, especially a randomised controlled trial, is especially valuable.

- Consistency between epidemiological and other forms of scientific investigation.

- The existence of a plausible biological explanation for a causal relationship.

A technique which is being used increasingly to resolve questions of causality is *meta-analysis*, in which statistical methods are used to pool the results of two or more studies. Meta-analysis is especially useful where individual studies are too small to give statistically conclusive results. An explanation of the technique is given by Greenland (1987).

Exposure assessment in epidemiology

The key issue in occupational epidemiology is the assessment of workplace exposures. The need to understand workplace exposures creates an important interface between toxicology and epidemiology, and leads to a consideration of at least three major topics. The first is the use of toxicological methods in the assessment of workplace exposures for epidemiological investigations. The second is the contribution of epidemiology, especially descriptive epidemiology, in generating causal hypotheses that lead to toxicological investigation of workplace exposures. The third is the joint use of epidemiological and toxicological methods in quantitative risk assessment.

For many agents the workplace is the only setting in which the magnitude and duration of exposure are sufficient to cause adverse health effects. Occupational epidemiological practice is therefore preoccupied with the comparison of disease occurrence among groups of workers classified by their levels of exposure to presumed toxicants. The accuracy and completeness of occupational exposure data are fundamental to this.

The relevant characteristics of exposure for the epidemiological evaluation of either acute or chronic effects are its *intensity* or *concentration*, and its *duration*. *Cumulative exposure* is the summation of exposure over time. Measurements of exposure provide estimates of the *dose* of a substance absorbed, or the *burden*, which is the amount of the substance within the body or within a particular organ. Reliable estimates of dose and burden are unusual in epidemiology, and use is often made of proxy measures such as the average exposure intensity and/or the cumulative exposure.

Biological measures of individual exposure to toxicants are increasingly used in many workplaces. However, the assessment of exposure in epidemiological investigations still usually relies on occupational hygiene records, work history records, or sometimes simply records of duration of employment in workplaces where particular agents were known to have existed. The magnitude and duration of individual exposures are then reconstructed from these records, and are often very approximate. Poor approximations give rise to measurement error, particularly non-differential measurement error, which, as noted above, tends to conceal associations between exposures and their putative health effects. Furthermore, many occupational epidemiological investigations are concerned with rare diseases and their possible association with low levels of exposure to toxicants. Such associations are easily obscured by the imperfections of traditional exposure measurement techniques.

In recent years advances in molecular biology have enabled the detection of subtle changes in molecular processes attributable to exposure to toxicants. These techniques offer opportunities for epidemiologists and toxicologists to improve the application of epidemiological methods in the study of the health effects of occupational exposures.

References

Armitage, P. and Berry, G., 1987, *Statistical Methods in Medical Research*. Oxford: Blackwell Scientific.

Battista, G., Cavalluci, F., Comba, P., *et al.*, 1983, A case-referent study on nasal cancer and exposure to wood dust in the province of Siena, Italy, *Scand. J. Work Environ. Health*, **9**, 25–9.

Eylenbosch, W. J. and Noah, N. D. (Eds), 1988, *Surveillance in Health and Disease*. Oxford: Oxford University Press.

Greenland, S., 1987, Qualitative methods in the review of epidemiologic literature, *Epidemiol. Rev.*, **6**, 1–30.

Infante, P. F., Wagoner, J. K., Rinsky, R. A. and Young, R. J., 1977, Leukaemia in benzene workers, *Lancet*, **ii**, 76–8.

Jarup, L. and Pershagen, G., 1991, Arsenic exposure, smoking and lung cancer in smelter workers—a case-control study, *Am. J. Epidemiol.*, **134**, 545–51.

Merler, E., Baldasseroni, A., Laria, R., *et al.*, 1986, On the association between exposure to leather dust and nasal cancer: further evidence from a case-control study, *Br. J. Ind. Med.*, **43**, 91–5.

Nurminen, M. and Hernberg, S., 1985, Effect of intervention on the cardiovascular mortality of workers exposed to carbon disulphide: a 15 year follow up, *Br. J. Ind. Med.*, **42**, 32–5.

Sackett, D. L., 1979, Bias in analytic research. *J. Chronic Dis.*, **32**, 51–63.

Venables, K. M., Dally, M. B., Burge, P. S., *et al.*, 1985, Occupational asthma in a steel coating plant, *Br. J. Ind. Med.*, **42**, 517–24.

Wagner, J. C., Sleggs, C. A. and Marchand, P., 1960, Diffuse pleural mesothelioma and asbestos exposure in the North Western Cape Province, *Br. J. Ind. Med.*, **17**, 260–71.

Uses of Toxicological Data

Chapter 18

Managing Workplace Chemical Safety

C. Winder and C. Vickers

Introduction

Chemicals are found in virtually all workplaces to a greater or lesser extent. Using this chapter as a guide in the first instance, one should be able to gain awareness of the different aspects relating to managing chemicals in the workplace.

Basic principles of chemical safety

There are only two factors that affect safety:

● Inherent properties, e.g. toxicity, flammability and corrosiveness.

● Factors relating to exposure, e.g. the probability, duration, frequency and intensity of exposure.

Approaches to chemical safety

There are really only four approaches to chemical control (see Table 18.1). These approaches apply equally well at the national or workplace levels.

Table 18.1. Approaches to chemical safety

Prohibit chemicals
● Any risk unacceptable
● No risk
● No benefits

Example: the US Delaney Amendment to the Food and Drugs Act (1976), which prohibits the introduction of any carcinogen into the USA

Check all chemicals
● Mandatory evaluation of hazard
● Resource intensive
● Risk minimisation

Example: in Australia, all pharmaceutical substances require chemical, toxicological and clinical evaluation by law (Therapeutic Goods Act 1966).

Table 18.1. (*Contd.*)

Screen all chemicals, check all suspect chemicals
● Risk–benefit analysis required
● Allows stepwise decision-making

Example: assessment of the environmental effects of agricultural chemicals.

Allow chemicals
● Ignore the hazard
● Accept the risk

Example: occupational or domestic exposure to tobacco smoke (in situations where prohibition of chemicals has not been implemented).

Components of a chemical safety programme

It is important to recognise that most, if not all, chemical substances can be handled and used safely, providing that: (1) the hazards are known and understood; (2) correct handling and use procedures are in place and adhered to; (3) the correct equipment to handle and use chemicals is available, used and maintained; (4) workers are informed about hazards and trained in correct procedures; and (5) prompt action is taken to control and minimise problems that do arise. A comprehensive chemical safety programme should incorporate activities in a number of areas, as shown in Table 18.2.

Table 18.2. Components in a programme for the management of chemical safety

● Assessment of workplace hazards
● Information and training
● Control of exposure
● Procedures for the workforce to deal with minor emergencies
● Requirements of special groups, such as the emergency services
● Disposal
● Monitoring

Workplace assessment

Assessment of the hazards and risks associated with the use of chemicals and the nature and cause of chemical-related injury and disease is an important factor in prevention. The purpose of assessment is to evaluate the risks to health arising from work involving the use of hazardous substances and to determine appropriate measures to protect the health and safety of employees. Assessment entails a process that identifies existing and potential hazards, evaluates the nature of the hazard and provides appropriate measures for their control. Workplace assessment of new chemicals and those already in use, and control of chemical inventories are important in controlling exposure.

Step 1: The materials inventory

MATERIALS ALREADY IN USE

As a first step, an inventory of all the chemical materials at the workplace should be made. Such an information base should contain at least a minimum amount of information and, as a first stage, this should be the name, manufacturer, approximate amounts in stock and workplace location. As some chemical hazards will only be produced during processing, it may also be necessary to create a process or reaction inventory as a subset of the materials inventory.

Once these materials have been identified, it may become necessary to develop priorities for action. Such priorities might include: (1) investigation of less hazardous alternatives; (2) action on chemicals that have poorly identified hazards; (3) development of policies for chemicals in use, where the present procedures are deemed inadequate; and (4) requirements for monitoring.

Options for creation of the information base include systems on computer, and a number of software systems are commercially available. However, sophisticated systems may not be necessary for workplaces where only a few chemicals are in use. Whatever system is used, a mechanism should be developed that allows review of the materials inventory on a periodic basis.

NEW MATERIALS

As part of the development of an information base, a process should be developed which identifies new materials entering the workplace, so that these can be targeted for assessment and action. Once in use, regular monitoring of exposure patterns may be required.

Step 2: The walk-through survey

If such systems are not already in place, an initial survey will be necessary to reinforce the contents of the materials inventory. Questions to be answered include those listed in Table 18.3. This initial survey should be comprehensive, and take into account the whole workplace, including places where extensive chemical use is not expected, such as offices (photocopier chemicals) and lunch rooms (cleaning materials). It is usual to find materials missed in the first stage.

In areas where chemicals are used, especially in manufacturing areas, it will also be necessary to consider the fate of materials. For example, a production process might use raw materials easily identified. Problem areas may be identified in the survey by observing work practices and making note of smells, dusts, smoke, waste materials and so on.

The minimum information required from the survey would include: (1) the names and manufacturers of the chemicals; (2) what information is already available; (3) how the product is handled and used; and (4) what controls are used to control hazard.

Table 18.3. Questions to ask on the walk-through

- What materials are present?
- Where are they located?
- What handling procedures exist (storage, decanting)?
- On average, what quantities are used?
- What labels, MSDS or other information is available on hazard?
- How are the materials used?
- How often are the materials used?
- What are the likely hazards?
- What controls are used to contain or mitigate exposure?
- What disposal procedures are used?

MSDS, material safety data sheet.

Conditions in a workplace change with time. Inspection of all areas of the plant should be made on a regular basis to identify and eliminate foreseeable chemical (and other) problems. This should include review of all control measures in place and procedures for their maintenance.

While nothing will be better that accurate knowledge of local conditions and hazards, safety audits will be facilitated by the use of appropriately designed check-lists. Check-lists aid in auditing activities, assist in the identification of hazards, permit on-the-spot recording of findings and comments, and can provide a report of the audit. Check-lists can also be tailored or developed for specific workplace applications.

Step 3: The chemicals register

While the materials inventory can be regarded as an information system, it is really only an interim measure until a better information resource can be developed. This information resource is the chemicals register which, if appropriately indexed and catalogued: (1) can be either a paper or computer database; (2) should provide, as a minimum, a central listing of all substances which are used in the workplace together with basic information such as the material safety data sheet (MSDS) (see below); (3) should be used as a tool to manage substances used at work; and (4) is a source of information.

There is currently no requirement for workplaces to have a chemicals register, and therefore there is great variability in the registers that do exist. However, using the basic information collected as part of the materials inventory and walk-through survey, a start on a chemicals register can be made.

Step 4: The assessment

The first three stages of managing chemical safety at work have been about finding out what hazards and hazardous processes and practices exist at the workplace. The next stage is about hazard control. This process consists of three phases: recognition, evaluation and control.

RECOGNITION

The recognition of hazards depends on one fact: *a chemical must make contact with, or be absorbed into, the human body to induce an effect.*

When identifying actual or potential problems, the following questions should be answered:

- How likely is it that a chemical will be released from the process or practice in which it is used?

- If release is likely, and control technology cannot be easily improved, what will be the nature, extent, intensity and duration of the resulting contamination?

EVALUATION

The next phase is the evaluation phase, where a systematic approach to assessing the risks involved in particular work needs to be established. The questions to be answered are:

- How will the released chemical/contamination make contact with, or be absorbed into the human body, by what routes and in what amounts? If absorption does occur, what are the consequences?

The information obtained can then be used to evaluate the hazards associated with work involving hazardous chemicals. Risk should be evaluated taking into account: (1) the hazardous substances involved and the possibility of safer alternatives; (2) the routes of exposure; (3) the duration, intensity and frequency of exposure; (4) the nature and severity of potential health effects; (5) the likelihood of potential health effects at the exposures observed; and (6) the economic and technical feasibility of alternative control measures.

As well as assessment of the workers involved directly in hazardous tasks, consideration must also be given to people who work nearby, who may come into contact inadvertently. This may occur through unplanned exposure or failure of control measures.

CONTROL

Finally, the assessment should make recommendations as to how the hazard can be controlled or the risk minimised. If the assessment process determines that the risk is insignificant and it is not reasonably foreseeable that it could increase in future, then it can be concluded that precautions or controls are not necessary, or that existing procedures are adequate, then no further action will be necessary.

If the assessment process determines that the risk is significant and it makes recommendations for control measures to be modified or introduced, or for new practices to be developed, then these should be given consideration in consultation with employer and employees. The role of any health and safety representatives or committees in this process is important.

Information and training

Workplace information sources

The range of chemicals and chemical products and the various hazards leads to differences in safe handling practices in the workplace. It is therefore important to ensure that the correct information is available on chemical hazards and their control.

At the workplace level, it is not normally a question of what information is available, rather it is a question of getting the existing information on chemical hazards and control measures to the right people. As a first step, information should be obtained from the employer and, failing provision of adequate information from this source, it should be obtained from the manufacturer, importer or supplier.

The basis of a workplace information transfer system is formed by: (1) the label; (2) the material safety data sheet (MSDS); (3) other information sources such as publicity pamphlets, technical bulletins, directions for use, and safety manuals; (4) warnings and placards on hazardous installations and processes; and (5) training and education.

LABELS FOR CHEMICAL PACKAGES

The label nearly always represents the first (and often only) source of information on hazard and control to the user. Physically, the label should have a number of characteristics, including robustness, strong attachment to the container and resistance to degradation by age or by spillage of the contents.

Table 18.4. Information guidelines for good labelling practice

The minimum information on a label includes:

- The information required by legislation
- Signal words or symbols on primary hazards
- Identification information, such as product name and hazardous ingredients
- Directions for safe use
- Risk phrases, such as 'Reacts violently with water'
- Safety phrases, such as 'Avoid contact with eyes'
- First aid instructions
- Details of the manufacturer or supplier

Other information that may be supplied includes:

- Expiry date
- Environmental information, such as 'Do not dispose waste materials into water supply'

One further inclusion is to refer the user to the material safety data sheet for more information

The label should identify the contents of the package or container and should draw attention of people handling or using the chemical to significant hazards. In addition, the most severe hazards should be highlighted by the use of suitable warning symbols or signal words (such as 'poison').

Issues which must be considered include legislative requirements, what needs to be labelled, how much detail is required, the needs of individuals who cannot read the label because of language or literacy problems and how often labels should be revised. Some of these have immediate application to the workplace (see Table 18.4).

The material safety data sheet

WORKER'S RIGHT TO KNOW
The issue of provision of information to workers under the concept of 'right to know' has been established in many countries. This has be extended even further in countries such as the USA, where 'community right to know' exists as well as 'worker right to know'. In the past, the minimum amount of information that should be available to users has been inconsistent for chemical hazards.

While the starting point for the safe use of a chemical is usually the label, it cannot always supply all the information workers need. Material safety data sheets (MSDSs) are a convenient, standard form for providing more detailed health and safety information. Most occupational health and safety legislation now requires that specific information on hazard be given to employees at risk. The MSDS is the appropriate form of disseminating information on chemical hazard.

GENERAL PROVISIONS
An MSDS should be: (1) product based; (2) understandable to handlers and users; (3) freely available in the workplace; and (4) updated as necessary. Access to information on a MSDS should be facilitated by using a standardised format and by differentiation of sections by distinctive blocking of headings.

MSDS APPLICATIONS
MSDSs must be available to all workers and users. The most appropriate way in which this can be facilitated is by their inclusion into a prominently sited Chemicals Register which all workers know how to use. MSDSs can be used in the development of more suitable control measures and workplace emergency action plans, where chemical hazards exist. MSDSs should be used in worker training programmes. Finally, MSDSs can be used to develop policies on purchasing safer alternative products.

In summary, MSDSs should enable users to: (1) understand safety recommendations and their rationale; (2) be aware of the results of failure to comply with these recommendations; (3) recognise symptoms of overexposure; and (4) take part in informed discussions between employers and employees (see Table 18.5).

Table 18.5. Information guidelines for inclusion on an MSDS

The minimum information on an MSDS includes:
- Details of the manufacturer or supplier
- Product identification, including:
    (a) product/trade name and any other relevant names/codes;
    (b) major uses;
    (c) physical properties;
    (d) ingredients, including all hazardous ingredients
- Health hazards, including short- and long-term effects by appropriate routes of exposure
- First aid advice which can be given by untrained people, such as: 'Remove affected person from exposure'
- Advice to medically trained personnel, including possible existing health conditions which may be exacerbated by exposure
- Precautions for users, such as:
    (a) any relevant exposure standards;
    (b) the correct engineering controls that should be employed, such as process enclosure or ventilation;
    (c) personal protective requirements;
    (d) information on flammability, reactivity, etc.
- Safe handling information for handlers of the product, such as transport, stores and emergency services personnel, aimed at handling problems such as spills, fires, disposal, etc.
- A Contact Point at the manufacturer/supplier, in case further information is required
- The date of the MSDS

Other information that may also be included:
- Environmental information
- Specific toxicity information (such as LD_{50} values)
- Reference sources
- MSDS identification, such as page numbers, MSDS number

Warnings and placards

Placards are signs that provide warning of chemical hazards. They can be posted on vehicles transporting dangerous materials, where chemicals are stored and where they are used. Warnings and placards alert people at the workplace, the emergency services and the general public about the presence, location and nature of hazards. Finally, they can provide information about the correct response to and contacts in an emergency.

Training

The training of workers is an integral part of a preventive strategy. Employees should be provided with the knowledge and skills needed to use the control measures and emergency procedures provided for their protection. Training and education should also enable participation in decisions about the use of substances at work.

TYPES OF TRAINING
Training should include: (1) induction training (before a worker is exposed to any hazard); (2) on-the-job training; and (3) periodic refresher training to advise of any significant changes to processes or operations, and to maintain knowledge and awareness.

WHO SHOULD BE TRAINED?
Training should be provided for the range of employees, including operators, stores personnel, the emergency action team. Supervisors and management also need training. Each group will have its own training needs. For example, differences in literacy must be considered.

ELEMENTS OF A TRAINING PROGRAMME
Training programmes will incorporate a number of essential elements, although the amount of detail and extent of training will depend on the nature of the hazard, the complexities of the work and the available control measures (see Table 18.6).

Table 18.6. Essential elements of a training programme

- Relevant statutory provisions
- Employer and employee rights, and collective responsibilities
- Information about workplace hazards, including chemicals, processes and routes of exposure
- Specific information on hazards, such as chemicals registers, workplace safety manuals, labels and MSDS
- The workplace assessment process
- Available control measures, the reasons for their use (including risks to health), their proper use and maintenance
- The proper use of personal protection, including fit, routine cleaning and maintenance, and any special decontamination procedures
- Correct work practices and procedures in all aspects of chemical use
- The importance of minimising potential and actual exposure by good workplace practices and personal hygiene standards
- Emergency procedures
- First aid and incident reporting procedures
- The nature and reasons for any monitoring, personal monitoring and health surveillance, including employee rights to consultation and access to medical records
- Disposal procedures

MSDS, material safety data sheet.

Training programmes should also be: (1) provided without loss of income to the employee and without the requirement to work additional hours;

(2) documented, with the names of trainees, dates of attendance, matters covered and names of the trainers as a minimum; (3) evaluated to ensure that the employees have an adequate understanding of the matters covered; and (4) reviewed periodically to ensure relevancy.

Instruction should be reinforced by distribution of written instructions relevant to the workplace. Such information should, as far as is practical, be in the language of the worker.

Control of exposure

A major problem with risk management is the lack of data on the hazards of many chemicals. In the past decade or so, approximately 4 million new chemicals have been prepared and identified, although three-quarters of these have been cited only once in the literature. However, of the 70 000 or so chemicals in use at work, exposure standards exist for only about 700 (or 1%). Moreover, multiple exposures, or exposures to mixtures are more common than single exposures.

Control of occupational hazards is especially important for exposures to chemicals and a prime objective of a workplace chemicals safety management programme is to control exposures to chemicals to levels at which the risk of adverse effects to health is acceptably low. This is best accomplished by making the workplace fit the worker, not the worker fit the workplace. Consistent with this principle, there is a clear hierarchy of control measures which may be implemented in workplaces where chemicals are handled or used (see Table 18.7). This hierarchy applies to both design of new workplace systems, and assessment and modification of existing conditions.

Table 18.7. A hierarchy of control measures

- Elimination
- Substitution with less hazardous materials or processes
- Minimisation of inventories
- Engineering controls at source, such as automation or process enclosure
- Engineering controls to reduce exposure, such as segregation, partial enclosure, mechanical handling, suppression methods or ventilation
- Administrative controls, such as safe working procedures, job rotation, good housekeeping
- Personnel procedures, such as adequate supervision, information dissemination and training
- Personal protection

Elimination

The simplest way to deal with a hazard is to get rid of it. Though not often an option, it is important to ensure that the option of elimination has at least been considered. The most effective risk control measures are those taken at the design stage in the cases of processes, and the purchasing stage in the case of materials. Elimination is an appropriate option at the design stage, and can apply to choice of materials, choice of hardware, building and equipment specifications, etc.

Substitution

It is often possible to replace relatively hazardous materials or processes with safer alternatives which offer the same general properties. Substitution may also include altering synthetic routes for a chemical substance, to avoid the use, or production of toxic intermediates. Consideration must also be given not only to the toxicity of reactants, intermediates, products, and wastes, but also to any impurities or contaminants which may arise.

Minimisation of inventories

An important principle in workplaces where chemicals are used is to reduce the inventory of materials as much as possible. This can be done by reducing the amounts being stored and the number of different chemicals being stored. Routine inventory audits, and disposal of off-specification, contaminated, out of date or no longer used stock will assist in this process.

Engineering controls at source

Control at source measures are those which stop hazardous exposures before they reach the workplace (and the worker). Examples of control measures include isolation, segregation of hazardous equipment or process away from work areas, automation, process enclosure, mechanical handling, special storage facilities such as bulk tanks, and use of welded piping instead of screwed joints. Control technology must be designed and maintained properly to ensure maximum performance.

Engineering controls to reduce exposure

These are measures which reduce hazardous exposures before they reach the worker. Examples of control measures include partial or temporary enclosure, spray booths, fume cupboards, glove boxes, dilution or local exhaust ventilation, bunding, dust suppression, prewetting. Again, engineering controls must be maintained properly to ensure maximum performance.

Administrative controls

Controls which rely on human behaviour are controls which minimise hazard by the expectation that the exposed person will undertake certain safe procedures. As human beings can be unreliable, administrative controls can also be unreliable. Examples include job rotation/multiskilling, minimising the numbers of people permitted access to the hazard, codes of practice, standardised work practices and safe working procedures, permits to work, and good housekeeping.

GOOD HOUSEKEEPING
Elements of good housekeeping and safe work practices that can be adopted at most, if not all, workplaces include: (1) safe storage and disposal; (2) storing small volumes in safety cans; (3) keeping only 1 days supply of a chemical at the work area; (4) keeping lids on containers when they are not in use; (5) prohibiting eating, drinking and smoking in contaminated areas; (6) regular cleaning of contamination from floors, walls and surfaces; (7) prompt clean-up of spills; (8) keeping used or chemical contaminated materials in covered containers; (9) disposing of unused chemicals or contaminated materials in covered, labelled containers; and (10) decanting and relabelling procedures.

Personal procedures

These are procedures which result in workers who are adequately informed, trained and supervised. The main approaches include the provision of information on hazard, training of workers to do their job properly, and development of an appropriate 'safety culture' through proper supervision.

Personal protection

These are controls that place a barrier between the hazard and the worker at the level of the worker. Preference should always be given to safe-workplace rather than safe-worker policies. Use of personal protection represents the safe-worker policy and, therefore, only offers protection to the wearer.

Some hazards are local (such as splashing of chemicals) and it is difficult to engineer out the hazard. Exposure to hazards may be so dangerous in some operations (such as maintenance or dealing with spills) that they require high levels of personal protection (such as respiratory protection). Some situations where personal protection can be used include those listed in Table 18.8.

A number of problems relate to the use of personal protection: (1) it is uncomfortable to use (especially in hot conditions); (2) it reduces communication and visibility; (3) it can lead to health problems such as heat stress and dermatitis; and, importantly (4) its use often inhibits the introduction of more appropriate engineering controls. The use of such controls should always be a last resort, and should never form the basis of a long-term control programme.

Table 18.8. Situations where personal protective equipment can be used

- Situations where, for one reason of another, the control measures are not reasonably practicable
- Jobs where close contact with the source of hazard is required
- Hazardous tasks of short duration
- Hazardous tasks that have to be undertaken occasionally
- Jobs in confined spaces
- Jobs where the task is very variable, or carried out in different locations
- Maintenance of plant and processes using hazardous materials
- Dealing with emergency situations, such as escape, rescue, spills, leaks or fires
- As an interim measure, until better control measures can be instituted

Supervision is an important part of any personal protection programme and should include: clear delegation of responsibility, selection, fit, use, maintenance and cleaning. This should be supplemented by appropriate training, including written instructions and procedures for compliance and situations of non-compliance. Finally, all personal protective equipment should be adequately maintained to ensure it is up to specification.

Is the programme working?

Workplaces are constantly changing. While there is no simple rule that may be used to determine the specific controls measures that may be feasible, only routine assessment of existing conditions may suggest changes which will lead to improvements in health and safety.

Emergencies

Prevention and management of chemical incidents requires: (1) preplanning; (2) information systems, such as placards and emergency plans; (3) training of the emergency response team; and (4) consultation with the emergency services.

The workplace level

Workplace emergencies involving chemical substances can result in injury to workers and emergency response personnel, interruption of business, bankruptcy, loss of markets, environmental damage, require costly decontamination and clean-up, have the potential for compensation or public liability, public concern and loss of confidence. Therefore, the design and management of plant and comprehensive emergency plans at the company level are crucial.

An incident may arise as a result of: (1) inadequate hardware, e.g. inadequate segregation of incompatible materials; (2) inadequate workpractices; or (3) inadequate emergency planning.

Procedures to minimise the likelihood of emergencies such as accidents, fire, explosion, spills, leaks, natural events (for example, storms or floods) include:

● Adequate building and facility design, including access for the emergency services, bunds, availability of safety equipment and water, sumps for firewater.

● Adequate security.

● Correct handling, storage and segregation.

● Provision of safety equipment such as smoke/fire/gas detectors, extinguishers, alarms, absorbants, personal protection.

● Special storage for explosives and flammables.

● Secure storage for radioactive materials, poisons and infectious agents.

● Correct procedures for the use of chemicals, including decanting and relabelling from larger containers.

● Correct procedures for the disposal of chemicals, their containers or contaminated materials.

An emergency plan detailing the action to be taken in all possible emergency situations should be accessible to all staff and updated regularly (see Table 18.9).

Table 18.9. Elements of a workplace emergency plan

● Who are the people responsible for dealing with emergency situations?
● What should people do in the case of an emergency?
● What equipment is required (extinguishers, protective clothing, breathing apparatus, absorbants)?
● When and how should evacuation be carried out?
● Regular simulations should be carried out, which:
  (a) inform workers about emergency procedures such as drills and evacuation;
  (b) trial the appropriate protection and equipment to be used;
  (c) train emergency response staff in emergency procedures such as fire fighting and evacuation of the injured
● Procedures for incidents involving first aid, including the names of qualified first aiders and reporting procedures
● Procedures for fires and explosions, the types of extinguishers to be used and when the fire authorities should be contacted
● Procedures for spills and leaks, whether to contain, absorb or dilute, and when to contact the emergency services
● What decontamination and clean-up procedures should be carried out?

The emergency services level

The emergency services are not part of the normal workplace activities. However, their involvement at the workplace in the case of an emergency is usually serious and immediate. Therefore, they need clean, accurate and concise information on chemical hazards, which meets their particular requirements. This can be assisted by the use of standard placards (see above) or by interlinkages between the authorities and the workplace.

A summarised list of hazardous materials by dangerous goods class, average quantities and location is of more use to the emergency services than the detailed data usually available from, for example, stores inventories. This summary information, or 'manifest', is particularly useful for workplaces where significant numbers or amounts of chemical substances are stored or used.

Manifests should contain information on at least: (1) a list of each category of hazardous substance by UN Dangerous Goods Class; (2) substances in Dangerous Goods Class 2.3 (poison gases) and Packaging group I should be individually itemised by correct technical name and UN Number; (3) the maximum anticipated quantities of these materials stored; and (4) a site plan showing the location of each category of hazardous substance.

While information on manifests is predominantly needed by the emergency services in order to select the most appropriate emergency action, the information may also be of use to others. For example, manifests can be used in the training and education of workers, can assist in the rationalisation of stores, and may be used as a basis for informing the public about hazards on site.

Disposal

The control of pollution caused by chemical wastes is a major concern. Wastes can be in a variety of forms, each with their own hazards. A programme for the disposal of all hazardous waste materials forms an elementary part of a chemical safety management programme. Options for waste disposal should be spelt out for each hazardous material or process stream. Options include:

- *Recycling and recovery*—these are often proposed as pollution-control measures, and many aspects of chemical manufacturing may be regarded as 'recycling' methods. For example, many metals, some solvents and oils are commonly recycled.

- *Separation of waste*—minimisation of waste costs and maximisation of resources requires appropriate separation of waste materials into recyclables, material that can be disposed through sewerage or local refuse collections and materials that must be otherwise disposed of.

- *Disposal of liquids*—it is probable that water authorities will allow some liquid waste into municipal sewerage, and local refuse collection agencies will allow some industrial waste for disposal at landfill sites. However, special waste needs specialised disposal services.

- *Waste treatment*—sometimes, it is possible to neutralise waste before disposal. For example, acid wastes can be mixed with alkaline wastes.

- *Specialised treatment*—this usually requires collection by contractors and treatment elsewhere.

Monitoring

Occupational disease and injury are prevented by minimising worker exposure. Workplace monitoring is used to check the effectiveness of exposure control measures. It can be of a number of types, but is essentially either measurement of contaminants in the workplace or at the worker level.

The pathway from exposure to production of adverse health effects involves a number of steps, and there is a number of important implications for occupational health management programmes in the type of monitoring chosen (see Table 18.10). It should be noted that, as the focus moves from the workplace to the worker, there is also a movement away from the cause of the problem. In cases where a general practitioner is faced with a patient with, say, a skin problem, the link between cause and effect may be broken if no information on occupational factors is obtained from the patient.

Table 18.10. Health hazards and monitoring

Type of hazard or effect	Type of action
Hazard in the workplace	Environmental monitoring
Hazard in contact with the worker	Personal monitoring
Hazard absorbed into the body	Biological monitoring of absorption
Early or minimal health effects	Biological monitoring of effects
Established illness or injury	Medical examination or screening

Workplace and personal monitoring

To assess the risk when using a hazardous chemical, it is necessary to: (1) measure its concentration in workplace air, preferably in the worker's breathing zone; (2) analyse the sample for the contaminants of concern; and (3) interpret the results in terms of accepted practices and standards. This information can be used to gauge whether changes need to be made in the way the chemical is handled or used. Personal monitoring of air in a worker's breathing zone is the most representative measure of individual exposure. Monitoring requires specialised knowledge of occupational hygiene and measuring equipment.

Health assessment

Health assessment encompasses both biological monitoring and medical surveillance.

BIOLOGICAL MONITORING

This consists of measuring blood, urine or exhaled gases from the worker. Monitoring of exposure (e.g. lead in the blood of lead workers) provides a measure of how much exposure has occurred. Monitoring of effect (e.g. measurement of liver function in solvent-exposed workers) provides a measure of how significant the exposure has been. Non-invasive measures are more acceptable than invasive measures, although there may be a trade-off between convenience and validity.

It should always be remembered that biological monitoring: (1) is not a means of prevention or protection; (2) will not reduce a hazard or risk; (3) should be conducted in conjunction with workplace environmental monitoring; (4) should not be used as the sole means of hazard identification; and (5) should not be used to direct resources away from more appropriate means of controlling exposure.

MEDICAL SURVEILLANCE

This can be considered as the observation of occupational health problems with the object of measuring the effectiveness of control programmes. It can therefore have a number of objectives: (1) it can make an initial assessment of fitness to work; (2) it can be used to evaluate the effect of worker exposure; (3) it can assess the fitness of an employee to continue to be exposed to a hazard; and (4) it will enable remedial action to be taken before adverse effects develop.

Health assessment requires special knowledge of occupational medicine, and a familiarity with exposure conditions and work circumstances of the examined worker.

Summary: The management of chemical safety

To be effective, health and safety activities must be integrated into the management functions of planning, organising, leading, coordinating, controlling, directing and evaluating workplace systems. This can take place at a number of levels, from the workplace level to the government level. The management of problems which address chemical safety should:

- Be aimed at reducing chemical-related occupational injury and disease.

- Be designed to provide an integrated structure to deal with all aspects of chemicals handling and use.

- Ensure a comprehensive approach to chemicals management.

Where chemical hazards are involved it is especially important to ensure that appropriate safety systems are incorporated into the workplace in a coherent management system and, if appropriately developed, such a system should answer the following questions with a 'yes':

- Do you have a materials inventory/chemicals register?

- Do you conduct routine safety audits (including chemical safety)?

- Do you inform employees about chemical hazards at your workplace?

- Do you train workers in dealing with chemical hazards?

- Do you routinely obtain material safety data sheets (MSDSs) for the chemical materials in your workplace?

- Do you ensure workers are aware of what MSDSs are and where they can be found?

- Do you have a system which evaluates the safety of all new products at your workplace?

- Is there adequate warning/placarding of chemical hazards and processes at your workplaces?

- Do you regularly maintain the technical measures (engineering controls, personal protection, etc.) used to control chemical hazards?

- Are there appropriate procedures for dealing with leaks, spills, fires, etc. (including investigating and reporting)?

- Do you dispose of chemicals appropriately?

- Do you have procedures for investigating incidents involving chemicals?

Bibliography

ACGIH, 1986, *Documentation of Threshold Limit Values and Biological Exposure Indices*. Cincinnati: American Conference of Governmental Industrial Hygienists.

Brickman, R., Jasanoff, S. and Ilgen, T., 1985, *Controlling Chemicals: The Politics of Regulation in Europe and the United States*. Ithaca, NY: Cornell University Press.

Carson, P. A. and Mumford, C. J., 1988, *The Safe Handling of Chemicals in Industry*, Vols 1 and 2. Harlow: Longman Scientific and Technical.

CCH, 1992, Management of chemical safety, in *Workplace Health and Safety Manual*. CCH International. Sydney.

Clayton, G. D., Clayton, F. E., Cralley, L. J. and Cralley L. V., 1978–1985, *Patty's Industrial Hygiene and Toxicology*, Vols 1–3. New York: Wiley.

Crone, H., 1986, *Chemicals and Society: A Guide to the New Chemical Age*. Cambridge: Cambridge University Press.

Ellenhorn, M. J. and Barceloux, G., 1987, *Medical Toxicology: Diagnosis and Treatment of Human Poisoning*. New York: Elsevier.

Frankl, M., 1979, *Chemical Risk: A Worker's Guide to Chemical Hazards and Data Sheets*. London: Pluto Press.

Halton, D. M., 1986, *How to Answer Questions about Hazardous Chemicals*. Hamilton, Ontario: Canadian Centre for Occupational Health and Safety.

Hammer, W., 1976, *Occupational Safety Management and Engineering*. Englewood Cliffs, NJ: Prentice Hall.

Harvey, B. (Ed.), 1980–, *Handbook of Occupational Hygiene*, Vols 1–3. Kingston upon Thames: Kluwer/Croner.

Lefevre, M. J. and Becker, E. I., 1982, *First Aid Manual for Chemical Accidents*. New York: Van Nostrand Reinhold.

NIOSH, 1981–, *Occupational Guidelines for Chemical Hazards*. Washington, DC: National Institute for Occupational Safety and Health.

NIOSH, 1985, *Pocket Guide to Chemical Hazards*. Washington, DC: National Institute for Occupational Safety and Health.

Ottoboni, M. A., 1984, *The Dose Makes the Poison: A Plain Language Guide to Toxicology*. Berkeley, CA: Vincente Books.

Sax, N. I. and Lewis Jr, R. J., 1988, *Dangerous Properties of Industrial Materials*, Vols 1–3. New York: Van Nostrand Reinhold.

Weiss, G., 1986, *Hazardous Chemicals Data Book*. New Jersey: Noyes.

Chapter 19

Working Examples in Occupational Toxicology

N. H. Stacey and C. Winder

Introduction

Toxicology and toxicological data have many uses relating to chemicals in the workplace. Toxicologists and others using data of a toxicological nature will be called upon to put the information to particular purposes. Tasks will vary from the relatively simple to the complex. Questions may be asked that can be quickly answered from one's knowledge to those where extensive searching of the literature and interpretation of data are required.

At the same time such tasks can be learning experiences and can readily be used to illustrate how an understanding of the basics of toxicology are so important in enabling one to provide cogent responses to issues or tasks raised.

It is the intention of this chapter to provide examples of some of the tasks/situations that befall those using toxicological information so that it can be more readily appreciated just how the information is used and also to show how the tasks rely on the basics of the science.

Requests for information on chemical-related problems

It is not uncommon to be asked to provide information of the toxicity of chemicals as it relates to specific workplace situations. Two examples will be considered. Firstly, in relation to a potential toxic injury suffered by a worker, and secondly a request for general information concerning the toxic properties of a chemical and how any regulations may affect the use of that chemical. Both situations are hypothetical, although they are similar to the sorts of requests that one may expect to receive.

Example 1

A letter is received from a company with the following text.

Safework Consultants
P. O. Box 1
Erehwon 12345

Dear Sir/Madam

I write to seek advice on the possible cause(s) of liver problems found in one of our workers.

Two weeks after returning from the Christmas/New Year break, during which tanks were cleaned and solvent replaced, the worker in question was found to have abnormal liver function tests following his regular 6 monthly screening test. Transaminases were moderately elevated while alkaline phosphatase and γ-glutamyl transpeptidase were essentially normal. The worker concerned has been with our company for 3 years and has not previously been found to have abnormal liver function tests. He has reported alcohol intake to be minimal—essentially social consumption over the weekend. The worker is one of six employed in our metal degreasing operation where the main chemical used is trichloroethylene. With regard to his coworkers, three had no abnormality in their liver function tests while one had mildly elevated γ-glutamyl transpeptidase and the other had borderline aspartate aminotransferase.

Periodic air monitoring carried out by an occupational hygienist has not indicated any atmospheric levels of trichloroethylene over the exposure standard of 50 ppm. There was a minor incident a few days prior to blood sampling, however, whereby some trichloroethylene was spilled on the floor. As a very rough estimate it seems that air concentrations may have been of the order of 150–250 ppm for about half an hour.

Please do not hesitate to contact me for further information if necessary. We look forward to receiving your advice at your earliest convenience.

Yours faithfully

Manager's name
Company

Response

A response itself will not be provided. There is no 'correct' answer, necessarily, to the problem raised. However, the steps taken and the kind of information sought are the important aspects. It should be appreciated that different individuals will approach this problem in different ways. For instance many will want to seek more information on a variety of points before responding. This is laudable and probably necessary but, for the purposes of this exercise where this is not possible, we can still identify the information that must be sought to provide a response to the request.

INFORMATION TO BE SOUGHT

- What are the tasks of a degreaser with regard to likely exposures?

- Is trichloroethylene hepatotoxic? Under what circumstances?

- How are the liver function tests to be interpreted with regard to chemical (and especially trichloroethylene) exposure?

- What is the basis for the exposure standard for trichloroethylene? Is is related to liver effects or to some other toxic response?

- Are there other potential hepatotoxicants to be found in this type of workplace?

- Could chemicals have been mislabelled, contaminated, etc?

- Is there a possibility of the toxicity being due to interaction with other chemicals—at work or otherwise?

Once information has been obtained on the above, a letter of reply can be drafted. It should be remembered that it is going to the manager and should be succinct and to the point. If it is felt that more information or investigations are required these should be stated, but at the same time provide as much information as possible. Recommendations should be clearly provided for an appropriate course of action. For example, one recommendation might be that the liver function tests be repeated. The reader may care to address the problem and draft a letter of reply.

ASPECTS TO BE ILLUSTRATED

Once completed and/or while going through the exercise the following basic aspects should have been invoked:

- Dose–effect.

- Extrapolation from animal data.

- Route of exposure.

- Duration of exposure.

- Disposition—absorption, distribution and excretion.

- Biotransformation.

- Toxicity versus hazard.

- Target organ toxicity.

- Toxicity by class of chemical.

- Use of information sources.

- Exposure standards—values and pitfalls.

- Use of regulatory control.

- Consideration of extraneous factors.

- Integration of toxicology, medicine and hygiene.

- Data interpretation and the importance of a thoughtful and considered approach.

Example 2

A letter is received from a Union requesting information as follows.

PP Consultants
GPO Box 000
Sydney 20001

Dear Sir/Madam

It has been brought to our attention that some of our members might be exposed to the chemical MOCA (methylene-*bis* (2-chloroaniline)) in the course of their work in polyurethane manufacture. We understand that this chemical may have cancer producing effects.

We therefore request that you provide a report to indicate whether or not these workers' health may be at risk and what steps might be taken to rectify the situation.

Yours faithfully

Union Official's name
Union

Response

Again the steps to be taken in order that a satisfactory response might be provided will be outlined, but an actual response not given. However, the interested reader is invited to draft a reply as an exercise in gathering, collating and interpreting toxicological information.

INFORMATION TO BE SOUGHT

- How is MOCA used in this industry?

- Are there physicochemical properties of MOCA that are relevant to potential exposure?

- What is the likelihood of exposure? Is there any evidence to suggest that it is a particular problem for this chemical?

- Is MOCA a carcinogen? What is the strength of evidence? Is there cause for concern?

- What might be done to rectify the situation if it is a problem? What are the options for:
  (a) elimination,
  (b) substitution,
  (c) containment,
  (d) safe working procedures,
  (e) ventilation and monitoring, or
  (f) personal protective equipment?

- What regulations cover the use of the chemical, if any?

Again, the letter of reply needs to be concise and address the issues raised in the request. Important aspects relevant to the use of this chemical should be raised. For example, in New South Wales, Australia, a licence is required for its use and there are conditions attached to this licence information relevant to the particular locate should be included.

ASPECTS TO BE ILLUSTRATED
Many of the basic aspects relevant to Example 1 are also relevant here. However, this exercise should highlight some additional matters, such as:

- Specific regulations exist covering particular chemicals in some jurisdictions.

- Consideration of product performance when addressing the use of chemicals.

- The importance of dermal absorption of some chemicals.

- The advantage of biological monitoring over environmental monitoring in some circumstances.

- The relevance of atmospheric standards for some chemicals as compared with biological exposure indices.

- The importance of considering all relevant toxicity data when deliberating on the use of a chemical.

- The necessity to consider various ways of dealing with a hazardous chemical.

Biological monitoring—processes and pitfalls

A programme for the biological monitoring of chlordimeform was evaluated (Kenyon, MPH(OH) treatise) and used as the basis for this exercise. It is provided to stimulate the reader's thinking about biological monitoring programmes and issues that arise from these. The reader is invited to proceed through the exercise in a step-by-step manner, and think about each step before proceeding to the next.

Exercise

Step 1

Chlordimeform is an insecticide that had extensive use in the cotton industry from about 1978 until 1986. Its use was discontinued due to association of a major metabolite with human bladder cancer which was consistent with the class of chemical and positive carcinogenicity results in experimental animals. During the period of its use it was required that workers participate in a programme to monitor exposure to the chemical.

Q.1. What possibilities can you think of for methods of monitoring exposure? Q.2. What do we need to know about the chemical to decide if such suggestions are feasible?

Step 2

Consider the information on the *disposition and detection of chlordimeform* as follows.

● Absorption—rapidly absorbed across skin, lung and gut.

● Distribution—essentially throughout body, including the central nervous system (CNS). No significant bioaccumulation.

● Biotransformation—several metabolites.

● Excretion—chlordimeform and metabolites are rapidly excreted by mammals.

● In humans, using a method that detects only those compounds that are hydrolysed to 4-chloro-*o*-toluidine, mean recovery from urine 72 h after absorption was 38%.

● Detectable residues were approaching zero in most subjects 36 h after absorption. Mean half-life was estimated to be 8.8 h.

Step 3

Consider the information on the *urine monitoring scheme* as follows.

● All chlordimeform workers were required to submit urine specimens for analysis. A spot sample was collected between 24 and 48 h after exposure ceased. The allowable level was 0.2 mgl^{-1}.

- Supervisors were responsible for collecting samples which were analysed within 96 h.

- Actions following detection of levels over the limit included:
  (a) immediate removal of the worker from further exposure to chlordimeform;
  (b) an incident report was completed detailing the circumstances causing the high exposure, if possible—it was the responsibility of the marketing companies to obtain this but sometimes a pesticides inspector was also involved in the investigation of such incidents;
  (c) appropriate remedial actions were required to be taken, including retraining of the offending worker if necessary;
  (d) the worker was not to resume work until permitted to do so by the Director of the Division of Occupational Health.

- During the operation of the scheme some changes were introduced, including, in 1983–1984:
  (a) incentive payments were offered by the marketing company with the intent of encouraging timely submission of correctly collected and labelled urine samples and to foster safe working habits. These incentive payments were:
  (i) $2 for each correctly filled and labelled urine sample collected 24–48 h after exposure; and
  (ii) $5 if the sample result was below 0.1 mg l^{-1}.
  (b) supervisors were also paid 10 cents per litre of product applied if samples were promptly collected and submitted, and work log books correctly maintained.

Q.3. Would you suggest any changes to the scheme?
Q.4. Does the information in Table 19.1 support your response to Q.3?

Table 19.1. Urine analysis results corrected to standard reference times

Worker No.	Time after exposure (h)	Chlordimeform metabolites (mg l^{-1})	Concentration (mg l^{-1})	
			at 8.0 h	at 24.0 h
1	31	0.73	5.35	1.13
2	34	0.85	8.08	2.02
3	36	0.27	3.05	0.76
4	38	1.20	16.12	4.03
5	48	0.31	9.9	2.48
6	15	0.26	0.48	0.12
7	3	0.79	0.51	0.13
8	46	0.16	4.30	1.07

Step 4

Look at Tables 19.2 and 19.3.

Q.5. What do they tell you about exposure?
Q.6. What are possible reasons for overexposure?

Table 19.2. Exposure level versus worker category

Category	Mean urine chlordimeform $mg l^{-1}$	
	1984–1985	1985–1986
Loader/mixer	0.62	0.52
Supervisor	0.41	0.14
Marker	0.13	0.17
Driver	0.17	0.13
Pilot	0.16	0.17

Table 19.3. Multiple exposures greater than $0.2 \, mg l^{-1}$ versus worker category in the 1985–1986 cotton season

Operator No.	Number of exposures $> 0.2 \, mg l^{-1}$		
	Loader/mixer/supervisor	Pilots	Driver/marker
1	2, 4, 8, 9	3, 7	2, 2, 2, 3, 3, 8
2	2, 2, 3, 8, 11	3	2, 2, 2, 4
3	2, 2, 3, 4, 6	2, 2	2, 2, 4
4	3, 6	2	3
5	4	2, 2	
6	13	3, 8	2, 2, 4
7	2, 2, 2		
8		5	

For information, the main causes stated were as follows.

● Exposures obtained from post-application maintenance. This was the most commonly reported cause in 1985–1986 (51 reports) and was commonly attributed to not wearing waterproof clothing when washing down vehicles and equipment. It appears that workers did not fully appreciate the degree to which aircraft and marker vehicles were contaminated and the ease with which chlordimeform was absorbed through the skin. This was despite emphasis on these facts in the training sessions. Many workers do not expect exposure to occur when they are not directly involved in mixing or spraying pesticides.

● Spray drift while marking was the second most common cause reported. This seemed to be a somewhat standard excuse and the 45 reports in

1985–1986 accounted for almost all the multiple high exposures detected in markers and drivers.

- No protective clothing worn (33 reports in 1985–1986) does not appear to be an acceptable reason. These situations should have been prevented by proper supervision.

- Accidental spillage on body accounted for a large proportion of the sample results exceeding 2.0 mgl^{-1}. Results of 2.3, 2.5, 2.5, 4.4, 11.1 and 12.3 mgl^{-1} were attributed to incidents which involved skin contact while uncoupling hoses, changing drum probes or removing a blocked filter (one instance).

- Exposure while repairing faulty equipment was reported 20 times in 1985–1986. It seems difficult to adopt adequate protective measures while repairing equipment in the work environment.

Less commonly reported reasons for high exposures were torn protective clothing, poor quality equipment, failing to wash after work and extended periods of general exposure. It is obvious that many of these high exposures could have been avoided by better attention to work hygiene and adherence to conditions stipulated in permits. It is disturbing that sporadic, relatively high exposures result from accidents.

Summary—lessons

- The toxicity of a chemical is important—Is comprehensive monitoring appropriate?
- How best to monitor?
- Importance of absorption (skin).
- Importance of biotransformation.
- Importance of kinetics (of excretion).
- Importance of assay procedure.
- Issues of 'penalty' of removing worker.
- Issue of incentive payments.
- Interpretation of results:
  (a) targeting of particular groups;
  (b) targeting of particular individuals.
- Reasons for overexposure.

Workplace reproductive hazards—exercise

Background

Your workplace safety committee notes that new evidence from Scandinavia has suggested that a material used extensively in your workplace may cause embryrotoxicity in pregnant animals at high doses and spontaneous abortions in workers.

Workplace

A factory manufacturing textiles/furniture.

Workers

78 in production areas (about two-thirds men); 32 in office areas (12 men and 20 women).

Process

Thick felt is glued to surface covers of furniture and mattresses with a flexible adhesive called 'Mutoglue'. To make the adhesive stick better and penetrate the material, the felt is immersed in a vat containing a watery solvent mixture called 'Mutosolv' for about 15 min before gluing. All processes are manual.

Chemical products

Mutoglue (and Mutosolv) was introduced about 2.5 years ago, as a replacement for an adhesive which contained *n*-hexane. The agent of concern is found in both Mutoglue (at a concentration of 0.4%) and Mutosolv (4%). Neither the label or the material safety data sheet (MSDS) mention anything about reproductive problems.

Exposed workers

The number of workers involved varies, depending on the size of the job (mattresses need more workers than chair covers), the number of items being made (the size of the order) and the amount of the material needing gluing. However, not more than 20 workers are used for any particular order, although probably most if not all manufacturing workers have been involved in gluing at some stage. Three factory workers and one office worker are known to be pregnant, and there are also at least two expectant fathers working in the factory.

Safety procedures

The factory has roof vents and ceiling fans which are used as dilution ventilation. Dust masks are used extensively by workers handling felt as it releases fibres and dust. All workers also wear gloves (bought from a local supermarket) when dipping felt into Mutosolv and when gluing with Mutoglue. No monitoring has been carried out in the factory since before the solvent adhesive was replaced, as it is considered that there is no need for it (the solvent has a faint chemical smell).

Exercise

What are the necessary steps to be taken to control the hazard by: (1) the safety officer; (2) the visiting occupational physician; and (3) a consultant occupational hygienist brought in to investigate the problem?

Writing material safety data sheets

Background

Below is a printout of a computer bibliographic database for a general solvent and chemical intermediate used in the chemical industry. It is sufficient for the purpose of this exercise to know that it is a chlorinated solvent.

COMPUTER DATABASE PRINTOUT: 79016

Identity
Name: 79016
CAS Number: ############
UN NUMBER: ####
Use(s): Chemical intermediate, solvent, agricultural excipient, industrial chemical, vapour degreasing

Chemico-physical properties

Appearance:	Clear, colourless liquid with a sweetish chloroform smell
Odour threshold:	21 ppm
Specific gravity:	1.5 at 20°C
Melting point:	− 85° C
Boiling point:	87°C
Refractive index:	1.48
Vapour pressure:	58 mmHg at 20°C; 77 mmHg at 25°C; 100 mmHg at 32°C
Vapour density:	4.53 (air = 1)
Flashpoint:	60°C
Flammability limits:	Upper 90%
	Lower 12.5%
Autoignition point:	410°C
Reactivity:	Reacts violently with Al, Ba, N_2O_4, Li, Mg, Na, Ti, alkalis, nitrates, liquid oxygen, ozone, anhydrous perchloric acid

Combustion products:		Hydrogen chloride, phosgene, carbon dioxide in the presence of complete combustion (carbon monoxide if oxygen supply limited) toxic smoke. Hazardous polymerisation will not occur		
Water solubility:		Practically insoluble		
Solvent solubility:		Soluble in most solvents		

Toxicity reports

SPECIES	ROUTE	TEST	PROTOCOL	RESULT
Toxic effects				
Rat	Oral	Acute tox.: TDLo*		2688 mgkg^{-1}
Rat	Oral	Acute tox.: TDLo		1140 mgkg^{-1}
Rat	Oral	Acute tox.: TDLo		36 000 mgkg^{-1}
Mouse	Oral	Chronic tox.: TDLo	77 weeks	455 000 mgkg^{-1}
Human	Oral	Case study.: TDLo		2143 mgkg^{-1}
Rabbit	Skin	Primary irritation	2 mg, 24 h	Severe irritant
Rabbit	Eye	Primary irritation	20 mg, 24 h	Moderate irritant
Rat	Inhal.	STRD tox.: TCLo$^+$	24 h/20 days	10 872 mgm^{-3}
Rat	Inhal.	STRD tox.: TCLo	4 h/17 days	604 mgm^{-3}
Rat	Inhal.	STRD tox.: TCLo	6 h/20 days	10 872 mgm^{-3}
Rat	Inhal.	STRD tox.: TCLo	4 h/14 days	604 mgm^{-3}
Mouse	Inhal.	STRD tox.: TCLo	7 h/5 days	604 mgm^{-3}
Mouse	Inhal.	STRD tox.: TCLo	24 h/4 weeks	906 mgm^{-3}
Rat	Inhal.	Chronic tox.: TCLo	7 h/2 years	906 mgm^{-3}
Mouse	Inhal.	Chronic tox.: TCLo	7 h/2 years	906 mgm^{-3}
Hamster	Inhal.	Chronic tox.: TCLo	6 h/77 weeks	604 mgm^{-3}
Rat	Inhal.	Acute tox.: TCLo		2688 mgm^{-3}
Human	Inhal.	Case study: TCLo	10 min	6900 mgm^{-3}
Human	Inhal.	Case study: TCLo	83 min	966 mgm^{-3}
Human	Inhal.	Case study: TCLo		812 mgm^{-3}
Human	Inhal.	Case study: TCLo	8 h	664 mgm^{-3}
Lowest lethal effects				
Rabbit	Oral	Acute tox.: LDLo§		7330 mgkg^{-1}
Human	Oral	Case study: LDLo		7000 mgkg^{-1}
Human	Inhal.	Case study: LCLo‡		17 516 mgm^{-3}
Rabbit	Skin	Acute tox.: LDLo		1800 mgkg^{-1}
Dog	Skin	Acute tox.: LDLo		150 mgkg^{-1}
Rat	Inhal.	Acute tox.: LCLo	4 h	48 321 mgm^{-3}
Rabbit	Inhal.	Acute tox.: LCLo		66 442 mgm^{-3}
Guinea-pig	Inhal.	Acute tox.: LCLo	40 min	224 694 mgm^{-3}
Cat	Inhal.	Acute tox.: LCLo	2 h	32 500 mgm^{-3}
Human	Inhal.	Case study: LCLo		17 516 mgm^{-3}
Dog	IV¶	Acute tox.: LDLo		150 mgkg^{-1}
Cat	IV¶	Acute tox.: LDLo		5864 mgkg^{-1}
Lethal effects				
Mouse	Oral	Acute tox.: LD$_{50}$		2402 mgkg^{-1}
Dog	Oral	Acute tox.: LD$_{50}$		1900 mgkg^{-1}
Mouse	Skin	Acute tox.: LD$_{50}$		16 000 mgkg^{-1}
Rabbit	Skin	Acute tox.: LD$_{50}$		>20 000 mgkg^{-1}
Rat	IP¶	Acute tox.: LD$_{50}$		1 282 mgkg^{-1}
Mouse	IV¶	Acute tox.: LD$_{50}$		33.9 mgkg^{-1}
Rat	Inhal.	Acute tox.: LD$_{50}$	4 h	51 039 mgm^{-3}

Genetic toxicity:

GENOTOXICITY ASSAY	GENETIC END-POINT	RESULT
E. coli	Point mutations	Weakly positive
S. cerevisiae	Gene conversion	Positive
S. cerevisiae	Reversion	Positive
D. melanogaster	Sex-linked lethal	Negative

RLV F344 Rat embryo	Cell transformation	Positive
Rat	Dominant lethal assay	Negative
Mouse	Dominant lethal assay	Negative
Mouse spot test	Sperm morphology	Positive

Carcinogenicity bioassays:

SPECIES	AGENCY	ROUTE	CONCLUSIONS
Rat	NCI, 1976	Gavage	No evidence
Mouse	NCI, 1976	Gavage	Clear evidence
Rat	–, 1980	Inhal.	No evidence
Mouse	–, 1980	Inhal.	No evidence
Hamster	–, 1980	Inhal.	No evidence
Rat	NTP, 1983	Feed	Inadequate study
Mouse	NTP, 1983	Gavage	Clear evidence
Rat	NTP, 1988	Gavage	Inadequate study

IARC EVALUATION
Human: inadequate (1979)
Animal: limited (1979)

---

* TDLo-Toxic dose low (i.e. the lowest dose recorded to produce toxic effects)
† TCLo-Toxic concentration low (i.e. lowest concentration recorded to produce toxic effects)
‡ LCLo-Lethal concentration low (i.e. lowest concentration recorded to produce lethal effects)
§ LDLo-Lethal dose low (i.e. lowest dose recorded to produce lethal effects)
¶ IV, Intravenous. IP, Intraperitoneal.

Exercise 1

● What is the significance of TD, LDLo, and LD_{50} data?

● What is the significance of data from non-occupational routes of exposure (for example, intraperitoneal and intravenous)?

● What do you do when there are a lot of data for the same species and a route of administration (for example, rat/inhalational), but the values are not consistent?

● What do you do for data from the same route but from different species?

● What is the significance of human data?

● How would you rate the genotoxicity data?

● What are the implications of the carcinogenicity data?

● What is your final toxicity rating of this material?

Exercise 2

Your company is marketing this chemical in a new product called 'Spot-Splott'. This is a formulated product containing 98.5% of this ingredient, and 1.5% of an organic surfactant, to be used as a cleaner for metal parts. Write an MSDS as part of your company's commitment to hazard communication to workers and customers. A fictitious MSDS is given in Appendix A19.1 to this chapter for reference to format. The contents should not be used as an acceptable guide. What sort of response do you think this MSDS will receive from your marketing people? What sort of response do you think this MSDS will receive from your customers?

Setting exposure standards

Background

This exercise is aimed at developing skills in evaluation material and being critical. The important points to bring out are:

● How much weight is given to toxicity data in the exposure standards setting process.

● How empirical data are used in the standards setting process.

● The contribution that each piece of data makes in the final decision.

Extract from an occupational toxicological hygiene publication on 79016

This material is a skin, eye and respiratory irritant to single exposures. It may be absorbed through the respiratory system or across the skin to produce conventional symptoms of solvent induced central nervous system depression.

Organ systems affected by prolonged and/or repeated exposure to this material include: (1) the central nervous system—euphoria, drowsiness, headaches, analgesia, anaesthesia; (2) the liver—degeneration, hepatocellular carcinomas (in mice only); (3) kidney—degeneration; (4) cardiovascular—skin redness and flushing, ventricular arrhythmias (at high exposures); (5) skin— irritation, vesication, paralysis of finger (following immersion); and (6) lung— tachypnoea. Some of these effects are exacerbated by alcohol consumption.

In workers, the main hazard is from inhalation of vapour, although significant exposure is possible if skin contact is substantial. Once absorbed, the chemical is rapidly partitioned into adipose tissue. Effects reported in different epidemiological studies of chronically exposed workers include:

● Subjective symptoms (vertigo, fatigue, headache) and experimental findings (short-term memory loss and increased misunderstanding) at 85 ppm (exposure data not expressed as a time weighted average).

● Intolerance to alcohol, tremors, giddiness and anxiety above 40 ppm.

Evidence is also available from controlled exposures of volunteers under laboratory conditions:

- Significantly decreased performance in visual perception and motor skill in volunteers at 1000 ppm, but not 300 or 100 ppm (2 h exposure).

- Significantly decreased performance in numerical ability in volunteers exposed to 100 ppm for 70 min.

- Drowsiness and upper airway irritation at 27 ppm, headache at 81 ppm, dizziness at 201 ppm (4 h exposure).

- Significantly decreased performance on a perception test, a complex reaction time test and manual dexterity test was found following two 4-h exposures separated by a 1.5 h interval at 110 ppm.

- In a repeated exposure experiment (7 h day^{-1}), slight fatigue and sleepiness were reported on day 5 above 20 ppm.

Exercise

Based on the data given in the above extract, and on the data in the MSDS writing exercise, establish an exposure standard for this material, and provide justification for the level. Is it possible to establish any short-term exposure limits? Does the fact that this chemical causes cancer in mice have any bearing on the standard setting process?

Managing chemical safety

Background

A company in the manufacturing sector uses a wide variety of hazardous chemicals in the production of its products. The company employs about 500 workers, including 150 office staff, 300 production workers (split into three 8.5-h shifts), 25 maintenance staff and the remainder as cleaners, laundry staff, canteen personnel and security officers. Other hazardous chemicals are also used by seven staff in a Quality Control Laboratory.

Systems for the control of chemicals have been developed in a completely reactive manner over the years, and include:

- The company has a dangerous goods licence for flammable liquids. Solvents are stored in a placarded flammable goods store, but other dangerous goods (including corrosives and poisons) are also present on site.

- An occupational health and safety committee, which has developed a health and safety policy, and spends a lot of time looking at accident reports and rehabilitation cases. While there is some concern about chemicals voiced by some workers, the committee does not know what to do about it, except think about developing some training.

Appendix A19.1

FICTITIOUS ACRYLICS LTD

(A Division of The Fictitious Chemicals Pty Ltd)

Material Safety Data Sheet May be used to comply OSHA's Hazard Communication Standard 29 CFR 1910.1200. Standard must be consulted for specific requirement.	**U.S. Department of Labor** Occupational Safety and Health Administration Non-Mandatory Form Form Approved OMB No. 1218-0072
IDENTITY *(As used on Label and List)* 　　FICTO GRITTO-FRITTO	*Note: Blank Spaces are not permitted. If any item is not applicable, or no information is available, the space must be marked to indicate that.*

Section I

Manufacturer's Name 　FICTITIOUS ACRYLICS PTY. LTD	Emergency Telephone Number 　USA:　1-012-345-6789
Address *(Number, Street, City, State and ZIP Code)* 　P.O. BOX FICTO 　WOOP WOOP NSW 9999 　AUSTRALIA	Telephone Number for Information 　Australia:61-1-234-5678
	Date prepared 　1/12/89
	Signature of Preparer *(optional)*

Section II - Hazardous Ingredients/Identity Information

Hazardous Components (Specific Chemical Identity: Common Name(s))	OSHA PEL	ACGIH TLV	Oher Limits Recommended	% *(optional)*
FICTO GRITTO-FRITTO: IS A WHITE ACRYLIC PASTE PRODUCT CONTAINING GRITS OF TITANIUM AND CALCITE				

Section III - Physical/Chemical Characteristics

Boiling Point	220 - 300 °F	Specific Gravity (H2O=1)	UNKNOWN
Vapor Pressure (mm Hg)	UNKNOWN	Melting Point	UNKNOWN
Vapor Density (air=1)	LIGHTER THAN AIR	Evaporation Rate (Butyl Acetate=1)	SLOWER THAN ETHER
Solubility in Water	TOTALLY SOLUBLE		
Appearance and Odour	ODOURLESS WHITE PASTE		

Section IV - Fire and Explosion Hazard Data

Flash Point (Method Used)		Flammble Limits	LEL	UEL
	NOT APPLICABLE	NOT APPLICABLE	UNKNOWN	UNKNOWN
Extinguishing Media	NOT APPLICABLE			
Special Fire Fighting Procedures	NOT APPLICABLE			

Section V - Reactivity Data

Stability	Unstable		Conditions to Avoid	NOT APPLICABLE
	Stable	X		NOT APPLICABLE

Incompatability *(Materials to Avoid)* NONE

Hazardous Decomposition Products or Byproducts   NONE

Hazardous	May Occur		Conditions to Avoid	NOT APPLICABLE
Polymerisation	May Not Occur	X		NOT APPLICABLE

Section VI - Health Hazard Data

Route(s) of Entry	Inhalation?	Skin?	Ingestion?
	NOT APPLICABLE	NOT APPLICABLE	NOT APPLICABLE

Health Hazards *(Acute and Chronic)*   NONE

Carcinogenicity	NTP?	IARC Monographs?	OSHA Regulated?
	NOT APPLICABLE	NOT APPLICABLE	NOT APPLICABLE

Signs and Symptoms of Exposure   NONE

Medical Conditions Generally Aggravated by Exposure   NONE

Emergency and First Aid Procedures   NONE

Section VII - Precautions for Safe Handling and Use

Steps to be Taken in Case Material is Released or Spilled DIKE AND CONTAIN SPILL WITH INERT MATERIALS (SAND, SAWDUST, ETC.) AND TRANSFER TO CONTAINERS FOR DISPOSAL. KEEP SPILL OUT OF OPEN BODIES OF WATER AND SEWERS. FLOORS MAY BE SLIPPERY.

Waste Disposal Method

Precautions to be Taken in Handling and Storing   NO PARTICULAR PRECAUTIONS

Other Precautions   NONE

Section VII - Control Measures

Respiratory Protection *(Specify Type)*	NONE NEEDED UNDER NORMAL		
	CONDITIONS OF USE		
Ventilation	Local Exhaust	NOT APPLICABLE	Special	NOT APPLICABLE
	Mechanical *(General)*	NOT APPLICABLE	Other	NOT APPLICABLE
Protective Gloves		NOT REQUIRED	Eye Protection	NOT REQUIRED
Other Protective Clothing or Equipment		NOT REQUIRED		

- Information on hazards of some products (MSDSs) is available in the production manager's office, the laboratory and the nurse's room. The responsibility for the purchase of materials below $500 resides with line management.

- Safety equipment is available:
  (a) some access to respirators for solvent exposure tasks (most workers do not use them);
  (b) all workers are issued with eye protection, although compliance is virtually non-existent;
  (c) first aid boxes, and trained first aiders; and
  (d) fire extinguishers, fire blankets, safety showers and eye-wash stations at selected locations throughout the factory.

- Visits of a visiting occupational health physician for 4 h per week.

- Visits of a waste contractor who removes:
  (a) two dumpsters of industrial waste per week; and
  (b) large numbers of 200-l drums of liquid waste (grease trap waste, acid waste and spent solvents in approximately equal amounts) about once every 6 months.

Chemical safety was added to the duties of the Quality Control Laboratory Manager about 5 years ago, but she is usually too busy to deal with anything other than urgent jobs. Overall, attitudes to safety are quite good, but most workers have little idea of the hazards of the materials they are using.

Exercise

The company has just been merged with a multinational company, which is introducing changes in the way the company is being run. As part of this process, new managers have been appointed in a number of areas, including personnel, production and safety. However, the workforce is largely unchanged, although concern is being expressed at the new changes.

You are the new Occupational Health and Safety Manager. You have inherited a department comprising a Rehabilitation Coordinator, a Safety Officer (who works part-time in the laboratory, and spends the rest of his time dealing with hazardous wastes) and two part-time Occupational Health Nurses (one from an agency). The possibility of new staff appointments in your department disappeared with the introduction of your position.

Q.1 What activities do you need to undertake to address the problems of chemical hazards in the short and long term?
Q.2 What systems, policies and programmes do you need to put in place to ensure that chemical safety issues are being effectively managed?

Chapter 20

Chemicals, Workplaces and the Law

C. Winder and J. Barter

Introduction

In many countries, legislative and administrative measures have been introduced to deal with chemical hazards. Whilst the origin of such measures can be traced back to the development by the courts of common law principles such as the law of nuisance, and to certain ancient statutes, the subject is essentially of recent origin. This, combined with the development of legislation in response to local, as well as international developments (for example, thalidomide, asbestos, and vinyl chloride) has meant that the legislative control of chemicals has developed of its own accord. As a result, it is a highly complex area.

Example: New South Wales, Australia

In 1991, the Public Interest Advisory Centre identified 72 pieces of legislation and 19 government departments involved in the regulation of toxic and hazardous chemicals in New South Wales (PIAC, 1991). Significant Acts in place for the control of chemicals include:

- Public Health Act 1902.

- Pure Food Act 1908.

- Construction and Safety Act 1912.

- Weights and Measures Act 1915.

- Local Government Act 1919.

- Stock Foods and Medicines Act 1940.

- Workers Compensation (Dust Diseases) Act 1942.

- Clean Air Act 1961.

- Factories, Shops and Industries Act 1962.

- Clean Waters Act 1970.

- Waste Disposal Act 1970.

- Therapeutic Goods and Cosmetics Act 1972.

- Dangerous Goods Act 1975.

- Pesticides Act 1978.

- Environmental Planning and Assessment Act 1979.

- Occupational Health and Safety Act 1983.

- Environmentally Hazardous Chemicals Act 1985.

- Ozone Protection Act 1989.

- Radiation Control Act 1990.

These statutes have developed against a background of jurisdictional uncertainty (particularly with regard to application of the Australian Constitution), reactive (rather than proactive) development of regulation, and an non-uniform approach to control. This complexity of legislation is not limited to one state or one nation. The Major Chemical Control Laws at the Federal level in the USA are as equally complex (see Table 20.1).

Table 20.1. Major American chemical control laws

Law	Federal agency administering/responsible*
Food, Drug and Cosmetic Act 1938	FDA
Food Additives Amendment 1958	FDA
Pesticide Residue Amendment 1954	EPA
Federal Hazardous Substances Act 1960	CPSC
Occupational Health and Safety Act 1970	OSHA
Consumer Products Safety Act 1972	CPSC
Federal Water Pollution Control Act Amendments 1972, 1977, 1987	EPA
Safe Drinking Water Act 1972 Reauthorised for 5 years—1986	EPA
Clean Air Act 1970 Amended 1977, 1990	EPA
Toxic Substances Control Act 1976 Amended 1981, 1984, 1986	EPA
Resource Conservation and Recovery Act 1976 Amended 1980, 1984	EPA
Federal Insecticide, Fungicide and Rodenticide Act 1976	EPA
Comprehensive Environmental Response, Compensation and Liability Act 1980	EPA
Hazard Communication Standard 1983 Amended 1988	OSHA
Superfund Amendments and Reauthorisation Act 1986	EPA

*FDA, Food and Drug Administration; EPA, Environmental Protection Agency; CPSC, Consumer Product Safety Commission; OSHA, Occupational Safety and Health Administration.

The scope of the problem

Numbers of chemical entities

To get some idea of the problem it is necessary to gain an appreciation of the numbers of chemical entities available. This is not too difficult, and it is possible to get a good idea of the numbers of chemical substances that are available in the world today. For instance, the Chemicals Abstract Service (CAS) allocates a uniquely identifying number to each new structure notified, and has allocated CAS registry numbers for approximately 5.5 million chemical entities. This therefore defines a 'universe' of known chemical entities.

Of these, the US National Toxicology Program (US NTP) estimated in 1984 that about 70 000 chemicals are in commercial use. These are broken down into categories of chemicals in Table 20.2. Although additional materials have entered commerce since 1984, many of the chemicals listed by the US NTP are no longer in use because of technological change, regulation and environmental concerns.

Table 20.2. Grouping of chemicals in commercial use in the USA, 1984

Chemical category	No. of chemicals
Therapeutic substances	1815
Cosmetics	3410
Agricultural chemicals	3350
Food additives	8620
Industrial chemicals	48523

The available information on chemicals

The category of industrial chemicals is by far the largest group. It is the category for which the least amount of knowledge on health and safety is available, with about 80% of these chemicals having insufficient information available to conduct any sort of health assessment. The US NTP also estimated the proportion of those chemicals for which a full, partial, minimal, below minimal or no toxicity information is available (see Table 20.3).

Table 20.3. The amount of toxicity information available on chemicals, 1984

Chemical category	Proportion of chemicals (%)				
	Full	Partial	Minimal	Below minimal	None
Therapeutic substances (1815)	18	18	3	36	25
Cosmetics (3410)	2	14	10	18	56
Agricultural chemicals (3350)	10	24	2	26	38
Food additives (8620)	5	14	1	34	46
Industrial chemicals (48523)	0	11	10	0	80

In recent years, there has been a significant increase in the availability and development of toxicological and environmental information as a result of both voluntary and regulatory required testing programmes and hazard communication initiatives in the USA and Europe. Most importantly, industrial chemicals are the category of chemicals to which people at work have the greatest potential for exposure. However, for the large numbers of industrial chemicals, the fact that so little is known about their health effects, and their current lack of real legislative control in Australia is a significant barrier to dealing with the problems that can occur, both at work and elsewhere.

Legal concepts of chemicals and the law

Traditionally, all governments have bodies of law applying within areas of their own jurisdiction. In many countries with legal systems based on the British model, this body of law is made up of:

- Common law (derived from operation of the courts);

- Statutory (or government derived legislation) law, comprising Primary Legislation (Acts) and Regulations.

- Non-statutory sources of law.

Common law

Basic duties and rights of suppliers, employers and workers have developed over time from case decisions in the courts. This is called 'common law' and in its broadest terms, places a responsibility on each person of legal age to act with care to each other. The operation of this responsibility is called 'duty of care'.

Employers

At the workplace, employers owe their employees a duty of care, and matters related to this duty of care are tested in the courts. Historically, under duty of care, an employer has an obligation to provide:

- A safe place of work.

- Safe materials, processes and tools to perform the work.

- Knowledge of work hazards, including those that are not immediately apparent but that may be encountered during performance of work.

- Competent supervisors and fellow employees.

● Rules and procedures by which all workers could perform safely, and means for their enforcement.

Suppliers

Under common law, suppliers of chemical substances owe their customers a duty of care relating to product safety and liability. This points to the supplier being the initial source of information on hazard and safe handling. The general duty of care of any supplier certainly includes notification to the purchaser that further information is available, and that accurate information is supplied when required.

Statute law

As well as common law, there is statute law, which are Acts of Parliament, Regulations and Orders, which are laid down by governments specifying certain responsibilities and rights.

Statute law for the control of chemicals falls into three broad categories:

● Legislation outlining general duties.

● Regulations which outline more specific duties.

● Legislation aimed at specific chemicals or groups of chemicals.

Legislation outlining general duties

Historically, restrictive type legislation has been used to regulate workplaces. However, modern occupational health and safety legislation has been moving towards legislation which involves the introduction of general duties for employers and employees, and participation in workplace self-regulation.

For example, in the UK, section 2 (2) (c) of the UK Health and Safety at Work Act (1974) places an obligation on every employer to, among other things, provide such information, instruction, training and supervision as is necessary to ensure, so far as is reasonably practicable, the health and safety of his or her employees.

In the USA, the Occupational Health and Safety Act (1970) places obligations on employers to provide working conditions that are safe for employees, and empowers the agency to prescribe mandatory occupational health and safety standards. Most OSHA health standards set maximum limits on employee exposure and prescribe changes in workplace procedures or equipment to achieve those levels.

All States in Australia have now enacted Robens-style occupational health and safety legislation. While the general duties are the same, the scope of the legislation and the precise wording of each State act varies.

This has important implications for workplaces where chemicals are used, and a number of concepts need to be observed.

GENERAL DUTY OF CARE

These general duties are similar from State to State, and include:

● The duty to ensure health, safety and welfare at work of employees.

● The provision and maintenance of safe plant and systems of work without risks to health.

● The provision of information and training.

● The provision and maintenance of a working environment that is safe and without risks to human health.

● Adequate facilitates for employee welfare at work.

RIGHT TO KNOW

The principles of worker right to know (as opposed to community right to know) are well developed in North America and the UK, and are explicitly outlined in Australian State occupational health and safety legislation.

In the UK, section 6 of the Health and Safety at Work Act 1974 created a duty for manufacturers, importers and suppliers of substances to be used at work to produce information on hazard of such substances and make such information available. Section 6 is presently under revision to ensure that this duty becomes more broadly applied—for example the provision of information and provision of updates.

In the USA, the main right-to-know legislation is the Federal Hazard Communication Standard, which was introduced into the manufacturing sector in 1983 and extended to include virtually all industry in 1988. This Act requires an assessment to determine if hazards are present in the workplace, and has provision for labelling, material safety data sheet dissemination and training programmes for workers exposed to hazardous industrial materials. Owing to constitutional provisions, Federal Acts take precedence over State laws in the USA, unless a sanction is given to a State Act at the Federal level, or a State Act successfully undergoes a constitutional challenge.

In Canada, the Workplace Hazardous Material Information System (WHMIS) became operational on 31 October 1988. Again, all hazardous industrial materials are required to have a label and material safety data sheet, and all employers will be required to devise a worker education programme.

In Australia, the general provisions relating to health, safety and welfare at work of all State occupational health and safety legislation noted above also outline a duty to provide such information, instruction, training and supervision to employees as may be necessary to ensure the health and safety at work of employees.

RISK MINIMISATION
The concept of reducing risks to health is a general duty, which also includes the concept of *as low as reasonably practicable*. This concept is incorporated into occupational health and safety legislation in many countries, including the USA, the UK, Canada and Australia. The concept of risk minimisation needs to be taken into account:

● The severity of the hazard or risk.

● The state of knowledge regarding:
   (a) the hazard or risk;
   (b) the ways of removing or mitigating that hazard or risk;
   (c) the availability and suitability of ways of removing the hazard or risk; and
   (d) the cost of removing the hazard or risk.

Regulations which outline more specific duties

Generally, these are called 'workplace hazardous substance regulations', which attempt to place obligations on manufacturers and employers to do something about chemical hazards at work.

USA
In the USA, the Federal Hazard Communication Standard (see above) is administered by the Occupational Health and Safety Act. This statute outlines requirements for manufacturers and importers as well as employers in the areas of assessment of hazards, information dissemination and training programmes. Specific requirements are:

● Chemical manufacturers and importers must:
   (a) determine the hazard(s) of each product; and
   (b) communicate hazard information and protective measures through material safety data sheets (MSDSs) and labels.

● Employers must:
   (a) identify and list chemicals in the workplace;
   (b) obtain MSDSs and labels;
   (c) develop and implement a written hazard communication programme, including training; and
   (d) communicate hazard information to employees.

UK

In the UK, the Health and Safety Executive introduced the Control of Substances Hazardous to Health (COSHH) Regulations under the Health and Safety at Work Act 1974. The regulations came into force on 1 October 1989. The new regulations:

- Place a responsibility on employers to do all that is reasonably practicable to ensure the safety of their employees and to protect them from harmful substances.

- Outline the essential requirements and a step-by-step approach for the control of hazardous substances and for protecting people exposed to them.

Employers are required to:

- Assess the risks to health arising from work and determine what precautions are needed.

- Introduce appropriate measures to prevent or control the risk.

- Ensure that control measures are used and that equipment is properly maintained and procedures observed.

- Where necessary, monitor the exposure of workers and carry out an appropriate form of health surveillance.

- Inform, instruct and train employees about the risks and precautions to be taken.

- Review and record.

It has been estimated that there are about 40 000 substances which are covered by COSHH. Many are used directly in manufacturing processes, some arise naturally, some are used in service functions, and some are given off as by-products of processes. The COSHH regulations cover virtually all substances hazardous to health.

AUSTRALIA

Worksafe Australia, through a State based Working Party, have developed COSHH-style model regulations for incorporation into State occupational health and safety legislation. A National Model Regulation to Control Workplace Hazardous Substances was published in June 1991. The Model Regulation outlines:

- Obligations of suppliers, employers and employees.

- Requirements for the provision of information on chemical hazards.

- Procedures for assessment, control, health surveillance, education and training, record keeping.

● Systems for the emergency services.

● Criteria for determining a hazardous substance.

The Model Regulation is now under consideration by a number of State occupational health and safety authorities for the development of State hazardous substances regulations to occupational health and safety legislation by the end of 1993.

Legislation aimed at specific chemicals

Acts of Parliament and regulations have been passed that deal with:

1. Specific chemicals (such as regulations for asbestos, lead or liquified petroleum gas). These tend to address the specific major hazards of these materials and how they should be contained or controlled.

2. Groups of chemicals (such as legislation poisons, dangerous goods, radioactive materials, pesticides). These tend to address specific matters such as labelling, storage and packaging, though they may cover other issues, such as point of sale considerations and security.

3. The location of chemicals in use or disposal (such as legislation for factories and shops, occupational health and safety, construction and safety, clean air or clean waters). These tend to address more general issues, such as duty of care.

For example, with regard to (1) above, in the USA, specific OSHA health standards have been developed for the workplace control of the following toxic and hazardous substances:

● Air contaminants (650 substances).

● Asbestos, tremolite, anthophyllite and actinolite.

● Coal-tar pitch volatiles.

● 4-Nitrobiphenyl.

● α-Naphthylamine;

● Methylchloromethyl ether;

● 3,3′-Dichlorobenzidine (and its salts).

● bis(Chloromethyl) ether;

● β-Naphthylamine.

● Benzidine.

● 4-Aminodiphenyl.

- Ethylenimine.

- β-Propiolactone.

- 2-Aminofluorene.

- 4-Dimethylaminoazobenzene.

- *N*-Nitrosodimethylamine.

- Vinyl chloride.

- Inorganic arsenic.

- Lead.

- Benzene.

- Coke-oven emissions.

- Cotton dust.

- 1,2-Dibromo-3-propane.

- Acrylonitrile.

- Ethylene oxide.

- Formaldehyde.

Legislation of this type tends to be developed in an *ad hoc* fashion by various government departments with responsibilities for various matters, including public health, occupational health and safety, environmental protection, pollution control, and transport.

LEGISLATION FOR THE NOTIFICATION AND ASSESSMENT OF CHEMICALS
In the past, notification and assessment of certain categories of chemicals has been introduced in response to specific public health or environmental concerns. For example, in Australia, the Federal Therapeutic Drugs Act 1966 was introduced following the thalidomide tragedy, where specific requirements for new therapeutic substances where made mandatory. Similarly, all States enacted Pesticides Acts and Dangerous Goods legislation in the 1970s following increasing concern about chemicals in the environment.

It can be argued that obtaining information relating to this sort of exposure is important because:

- Therapeutic substances are deliberately ingested.

- Cosmetics are applied to the skin or mucous membranes.

- Food additives are present in food, sometimes in large quantities.

- Agricultural chemicals often find their way into food chains either as contaminants or by design.

Therefore, there is a specific need to have health and safety information available.

In the USA, both the Food and Drug Administration (FDA) and the Environmental Protection Agency (EPA) have enabling legislation to require notification and assessment for certain chemicals. The Food, Drug and Cosmetic Act empowers the FDA to require notification and assessment of the sponsor prior to marketing for human drugs, animal drugs which will leave residues in food, and new food additives. The Federal Insecticide, Fungicide and Rodenticide Act (FIFRA) requires registration of pesticide products with the EPA prior to marketing. The EPA requires extensive data, provided by the registrant, to assess the acceptability of the proposed use of the product. The Toxic Substances Control Act (TSCA) requires manufacturers or processors of new industrial chemicals to notify the EPA prior to the production of the material and submit any data that the notifier possesses.

Although it does not have pre-market authority or the power to require testing for all new chemicals, the EPA can request additional information. For existing chemicals, the TSCA empowers the EPA to require testing if the use of the chemical may pose unreasonable risks to human health or the environment.

REGULATION OF WORKPLACE CHEMICALS
Regulation of industrial chemicals has traditionally been slow compared with other categories of chemicals, such as therapeutic drugs and pesticides. Human exposure to industrial chemicals may appear less widespread and related to workplace exposures, pollution of atmosphere or water, or as a result of low exposure to small sectors of the population. However, countries like Switzerland, New Zealand and Sweden had limited schemes for the assessment of some industrial chemicals in the early 1970s.

USA
The Toxic Substances Control Act (TSCA) represents the broadest effort to control chemical hazards. TSCA applies to all chemical substances manufactured or processed in, or imported into, the USA except for substances regulated under other legislation (drugs, pesticides, and so on). Under the law, the EPA is given three main powers:

- The EPA is empowered to restrict the manufacture, processing, distribution, use or disposal of a chemical substance when there is reasonable basis to conclude that this activity presents an unreasonable risk of injury to health or the environment.

- If the EPA suspects that a chemical may present an unreasonable risk, but lacks sufficient data to take action, it is empowered to require necessary testing to provide needed data.

- Any manufacturer of a new chemical must notify the EPA prior to manufacture and provide the agency with any data that it possesses which show that the material does not present an unreasonable risk.

The TSCA has a number of provisions relevant to the control of industrial chemicals:

- The generation of an inventory of existing chemicals (the TSCA inventory), which currently contains about 70 000 chemical entities (although the inventory excludes polymers).

- It requires premanufacture notification (at least 45 days before manufacture) to the US EPA of new industrial chemicals.

- All health and safety data in the notifier's possession must be forwarded to the US EPA with the premanufacture notification.

- It requires reporting and record keeping on chemicals substances.

- It requires notification if there is any indication of an increase or change in risk with regard to notified chemicals.

- It requires notification if there is a significant new use for notified chemicals.

The operation of TSCA in regulation of industrial chemicals has been somewhat problematic. Although it was originally considered that the EPA would mandate testing through public rule-making, this process proved to be burdensome and lacked flexibility. Initially, an informal process evolved, in which manufacturers or processors conducted studies agreed upon with the EPA as necessary to resolve issues. However, a legal challenge to this process produced a decision that the EPA could not engage in negotiated test programmes. At present, companies can enter into consent agreements with the EPA as an alternative to the development of formal test rules. Much of the recent extensive testing of existing chemicals has been conducted in response to proposed or final TSCA test rules as well as other voluntary testing initiatives.

The European Community
The European Community (EC) comprises 12 Member States, each with its own existing chemicals control legislation. Therefore, the role of the EC has been to harmonise such legislation, to avoid commercial and administrative chaos, and to prevent technical and other non-tariff barriers to trade.

The first initiative in this area was EC Directive 67/548/EEC, of 27 June 1967, to approximate the laws, regulations and administrative provisions of Member States relating to the classification, packaging and labelling of dangerous substances. To date, this Directive has been amended on 16 occasions. The most important of these is the Sixth Amendment, passed on

18 September 1979 (EC Directive 79/831/EEC). The Sixth Amendment outlines procedures for:

- An inventory of existing chemical substances (EINECS, containing approximately 117 000 substances, including polymers).

- Testing of new chemical substances, including a specific set of toxicity tests.

- Premarket notification (at least 45 days before a new substance is placed on the EC market) which must include prescribed information on health and safety.

- Classification of the substance.

- Labelling of the substance.

- Packaging of the substance.

The Sixth Amendment is similar to the TSCA by requiring that notifiers provide all the health and safety information in their possession, but extends the provisions of the TSCA by requiring at least a specific set of data (a minimum premarketing dataset). Assessment agencies can ask for more information if the data they receive are insufficient to establish a clearance. This places onus of proof of safety back to notifying companies.

Clearance of a chemical is considered effective in all Member States, following clearance of a chemical by one National Competent Assessment Authority, forwarding of the assessment report to the EC, and circulation to all Member States.

The EC is currently engaged in an initiative to require manufacturers of certain existing industrial chemicals to develop test programmes designed to provide a basic dataset for those materials.

Australia

The lack of legislative control of industrial chemicals is now being addressed in Australia, and the Australian and New Zealand Environment Council (ANZEC) (formerly called the Australian Environment Council (AEC)), in conjunction with the Department of Arts, Sport, the Environment, Tourism and the Territories (DASETT) began developing a scheme for the notification and assessment of industrial chemicals from about 1977. Since 1981, DASETT has operated a voluntary interim notification and assessment scheme, so that industry and government can develop the administrative mechanisms, expertise and attitudes required for a mandatory scheme. The AEC published the Discussion Paper on the Proposed National Chemicals Notification and Assessment Scheme (now known as NICNAS) in June 1984.

Following Federal Cabinet agreement in 1984 and again in 1986, the responsibility for operation of the National Industrial Chemicals Notification and Assessment Scheme (NICNAS) passed from DASETT to the National Occupational Health and Safety Commission (Worksafe Australia) at the end of the development phase (mid-1990). A number of key issues relate to NICNAS, which is partly based on Organisation for Economic Cooperation and Development (OECD) principles. The scheme requires manufacturers or importers of industrial chemicals new to Australia to notify Worksafe that such a chemical is being introduced, and submit a package of data that will allow an objective assessment of health and safety to humans and the environment. The distinction between new and existing chemicals will be made by reference to a published list of chemicals in use in Australia, called the Australian Inventory of Chemicals Substances (AICS 1992).

While it has been estimated that there are about 70 000 industrial chemicals in existence (excluding polymers) in the USA, AICS will contain just about two-thirds this number (about 40 000). The moderately small size of AICS is due to a number of factors, including the size of the chemical industry in Australia and the number of obsolete chemicals on overseas inventories which are no longer in use. For comparison, the US Toxic Substances Control Act (TSCA) Inventory contains over 70 000 chemicals, and the European Inventory (EINECS) contains over 110 000 chemicals.

Federal legislation for the new scheme, the Industrial Chemicals (Notification and Assessment) Act (1990) became operational in July 1990. A programme for priority existing chemicals commenced in 1992.

Non-statutory sources of law

The process of developing and adopting legally enforceable workplace standards for particular materials is usually cumbersome, requires a long time, often requires detailed consultation and, if enacted, is slow to respond to new information. The generic carcinogen standard introduced by OSHA is a case in point. Frequently, workplace practices and exposure levels are controlled by employers on the basis of voluntary non-enforceable activities determined by independent groups of health professionals (for example, the American Conference of Government Industrial Hygienists (ACGIH) threshold limit values (TLVs) or the American Industrial Hygiene Association WHEELS) or by health professionals from industry groups or individual companies. Occasionally, sources of detailed technical requirements on material relevant to a law can be incorporated into legislation.

For example, when OSHA first promulgated the Air Contaminants Standard in 1971, it established permissible exposure limits (PELs) for a large number of materials by invoking the 1968 list of ACGIH TLVs for these materials. Similarly, when the Air Contaminants Standard was updated, OSHA again incorporated the current TLVs for a large number of materials.

Other examples of non-statutory sources include:

- Workplace exposure standards, such as the TLVs recommended by the ACGIH (1986).

- Biological exposure indices, such as the recommended blood lead level in lead workers recommended in the Victorian Lead Control Regulation, or the ACGIH biological exposure indices (BEIs).

- Performance standards, such as the strategic recommendation of the Worksafe Australia National Strategy for the Prevention of Occupational Skin Disorders which has an aim 'to reduce the incidence and severity of occupational skin disorders in Australia'.

- Codes of practice and guidance, such as AS 2865 Safe Working in a Confined Space or the Worksafe Australia Code of Practice for the Removal of Asbestos or the Worksafe Australia Guidance Note for Completion of a Material Safety Data Sheet or the Australian National Health and Medical Research Council Code of Practice for vinyl chloride. These outline general provisions which will assist in reaching a desirable standard.

- Materials, equipment and process specifications, such as AS 1692 Tanks for Flammable and Combustible Liquids or AS 2161 Industrial Safety Gloves and Mittens, which are more specific recommendations which tightly define how to reach an appropriate level of compliance.

These documents fall under the general name of 'standards'.

Examples of chemicals control legislation

Notwithstanding this complexity and uncertainty, there are numerous pieces of legislation which have a significant impact on hazardous materials.

Clean air acts

These are concerned with preventing and minimising air pollution from premises, mobile equipment and motor vehicles. They usually provide for licensing of premises scheduled under the act which will be allowed to discharge pollution to air (making it a 'dirty air act'). A basic premise of such acts is the prescription of emission standards and control equipment. Where no standards exist, the 'best practicable means' approach is usually adopted.

Factories, shops and/or industries acts

These tend to be broad-based acts, covering a range of industrial activities. In the area of hazardous substances control, these acts often have a number of specific regulations, including those for the control of:

- Lead.

- Asbestos.

- Abrasives.

- Welding.

- Electroplating.

- Spray painting.

- Synthetic mineral fibres.

- Pest controllers.

- Foundries.

Poisons acts

This legislation usually provides for the classification (scheduling), labelling, packaging and sale of poisons, including:

- Natural poisons.

- Therapeutic poisons (prescription drugs, drugs of dependence and drugs of abuse).

- Domestic, agricultural and industrial poisons.

Regulations under this sort of legislation may control for certain groups of poisons, such as carcinogens or teratogens.

Clean waters acts

These acts usually complement clean air acts, and provide for the prevention, control or mitigation of water pollution. The definition of 'water pollution' is crucial in this legislation, as it may be quite broad, for example the introduction of any matter into fresh or marine water to cause a change in its physical, chemical or biological condition. This legislation also usually allows for the licensing of premises that discharge to sewers, drains, watercourse or ground water.

Therapeutic goods and/or cosmetics acts

Aimed at particular sectors of the chemical industry, rather than a chemical or group of chemicals, this legislation aims to regulate the manufacture, distribution and advertising of therapeutic goods or devices and/or cosmetics. The legislation also usually imposes quality and quantity standards on these products.

Consumer protection/trade practices acts

These provide protection for consumers of among other things, chemicals. Under such acts, products can only be supplied which comply with approved safety standards. These standards include contents, packaging, warnings, disclosure of product information. It is likely that chemicals falling into the jurisdiction of one or more pieces of legislation (cosmetics, drugs, domestic pesticides, foods) will also be covered by this statute.

Dangerous goods acts

These are acts for the transport of hazardous chemicals, which have a high degree of conformity world-wide. The reason for this is that they are, in the main, based on the recommendations of the United Nations (UN) Committee of Experts on the Transport of Dangerous Goods covering the classification of hazardous materials, standards for labelling and packaging, minimal information and documentation requirements, and so on. These include a numbering system for identification of specific chemicals or groups of chemicals with the same hazards (the UN Number), a classification system according to the predominant hazard of the material (the Dangerous Goods Class) and a system for recognising the degree of danger or risk (the Packaging Group). Most dangerous goods transport systems use the UN system, or derivatives of it, and national legislation follows accordingly. (The UN recommendations are incorporated into regulations and standards of a number of international and national organisations, including air transport, maritime transport and road transport agencies.)

For example, in Australia, the Federal Government has released the document The Australian Code for the Transport of Dangerous Goods by Road and Rail to provide handlers of dangerous materials with guidance on how certain substances should be packaged, labelled, transported and, in some cases, stored. The Australian Dangerous Goods Code incorporates all of the recommendations made by the UN Committee of Experts on Dangerous Goods. This Code is incorporated into State legislation in all States in Australia.

Pesticides acts

Of all the legislation to control chemicals, pesticides acts tend to be the most variable, depending on jurisdictional needs and political influences. These acts are aimed at agricultural chemicals and (sometimes) veterinary drugs (these may have their own controls, such as stock medicine or animal husbandry acts) and control a number of pesticide activities including possibly:

● The assessment of pesticides for human or animal health and for environmental protection.

- Determination of allowable levels of pesticide residues in foods.

- The registration of pesticides.

- Approval of labels.

- Approval of containers.

- Issue of permits for the sale of unregistered pesticides.

- Control of the supply, sale, date marking and possession of pesticides.

- The use of pesticides, including storage, personal controls during use, recommended application rates, disposal of used product or containers.

- Re-entry periods to areas where pesticides have been applied.

- Development of analytical methods to assure that food items do not contain higher that allowable levels of pesticide residues.

- The prohibition or prevention of certain food items containing prohibited residues from being available for consumption.

For example, in the USA, the Federal Insecticide, Fungicide and Rodenticide Act (FIFRA) was enacted in 1976. This law was intended to control nearly all aspects of the development, assessment and use of pesticide products. These products are regulated on the basis of each specific intended use (for example, herbicides on soybeans, termiticides for domestic dwellings, and insecticides for ornamental plants), and data must be developed for each to allow assessment of potential effects of the pesticide on human health, animal health and the environment. The applicant for registration of the pesticide product is responsible for all data development, and the EPA conducts the assessment. Labels for pesticides must be approved by the agency and contain specific information and warnings to ensure safe use of the product in all intended applications. For pesticide uses which will result in residues on raw agricultural commodities, sufficient data must be developed to enable the EPA to approve an allowable level of residue; that is, to establish a tolerance. Interestingly, the legal basis for the EPA to require these data is not derived from FIFRA, but rather from the 1954 amendment to the Food, Drug and Cosmetics Act.

Occupational health and safety acts

This legislation, if introduced after 1973, tends to follow a model of enabling statute, which puts general obligations, duties and rights on a legal basis. This is a fundamentally different approach to the older style 'prescriptive' legislation, such as the factories and shops acts (see above), which only sought to regulate specified industries and processes. Occupational health and safety legislation requires employers to ensure the health, safety and welfare of their employees and other persons at work. This duty of care sometimes (but not always) extends to manufacturers and suppliers of materials and production plant to workplaces.

There are also usually a number of chemically related regulations or non-statutory codes of practice to such acts, similar to those found under the factories and shops acts (see above). However, one regulation which has a major impact on the control of chemicals in the workplace are hazardous substances regulations, which explicate employer obligations to workers. For example, in the UK there is the Control of Substances Hazardous to Health Regulations 1989, which impose a number of obligations on employers who use hazardous chemicals (see above).

Waste disposal/environmentally hazardous chemicals acts

This legislation covers chemicals or chemical wastes considered to be environmentally hazardous, and may be subject to control by licensing or prohibition. It also sometimes provides for the restoration of premises contaminated by chemicals or chemical wastes.

Aerial spraying control acts

These control the licensing of pilots and aircraft for pesticide spraying. The statutes normally cover orders for the concentration of chemical applied, the type of aircraft and application equipment used, the land where the chemical is to be applied, and the climatic conditions during spraying. Some, but not all, statutes also contain provision to cover hazard communication to third parties. In the USA, aerial application of pesticides is regulated by the Federal Aviation Administration.

Radiation control acts

This legislation is concerned with the regulation of radioactive materials and radiation apparatus, including:

- Licensing of premises (such as nuclear reactors and facilities, but also possibly X-ray installations).

- The transport, storage, use and safe disposal of any radioactive waste products from manufacture, production, treatment and storage of radioactive substances.

Hazard communication legislation

See above for the conditions of the US Federal Hazard Communication Standard, which has become the model on which most of this legislation is based.

Major hazards acts

These require the control of major hazards (rather than the siting or location of major hazards, which tend to be controlled under planning legislation). These vary considerably, depending on the country in which they are enacted. Examples include the EC Seveso directive, the UK CIMAK regulations. A draft Control of Major Hazards Standard was released for public comment in Australia at the end of 1992.

Case study: chemicals and the law in Australia

Existing responsibilities

The regulatory control of chemicals in Australia is essentially a State Government responsibility, though the States generally look to the Commonwealth Government for overall assessment of health and safety and, where possible, coordination of inter-State uniformity.

Certain chemicals fall more obviously into the activities of specific Commonwealth Departments or regulatory agencies and therefore in the past their control has been incorporated into the responsibilities of such bodies. Examples include the assessment of therapeutic substances at the Commonwealth Department of Community Services and Health and the clearance of agricultural chemicals by the Commonwealth Department of Primary Industry and Energy. This division of responsibilities has been more traditional than rational. The primary regulatory responsibility for each category of chemicals at the Commonwealth level in Australia is:

● Therapeutic substances—Therapeutics Division, Commonwealth Department of Health, Housing and Community Services.

● Food additives—the Food Standards Council.

● Agricultural chemicals/veterinary drugs—Australian Agricultural Council (with assessment for health and safety being carried out by NHMRC).

● Consumer products (including cosmetics and toiletries)—the Bureau of Consumer Affairs, Attorney Generals Department (with assessment of health and safety probably being carried out by the NHMRC).

● Industrial chemicals—no agency until 1990, then Worksafe Australia, following enactment of the NICNAS legislation.

However, there has been some problem in this approach in that other agencies with an interest in the use of certain chemicals had little input to the decision-making process. An example of this is the environmental concerns of pesticides. The responsibility for the assessment of the environmental effects of chemicals lies with the Department of Arts, Sport, the Environment, Tourism and the Territories (DASETT), though the functional responsibility for clearance of pesticides lies with the Commonwealth Department of Primary Industry and Energy.

Therefore overlaid on these jurisdictional responsibilities are the further divisions of departmental interests. In the past, it has been difficult to incorporate these interests with any consistency.

Australian initiatives in the control of chemicals

A major impetus in the attitude the Commonwealth Government took towards the control of chemicals stemmed from publication of the House of Representatives Standing Committee on Environment and Conservation 1982 Second Report on the Inquiry into Hazardous Chemicals (SCEC 1982). Among its 35 recommendations were:

- Expansion of NHMRC and AEC assessment capabilities for public health and environmental assessment respectively.

- Formation of a national occupational health and safety authority.

- Mandatory notification and assessment for all new chemicals.

- To ensure the comprehensiveness and coordination of assessment and regulatory processes for hazardous chemicals.

The last of these listed recommendations has engendered better communication with cross-representation on expert and technical bodies of the various regulatory agencies. As a result, the relevant competent assessment authorities are now involved in the assessment processes of all other bodies. In this way coordination of the assessment process is ensured.

The second of the recommendations listed above saw the formation of the National Occupational Health and Safety Commission (Worksafe Australia).

The third of the listed recommendations has seen the development and improvement of schemes for the evaluation of health and safety of chemical substances prior to introduction to Australia. These include:

- The responsibility for assessment of occupational health and safety concerns of exposure to all chemicals passed from the NHMRC to the National Occupational Health and Safety Commission in 1983.

- The Therapeutic Goods Act 1966 has been revised and amended and a Therapeutic Goods Administration was established in 1990.

- The non-uniformity of State Pesticide and Stock Medicines registration processes and the informal nature of the clearance of agricultural chemicals and veterinary drugs is being addressed by specific

Commonwealth legislation introduced by the Minister for Primary Industry and Energy in 1989, and proposed State–Commonwealth agreements making clearance a condition of State registration. It is envisaged that this legislation, the Agricultural and Veterinary Chemicals Act 1989 will be used to develop a national pesticides registration scheme by the mid-1990s.

● The non-uniformity of State Food Standards legislation has been targeted by the Australian Food Standards Council, which comprises the Commonwealth, State and Territory Ministers of Health. This is to provide a mechanism for implementation of uniform food standard regulations. The NHMRC have issued Model Food Standard Regulations which can be used by State Governments to develop 'harmonised' legislation.

● The responsibility for consumer protection (that is, food additives and cosmetics), formerly a public health function of the NHMRC, has passed to the Bureau of Consumer Affairs in the Attorney General's Department. Some uncertainties remain as to assessment of consumer chemicals.

Publication of the House of Representatives Report on Hazardous Chemicals highlighted the various interests and responsibilities of different regulatory bodies at the Commonwealth level. While there are three separate assessment interests (public health, environment and occupational health and safety), in fact there are (in 1988) 10 separate interests in seven separate ministerial portfolios with an interest in controlling chemicals (see Table 20.4). This has produced a regulatory system which covers three tiers of government (Federal, State and Local Government), and which is unintegrated, fractured and complex.

Table 20.4. The ten interests and the ministerial portfolios with which they are connected for the control of chemicals in Australia (1993).

Interest	Jurisdiction/portfolio
Agriculture	Primary Industry and Energy
Consumer safety	Attorney General
Customs	Industry, Technology and Commerce
Environment	Arts, Sport, Environment Tourism and Territories
Industrial relations	Industrial Relations
Legal	Attorney General
Occupational health and safety	Industrial Relations
Public health	Health, Housing and Community Services
Trade	Industry, Technology and Commerce
Transport	Transport and Communications

Summary

From this, there are four different approaches to the application of the law in the control of chemicals.

Primary legislation

In Australia this can take place at three separate levels:

- The local government or state level, where State Governments can enact specific legislation as part of their jurisdictional responsibilities.
  Example: New Jersey Right to Know Act.

- At the national level. In countries which do not have a federal or provincial system of government (such as the UK or New Zealand) this is a fairly straightforward process, subject to the systems in place in that country. In countries which have a less centralised structure, such as the USA, Canada, Australia and Germany, systems for enacting legislation are dependent on constitutional demarcations and administrative arrangements between national and local levels. Nationally imposed law can be picked up or modified by other jurisdictions within the country, depending on priorities. However, they can produce a chronic problem (particularly in countries with constitutions that devolve power to state governments, such as Australia), of non-uniformity of legislation within the different States.
  Example: the Canadian Workplace Hazardous Materials Information System.

- Finally, there is the international level, at which national governments can pick up internationally derived recommendations.
  Example: The EC Sixth Amendment.

Regulation

These are regulations introduced under various statutes.

Recourse to common law

This would be made through the courts. There are a number of legal doctrines which have affected workplace chemical safety in the past. These include 'voluntary assumption of risk' (implied by accepting the job), 'contributory negligence' and 'acceptable risk'. However, a number of judicial decisions and legislative changes have tended to restrict or eliminate the scope of these doctrines. And ultimately, they are subject to the whims and vagaries of judges or juries.

Consensus approaches

Lastly, a fourth approach is also worthy of consideration, in which development of traditional restrictive legislation based controls are moving away to a less prescriptive approach, incorporating tripartite development of standards and preventive strategies with more emphasis on consultation. These may or may not be incorporated into statute.

Bibliography

ACGIH, 1986, *Documentation of Threshold Limit Values and Biological Exposure Indices*, 5th Edn. Cincinnati, OH: The American Conference of Governmental Industrial Hygienists.

AEC, 1984, *Discussion Paper on the Proposed National Chemicals Notification and Assessment Scheme*. Canberra: Australian Environment Council.

ATAC, 1992, *Australian Code for the Transport of Dangerous Goods by Road and Rail*. Canberra: Australian Transport Advisory Council/Australian Government Printing Service.

CEC, 1987, *Legislation on Dangerous Substances: Classification and Labelling in the European Communities*. Luxembourg: Commission of the European Communities.

DFG, 1983, *Maximum Concentrations at the Workplace and Biological Tolerance Values for Working Materials*. Weinheim: Deutsche Forschuggemeinschaft.

Doull, J., 1984, The past, present and future of toxicology, *Pharmacol. Rev.*, **36**, 155–85.

Druley, R. M. and Ordway, G. L., 1981, *The Toxic Substances Control Act*, revised edition. Washington, DC: Bureau of National Affairs.

NAS, 1984, *Toxicity Testing: Strategies to Determine Needs and Priorities*. National Toxicology Program, National Academy of Science. Washington, DC: National Academy Press.

NHMRC, 1987, *Standard for the Uniform Scheduling of Drugs and Poisons*. Commonwealth Department of Community Services and Health/National Health and Medical Research Council. Canberra: Australian Government Printing Service.

PIAC, 1991, Toxic Maze. Public Interest Advisory Centre, Sydney.

SCEC, 1982, *Hazardous Chemicals. Second Report on the Enquiry into Hazardous Chemicals of the House of Representatives Standing Committee on Environment and Conservation*. Canberra: AGPS.

UK HSE, 1989, *Control of Substances Hazardous to Health Regulations*. UK Health and Safety Executive.

US OSHA, 1983, *Hazard Communication Standard 29 CFR 1910.1200*. US Occupational Safety and Health Administration. Federal Register.

WHMIS, 1985, *Workplace Hazardous Material Information System*. Ottawa: Labour Canada.

Worksafe Australia, 1987, *Asbestos: Draft Code of Practice and Guidance Notes*. Sydney: National Occupational Health and Safety Commission.

Index

ABS 213
absorption 25–6, 37, 271, 272
  metals 166, 168–73
  monitorinig techniques 278
  percutaneous 91–3, 102
acetone 93
acne 99, 191
acrylamide 55–7, 219, 221–2
acrylic 213, 216, 219
acrylonitrile 219, 222
adipates 226–7
adsorption monitoring 278–82
aflatoxin 156–7
age, effects of 56, 108, 151
alcohol 42, 53, 56, 188, 223
  cancer 150, 152, 155–8, 319
  reproductive system 107, 108, 111, 116
alcohols (solvents) 206, 207, 211
aldehydes 73
alkyl compounds 165
alkyl lead compounds 53
allergic contact dermatitis 96–7, 102,
    103, 247
  pesticides 191–2
allergic reactions 31, 63, 84, 94
  dust 259, 260, 263
allylamine 68
aluminium 166–7
Ames test 130
amides 194
amines 149, 278
ammonia 233, 238–9, 242–3
anaemia 48, 169, 299
  aplastic 59–60, 208
  haematotoxicity 59–62
  solvents 210, 211
analgesics 47
aniline 60, 118
antibiotics 47, 49
antimony 69, 167
ANTU 195

aplastic anaemia 59–60, 208
apoptosis 40, 41, 44
argon 233
arsenic 45, 50, 51, 55, 194
  carcinogenicity 154, 156, 259
  cardiotoxicity 68–9
  epidemiological example 312
  gastrointestinal tract 71, 73
  in hair 94
  haematotoxicity 59, 62
  reproductive system 118
  toxic effects 166, 167–8
arsine 60, 61, 69, 71
aryl hydrocarbon hydroxylase 94
asbestos 64, 83, 309
  asbestosis 258, 261–2
  carcinogenicity 4, 73, 154, 156, 159
  lung cancer 259, 261–2
  dust 251, 255–6, 258, 261–2
  legislation 375, 382
asphyxiation 83–4, 233–8
aspirin 61
Australian and New Zealand
    Environment
Council (ANZEC) 379
autoimmune conditions 63
azoospermia 112, 119, 195–6

benzene 64, 118, 208, 300, 301, 310
  cancer risk 153, 154, 156, 159
  haematopoietic system 57, 59–60, 62
  monitoring 283, 289
beryllium 40, 118, 166, 168
bias in studies 317–19, 320–1, 322–3
bile 69
  excretion of chemicals 38–40, 71
  excretion of metal 166, 171
  liver toxicity 40–3
bilharziasis 157
biological exposure indices (BEIs) 270,
    286, 353, 381

pesticides 179, 186
biological monitoring 9–10, 285–9,
    300, 303
  chemical safety 344, 345
  working example 353–7
biotransformation 7, 22, 25, 37, 82,
    271, 287
  by enzymes 7, 27–30, 38, 43, 47, 70,
    222
  in epidermis 91, 93–4
  n-hexane 209–10
  kidney 47, 49
  liver 27–9, 38–40, 43
  mercury 171
  plastics 222–3
birth defects 308
  see also teratogens
bladder cancer 149, 154–7, 158, 159, 354
  occupation 159–60
blood 57–62, 236, 299–300
  biological monitoring 286, 287–9, 345
bone marrow 58–61, 301
brain 51–2, 54, 167, 171, 235
  cancer 52, 155, 157
breast cancer 150, 154–5, 157
bromochloromethane 71
bronchitis 86, 87, 168

cadmium 21, 64–5, 68, 73, 165–6, 168,
  biological monitoring 286, 288
  excretion through skin 94
  kidney 45, 49, 50, 166
  plastic additive 225–6
cadmium oxide fume 259
calcium 174
calcium cyanide dust 54
cancer 5, 41, 149–61
  asbestos 4, 73, 154, 156, 159, 259,
    261–2
  bladder 149, 154–7, 158, 159, 354
  brain 52, 155, 157
  colorectal 73, 150–2, 157, 220
  diet 149, 150, 152, 153, 157
  epidemiology 308, 312, 319
  gastrointestinal 71, 154–5, 159
  genetic effects 123, 125, 151–3
  haematotoxicity 60
  kidney 48, 155, 158
  liver 41, 45, 153, 154–9, 223–4
  lung 149–53, 154–60, 168, 171–3,
    259–64, 312, 319
  mouth/pharynx 150, 154–5, 158
  occupations 52, 149, 159–60
  pesticides 192–3

reproductive system 118, 119
  scrotum 149
  skin 102, 149, 154–6, 157, 159, 160–1
  solvents 210–11
  study example 310–11, 312, 319
  working example 352–3, 354
  see also carcinogenicity
carbamates 53, 177, 184, 187
carbaryl 119
carbon dioxide 56, 234–5
carbon disulphide 119, 211, 281–2,
    300, 301
  cardiotoxicity 68, 69
  cohort study example 309–10
  nervous system toxicity 51, 53, 55, 57
carbon monoxide 118, 233, 235–7
  biological monitoring 286, 289
  cardiotoxicity 68, 69
  haematotoxicity 60, 61, 62
  nervous system toxicity 51, 53
carbon tetrachloride 50, 52
  liver 40, 41, 44, 301
carcinogenicity 83, 247, 259, 380, 382
  DNA tests 143–5
  experimental animals 8, 15
  genotoxicity 123–5, 126
  hepatitis 156, 157
  insecticides (working example) 181,
    354–7
  pesticides 180–2
  plastics 218–20, 224–5, 229–30
  prevention 149–61
  target organs 154–5
  see also cancer
cardiomyopathy 169
cardiovascular system 65–9, 168, 170
  cohort study example 309–10
  solvents 67, 210, 211, 300
case-control studies 310–11, 315–16,
    320, 322
central nervous system 21, 50–4,
    207–8, 300
  metals 170–3
  pesticides 51, 52, 56, 184–6
  plastics 221–3
cervix cancer 150, 154, 157
chance effect on studies 316–17
chelation and chelators 174–5, 303–4
chemical safety programme 330–45
chemicals Abstract Service (CAS) 369
chemotherapeutic drugs 59–60, 64, 68,
    172
chlodecane 56, 189
chloracne 99, 191

chlordimeform 353–7
chlorine 233, 239, 242, 243
chlorobenzene 73
chloroform 49, 50, 68, 301
chlorophenoxy compounds 191–3
chloroprene 118, 119
cholestasis 40–1
chromium 159, 165–6, 169, 288
chromosomal aberrations 142–3, 247, 248, 301
  cancer 151–3
  genotoxicity 125, 126–8
  tests for 132–42
  heritable translocation 141–2
  micronucleus 140–1
cigarettes *see* tobacco
cirrhosis 40, 41, 45
coal tar and skin cancer 149, 155, 156, 159
cobalt 165, 169
cohort studies 309–10, 313–15, 322
colorectal cancer 73, 150–2, 157, 220
confounding and confounders 319–21, 322
contact dermatitis 94–5, 101, 104, 171
  allergic 96–7, 102, 103, 191–2, 247
  epidemiological study example 313 14
control of chemical hazards 273, 291–2, 333–4, 346
  exposure 338–41
Control of Substances Hazardous to Health
  (COSHH) Regulations (UK) 374, 385
copper 165, 166
corrosives 95, 102
cosmetics 5, 100, 376, 382, 386
cross-sectional analytical studies 311–12, 316, 320, 322
crystalline silica 85–7
  dust 255–6, 258, 263–4
cumulative insult dermatitis 95–6, 101
cyanide 53, 61, 69, 222
cyclodienes 189, 190
cyclopentadienes 56
cyclophosphamide 64, 153, 156
cytopenia 59–60
cytotoxic drugs 118–19

DASETT (Australia) 379–80, 387
DBCP 119, 195–6
DDT 56, 189, 190
dermatitis 95–6, 101, 102–3, 169, 207, 300

pesticides 191–2
  see also contact dermatitis
dermis 89–91
descriptive toxicology defined 17
development 107–20, 170
diabetes 56, 65
1, 2-dibromoethane 196
dicarboximides 194
dichloroethane 54
diet
  cancer 149, 150, 152, 153, 157
  control of risk 158, 161
diethylene dioxide 301
diethylene glycol 301
diethylstilboestrol 118
diisocyanates 64
dimethyl formamide 44
dinitrophenols 196–7
dioxane 211
diquat 50, 193
disposal of chemicals 343–4, 346, 375, 385
disposition 24–30, 37, 165, 354
dithiocarbamates 54, 184, 186–7
DNA damage 60, 124, 126–8, 247, 248
  cancer 151–2
  tests 128–37, 143–5
dominant lethal test 126, 141
dose response 19–21, 41, 114, 115
drugs (social) 5, 107, 111, 116, 149
dust 251–64, 272
  case-control study example 310–11
  clearance 254
  deposition 252–4
  monitoring 274–8, 282–4
duty of care 370–1, 372, 385

EINECS 379, 380
elimination 271, 287
  see also excretion
emergencies 341–3
emphysema 84, 87, 168, 243
encephalic syndromes 51–2
Environmental Protection Agency (EPA)
  (USA) 377–8, 384
enzymes 57, 65, 70, 82, 94, 237, 299
  biotransformation 7, 27–30, 38, 43, 47, 70, 222
  liver 38, 42–4
epidermis 89–91, 93–4, 96
epoxies 103
erythropoiesis 58, 60
esters 206, 207, 211

ethanol 40, 223
ethers 206, 211
ethylene dibromide 196
ethylene oxide 118, 233, 247–8
excretion 25, 26–7, 30, 46, 77
  by liver 38–40, 71
  metals 165–6, 167–9, 171–3
  pesticides 185–6
  through skin 94
exhaled gases 286, 288–9, 345
exposure
  chemical safety 329–30, 333
  control 338–41
  lead 298–9
  monitoring 273–9, 331, 344–5,
    354–7
    biological 9–10, 285–9
    dust 274–8, 282–4
    epidemiology 289–91
    gases and vapours 277–85
    instruments 282–5
    passive sampling 281
  organic solvents 301–2
  responses 30–1
  routes 22–4, 37, 271–2, 286, 291, 333
  skin 23–4, 100–1, 103
  standards 81, 85, 270–2, 273, 338, 351,
    362–3
    asbestos 262
    legislation 380–1
    workplace 6–9, 16, 17
  teratogenicity 115–16
  workplace epidemiology 305–6, 309,
    313–16, 322–4
  see also biological exposure indices
extrapolation of data across species
  21–2
eyes 208, 244, 246
  plastics 218, 221, 228

FAM 284
Federal Hazard Communication
  Standard
  (USA) 372, 373, 385
fertility 108–13, 117, 118–19, 137
fctal malformations 108–9
  see also teratogens
fetotoxicity 219, 222, 223
fibreglass 260
fibrosis 40, 41, 45, 87
Ficks Law 91
fluoroacetic acid 195
fluorocarbons 67, 68
food additives 5, 113, 376–7, 386

Food and Drug Administration (FDA)
  (USA) 377
formaldehyde 118, 233, 245–7, 278
fungicides 177, 183, 187, 194, 196–7
  carcinogenicity 181–2
  dermatitis 192
  plastics 225
  tin 173

gases 82, 93, 233–48
  asphyxiants 233–8
  exposure 270, 272
  monitoring 277–85
  irritants 238–43
gastrointestinal tract 23–6, 69–73
  absorption 25–6, 271, 272
  cancer 71, 154–5, 159
  dusts 254–5, 260
  metal poisoning 166, 168–71, 174
    monitoring 286, 290
gene mutations
  cancer 123, 125, 151–3
  mitosis 137–9
  tests 133–7, 140–3
genotoxicity 123–45, 247, 248
  plastics 219, 224–5
glucuronidation 29
glycols 50, 206, 207, 211, 248, 301
gold 48, 50, 166
grain dusts 262–3

haematopoietic system 57–62, 169
  carcinogens 154–6, 159–60
haematuria 48
haemolysis 61
halogenated carbon compounds 300, 301
Health and Safety at Work Act (1974)
  (UK) 371–2, 374
helium 233
hepatitis 41, 118, 153, 156, 157
heptane 210
herbicides 62, 177, 187, 191–4, 196–7
  carcinogenicity 182
  dermatitis 191–2
  kidney toxicity 47, 50
heritable translocation test 141–2, 143
hexachlorobenzene 56, 73, 194
hexachlorocyclohexane 189, 190–1
hexachloroprene 118
hexacyclohexane 52
n-hexane 21, 55, 93, 208–10, 300
  biological monitoring 289
  working example 358–9
hexavalent chromium 103

hydrocarbons
  aromatic 149, 283, 301
  halogenated 69, 73
  kidney toxicity 47, 50
  solvents 205–7, 210
hydrocyanic acid 52
hydrofluoric acid 95
hydrogen 233, 234
hydrogen cyanide 196, 233, 237–8
hydrogen sulphide 69, 233, 243–4
hyperlipidaemia 65
hyperplasia 59
hypertension 48, 65, 69
hypoalbuminaemia 48
hypomethylation 151
hypoxia 49, 65–8, 72

idiosyncratic responses 31
immune cell infiltrate 40, 41
immune system 62–5
incidence of disease 306–7, 313–15
informational toxicology defined 17
insecticides 53, 177, 183–91, 196–7, 286
  carcinogenicity 181
  dermatitis 191
  working example 354–7
interaction between chemicals 77, 83, 312
intervention studies 312
inventory of chemicals 331, 339
iron 165, 166, 236
irritants 84, 95–6, 101, 105
  gases 238–43
ischaemia 47, 49, 66, 68, 236

kepone 119
ketones 206, 207, 210, 285
  methyl-*n*-butyl 55, 57, 300
kidneys 21, 45–50
  cancer 48, 155, 158
  excretion of chemicals 26–7, 173
  metals 47, 49, 50, 166–71, 173–4
  pesticides 47, 50, 193, 197
  plastics 219, 221
  solvents 47, 50, 210, 211, 301, 303

labels for chemicals 334–5
large bowel 150, 157
larynx 154–5, 158–9
lead 165–6, 169–70, 271
  biological monitoring 286, 288–9
  in bone 26, 114, 166
    cardiotoxicity 68, 69
  chelation 174
  excretion through skin 94

gastrointestinal toxicity 71, 73
haematotoxicity 59, 60–1, 62
kidney toxicity 45, 49, 50
legislation 375, 382
nervous system 51, 52, 54, 55, 57
occupational medicine 295, 297,
    298–300
plastic additive 225–6
reproductive system 118, 119, 170
lead arsenate 56
lead oxide 260
legislation 367–89
  Australia 367–8, 374–5, 379–80, 386–9
  common law 370–1, 389
  European Community 378–9, 389
  non-statutory law 380–1
  statute law 371–80
  UK 374
  USA 368, 373, 377–8
lethal dose 20, 361
leukaemia 59–62, 157, 310
  solvents 208, 301
lifestyle 149, 150
  reproductive system 107, 108, 111, 116
lindane 190–1
lipid peroxidation 43, 44
liquefied petroleum gas 259, 375
lithium 170
liver 22, 31, 38–45
  biotransformation 27–9, 38–40, 43
  cancer 41, 45, 153, 154–9, 223–4
  excretion into bile 38–40, 71
  metals 166, 168
  pesticides 193, 197
  plastics 219, 221, 223, 227
  solvents 44–5, 210, 211, 301, 303,
    350–2
local toxicity defined 37
lungs 77–87
  absorption 25–6
  anatomy 79–80
  cancer 149–53, 168, 171–3, 259–64,
    312, 319
  carcinogens 154–9
  occupation 159–60
  dusts 251–63
  excretion of chemicals 27
  irritant gases 242–3
  localised toxicological effect 258–60
  metals 167–9, 171–3
  monitoring exposure 275
  pesticides 193
  plastics 218
  route of exposure 23–4

solvents 210
lymphatic system 154–5, 160

manganese 51, 53, 119, 165, 170
material safety data sheets (MSDSs)
    101, 103, 332, 334, 335–6, 346, 373
  examples 359–62, 363–5, 366
mechanistic toxicology defined 17
mercury 60, 118, 165–6, 170–1, 295
  biological monitoring 288
  gastrointestinal toxicity 71, 73
  kidney toxicity 48, 49, 50, 166
  nervous system 51, 52, 55
metal fume fever 168, 170, 174
metals 55, 68, 73, 165–75
  kidney toxicity 47, 49, 50, 166–71,
    173–4
methaemoglobinuria 53
methane 233, 234, 235, 285
methanol 55, 208
methyl bromide 52, 53, 56, 300
methylchloroform 289
methylene dianiline 44
methylmercury 116, 165
microTIP 285
MINIRAM 284
MIRAN 285
mirex 189
mitosis 137–9
MOCA 352–3
monitoring 273–85, 289–91, 331,
    344–5, 354–7
  see also biological monitoring
mouth/pharynx cancer 150, 154–5, 158
mustard gas 124, 154, 156, 174
mutagenesis 123–45

National Model Regulation to Control
    Workplace
  Hazardous Substances (Australia)
    374–5
nematocides 183, 187, 195
neoplasia 84, 137, 150–2, 156
  liver 40, 41
nervous system 50–7, 207–9, 219, 221
  metals 167–8, 170–3
  see also central nervous system;
    peripheral nervous system
NHMRC 386, 387, 388
nickel 64, 68, 94, 159, 171–2
NICNAS (Australia) 379–80, 386
nitrobenzene 286
nitrocresols 52
nitrogen 233

nitrogen mustard 95
nitrogen oxides 233, 241, 243
nitroglycerin 68
nitrophenols 52
nitrosamines 73
noise 54, 107, 269, 273, 318
non-steroidal anti-inflammatory drugs
  (NSAIDs) 47

Occupational Health and Safety Act
    (1970)
  (USA) 371, 373, 375–6, 380
occurence of disease 306–7
ocular toxicity 208
oesophagus cancer 150, 155, 158
oestrogens 153
oliguria 48
oral contraceptives 116, 154
organic arsenicals 40
organic nitrates 68, 69
organic solvents *see* solvents
organochlorine compounds 52, 177,
    180, 188, 189–90
organophosphates 22, 69, 183–6, 286
organophosphate-induced delayed
    polyneuropathy
  (OPIDP) 184–6
organophosphorus compounds 52–4,
    56–7, 71, 177–9, 183–6
organotin compounds 51, 53, 56, 95,
    165, 226
orthoergic dermatitis 191–2
oxidative phosphorylation 84, 167,
    174, 196–7, 238
ozone 233, 240, 243

pancreas 155, 157, 158, 174
paraquat 31, 50, 193
parasites 157
parathion 179, 186
PBBs 56
PCBs 56, 114, 118
D-penicillamine 48
pentachlorophenol 179, 180, 197
pentane 210
peripheral nervous system 50–1, 54–7,
    172–3, 208–9
peripheral neuropathy 21, 208, 210,
    248, 299, 300
peritoneuum cancer 154
permissible exposure limits (PELs) 380
pesticides 5, 15, 167, 177–99, 291
  absorption 271
  aerial spraying 385

biological monitoring 288
cancer 192–3
carcinogenicity 180–2
classification 178
exposure 8, 179–83, 186
legislation 375–7, 382, 383–8
nervous system 51, 52, 56, 184–6
reproductive system 113, 116
study example 318–19
see also herbicides; insecticides
pharmacokinetic modelling 12
phenol 73, 288
phosgene 233, 242, 243
phosphate 165
phosphine 233, 244–5
phosphorus 40
phosphorylation 57
photoallergy 97–8
photochemical alteration 91, 93–4
photosensitisation 97–8
phototoxicity 97–8
phthaltes 226–7
plant regulators 183, 187
plastics 213–30
  additives 217, 225–8
  fumes 228–9
  monomers 216, 221–5
  polymers 214, 216, 217, 218–20
platinum 172
polyester 213
polyethylene 213, 216, 228
polyneuropathy 54–7, 184–6
polypropylene 213, 216, 220, 228
polystyrene 213, 216
polyurethane 213, 352–3
polyvinyl chloride 73, 213, 216, 218, 226
pneumoconiosis 169, 218, 255, 258
population monitoring 127–8
potassium 166, 172
potentiation 180
prevalence of disease 306, 316
product registration 125–7
propane 234, 235
propylene glycol 68
prostate 150, 155, 157
proteinuria 48–9, 168
pyrethroids 188–9
pyruvate 167

radiation 59–60, 62, 123, 143, 269, 385
  cancer 153, 156
  reproductive system 107, 118, 119
    ultraviolet 90, 94, 156, 160–1
radium 62

register of chemicals 332, 335, 346
regulatory toxicology defined 17–18
reproductive system 107–20, 137, 195–6
  lead 118, 119, 170
  occupation 117–18
  plastics 222
  solvents 116, 211, 301
  working example 358–9
respiratory system 77–87, 259, 311–12
  asbestos 261–2
  biological monitoring 286–7
  clearance 82, 86, 254
  dusts 252–5, 260, 262–3
  exposure standards 271–2
  gases 233, 242, 244–7
  plastics 218, 219, 221
  solvents 300, 303–4
  see also lungs
retinoblastoma 152
right to know 372–3, 389
risk 78, 338, 373
  cancer 149, 152–6, 157–8, 159–60, 161
  chemical safety 329–30, 333
  confounding 319–21, 322
  defined 18
  disease 306, 313–16
  monitoring 344–5
    skin toxicity 102–5
rodenticides 192, 194–5
rubella 116

scrotum cancer 149
selenium 165, 172, 308
sensitisation 83, 96–7, 98, 263
sex-linked recessive lethal test
  in *Drosophila* 126, 136–7, 143
sexual behaviour and cancer risk 149, 152
silicon oxide 85–7
silicosis 81, 258, 263, 264, 295
sister chromatid exchange (SCE)
    143–4, 247, 248
skin 80, 89–105, 246–8, 381
  absorption 25–6, 91–3, 102, 271, 272
  cancer 102, 149, 154–6, 157, 159, 160–1
  excretion 94
  exposure 23–4, 100–1, 103
  metals 167–9
  monitoring 286, 290
  plastics 221
  solvents 93, 207
smoking *see* tobacco
sodium hydroxide 95
solvents, organic 205–11
  absorption 271

biological monitoring 288
cardiotoxicity 67, 210, 211, 300
epidemiological example 311–12, 313–14
gastrointestinal toxicity 71, 73
kidney toxicity 47, 50, 210, 211, 301, 303
liver toxicity 44–5, 210, 211, 301, 303, 350–2
nervous system 21, 51, 53, 54, 55
occupational medicine 297, 300–3
reproductive system 116, 211, 301
skin toxicity 93, 207
specific locus test 143
spinal cord 51–2, 54
steatosis 40, 44
stomach cancer 150–1, 157
styrene 50, 56, 118, 224–5, 288, 289
sudden infant death syndrome 308
suicides with pesticides 178, 185
sulphuric acid 95
sulphur oxides 233, 239–40, 242–3
sunlight and cancer risk 152, 160–1

talc 255
teratogens 108–9, 113–16, 118, 119, 173, 382
pesticides 194
plastics 219, 222
testing of chemicals 31–3
testis cancer 154
tetrachlorethane 45, 52, 301
tetrachlorethylene 301
thalidomide 3, 114, 116, 194, 376
thallium 52, 56, 172–3
therapeutic drugs 56, 113, 116
legislation 376, 382, 386–7
see also chemotherapeutic drugs
thiols 166
threshold limit values (TLVs) 270–1, 286, 380–1
tin 95, 173
tobacco (including smoking)
carbon monoxide 236–7
cardiovascular toxicity 65, 69
formaldehyde 246
interaction with asbestos 83
interaction with other chemicals 77, 312
lung cancer 149–50, 152–3, 155–6, 259, 319
control of risk 157, 158–60
reproductive system 107, 108, 111, 116
toluene 55, 118, 206, 208, 283

biological monitoring 286, 288, 289
cardiovascular system 300
kidney damage 50, 301
toluene diisocyanate (TDI) 31, 119
toxaphene 189
toxic dose 20, 361
Toxic Substances Control Act (TSCA) (USA) 377–8, 379, 380
toxicokinetics 29–30
training for safety 336–8, 346, 373–4
transformation of mammalian cells 144–5
transport of hazardous goods 383
triazines 177, 193–4
trichloroethylene 50, 54, 55, 64, 301, 350–2
trinitrotoluene (TNT) 40, 41, 45, 59, 62
triorthocresol phosphate 52, 55–6, 300
triphenylphosphate 95
triphenyltin compounds 197–8

ultrasound 54
ultraviolet light 153, 240
radiation 90, 94, 156, 160–1
unscheduled DNA synthesis (UDS) 126, 127, 143–4
unsubstituted hydrocarbons 205
uranium 166, 173, 251
urine analysis 26–7, 45–9, 354–6
biological monitoring 286, 288, 345
urticaria 98–9, 198
US National Toxicology Program (US NTP) 369
uterus cancer 154

vanadium 173–4
vapours 272, 277–85
vibration 54, 107, 269
vinyl chloride 22, 40–1, 45, 118–19, 156, 159
liver cancer 223, 224

walk-through surveys 272–3, 331–2
Workplace Hazardous Material Information System (WHMIS) (Canada) 372, 389
Worksafe Australia 374, 380, 381, 386–7

xeroderma pigmentosum 153
xylene 206, 208, 283

zinc 165, 174
zinc oxide fumes 258